D1623892

PACS

A GUIDE TO THE DIGITAL REVOLUTION

Springer
New York
Berlin
Heidelberg
Barcelona
Hong Kong
London
Milan
Paris
Singapore
Tokyo

PACS

A GUIDE TO THE DIGITAL REVOLUTION

KEITH J. DREYER

AMIT MEHTA

JAMES H. THRALL

EDITORS

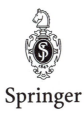

Springer

Keith J. Dreyer, DO, PhD
Amit Mehta, MD
James H. Thrall, MD
Department of Radiology
Massachusetts General Hospital
Boston, MA 02114, USA

Library of Congress Cataloging-in-Publication Data
Dreyer, Keith J.
PACS : a guide to the digital revolution / Keith J. Dreyer, Amit Mehta, James H. Thrall
p.   cm.
Includes bibliographical references and index.
ISBN 0-387-95291-8 (alk. paper)
1. Picture archiving and communication systems in medicine.   2. Diagnostic imaging.
I. Mehta, Amit.   II. Thrall, James H.   III. Title.
R857.P52 D74 2002
616.07′54—dc21   2001032835

Printed on acid-free paper.

Production coordinated by Chernow Editorial Services, Inc.
Book design by Steven Pisano.
Manufacturing supervised by Joe Quatela.
Typeset by Matrix Publishing Services, York, PA.
Printed and bound by Edwards Brothers, Inc., Ann Arbor, MI.
Printed in the United States of America.

9 8 7 6 5 4 3 2 1

ISBN 0-387-95291-8   SPIN 10838544

Springer-Verlag   New York Berlin Heidelberg
A member of BertelsmannSpringer Science+Business Media GmbH

To my parents and family who have always supported my efforts, my friends who have provided the humor, and my colleagues who have inspired and taught.
AM

To my close friends and family who have always been there through the years.
KJD

To my wife Jean, who manages information technology in our household and my children, Trevor and Keely, who have joined me in working in the digital world.
JHT

PREFACE

Radiologists have held a vision for practicing in an all-digital environment for well over twenty-five years. Now, as we enter the twenty-first century, radiology has progressed to the point where we have achieved the reality of this vision, and we are well underway toward an even larger goal—the all-digital healthcare enterprise.

The achievement of an all-digital radiology practice requires the acquisition of images in digital form, and the ability to view, archive, and transmit digital image data sets on a large scale, as well as the ability to interact with activities outside of departments of radiology by digital means. By beneficial coincidence at the time of this publication, all radiological modalities are now either intrinsically digital (MRI, CT, PET) or have been modified to allow direct digital image capture (nuclear medicine, ultrasound, conventional radiography, angiography, and mammography). This front-end digital acquisition capability sets the stage for the creation of the all-digital radiology department. This book begins with the capture of the digital image and encompasses all of the events from that point to completion of the radiological process.

While radiologists have been working toward the all-digital department, remarkable parallel developments have occurred in enterprise information systems and the networking capability that enables electronic interchange between departments of radiology and all other departments and services within a hospital or healthcare system. For twenty years, the dream in radiology focused on the ability to acquire digital images and manage them within departments of radiology. The challenge today—in the age of the Internet—has been extended to the integration of radiological activities with the rest of the care process across healthcare systems.

Leading institutions now offer clinicians the capability to use electronic order entry systems on their desktops, with autorouting of radiological requests through the hospital information system to the radiology information system. This is followed by further autorouting of study data to the relevant imaging device, then transmission of image data sets to the PACS for soft copy interpretation using voice recognition, and finally return of the image data sets and reports to the physician's desktop through connectivity from the RIS and PACS to the hospital information system and electronic medical record. When all of the elements are in place, the entire process occurs as an unbroken series of events protecting the integrity of patient data through electronic connectivity.

Picture Archiving and Communications Systems (PACS) are now part of the fundamental technological infrastructure supporting radiology practice in the digital age. Every radiologist and every department will be touched by the concepts embodied in PACS. Even those who do not become experts in the arcana of PACS will be well served to have a working knowledge of fundamental design elements and deployment strategies. Thus, this book is intended to provide information necessary for radiologists, computer scientists, and administrative personnel to understand PACS from a technical perspective, and to see its substantial potential benefits in the management of the departments of radiology and the delivery of image-based healthcare services.

We are all embarked on an exciting adventure as the practice of radiology is being redefined in the digital era. We wish our readers success in their undertakings with the hope that this book provides useful information of both a theoretical and practical nature to help guide them along the way.

CONTENTS

I

INTRODUCTORY CONCEPTS

INTRODUCTION

AMIT MEHTA

Information technology (IT) has become a critical contributor in the plans of healthcare institutions to reduce costs, improve efficiency, and provide better patient care. The effects of computer-based technologies are widespread in all aspects of medicine; especially within radiology. The advent of digital imaging has led to a revolution within the medical arena: the development of the Picture Archival and Communication System (PACS). PACS means very different things to different people. It is a unique technology in that it affects and applies to the practice of a broad range of individuals, including physicians—both radiologists and nonradiologists—technologists, administrators, vendors, and IT professionals. To some radiologists, PACS often does not extend past the system that acquires, delivers, and stores the medical images interpreted each day. For others it represents an incredible resource for research, education, and future developments. For referring physicians, it means easy remote access to the images of their patients as well as improved turnaround times and patient care. For technologists, it means streamlining operations and spending more time performing examinations and less on filming and placing stickers. For administrators, it means saved monies, personnel, and physical space, but also capital expenditure and cost-justification strategies.

Key elements form the infrastructure of a digital enterprise. First is the Radiology Information System (RIS). The RIS is responsible for all aspects of the workflow within a radiology department, from scheduling to billing to reporting. Second is the imaging network or the PACS. This technology encompasses such elements as workstations, archives, networks, and acquisition devices that enable the digital creation, transfer, and storage of medical data. This text will focus on the PACS aspect of the digital enterprise, as this in itself constitutes a large volume of information.

What is PACS? The term "Picture Archiving and Communication System" encompasses a broad range of technologies that enable digital radiology and the digital department. At its most fundamental level, PACS represents the integration of image acquisition devices, display workstations, and storage systems—all connected via a computer network. The early systems in the 1980s typically served single functions to solve single operational problems within a department. As the technology blossomed over the following two decades, more complicated and more encompassing systems were developed, with current offerings allowing complete conversion to digital acquisition, transfer, interpretation, storage, and transmission.

In discussion with leaders in the radiology community, it is evident that digital imaging and PACS specifically is becoming a revolution and most departments will perform digital radiology in one form or another. In the next decade, hundreds of hospitals will experience conversion to PACS and enterprise-level imaging. Because of its numerous benefits, the adoption of this technology is inevitable and a keen understanding of its key components can benefit every aspect of daily practice.

HOW TO USE THIS TEXT

This book is meant for radiologists, technologists, administrators, and IT professionals wishing to gain a better understanding of this emerging field. This does not preclude industry vendors or consultants and healthcare leaders who have an interest and modest knowledge of IT management issues. The information contained within this text brings together the expertise of many of the respected leaders in the field of PACS. It strives to provide a macroscopic perspective on aspects of the integrated digital radiology department, but ensures that microscopic details are not omitted. The format logically mirrors the processes one must understand in developing a plan or Request for Proposal (RFP) for PACS. Each chapter delivers a thorough and comprehensive review of a different but specific component of PACS technology.

ORGANIZATION

This book is divided into four broad categories:

I   Introductory Concepts
II   Computing Fundamentals
III Advanced Imaging Technologies
IV   Future Opportunities

Section I presents nontechnical issues that one must understand prior to implementing PACS. This includes the issues raised in this chapter in addition to issues surrounding financial integrity. In Chapter 2, Ms. Syrene Reilly and Dr. David Avrin begin with an overview of basic financial terminology and then explain issues associated with cost justification for transition to a digital department. They provide examples of various models to demonstrate cost savings and prepare you to understand the issues you may deal with when explaining and understanding PACS with a chief financial officer (CFO).

Section II provides the reader with the necessary technical understanding and information to maximize the benefit of the remainder of the book. Chapter 3 overviews the basics of computers and explains some of the terminology of digital imaging. This may be basic for many users, but imperative for others. If you are a veteran computer user, use this chapter as a reference for teaching your colleagues who are not as well versed.

In Chapter 4, Mr. Scott Rogala, Corporate Manager of Network Systems at Partners HealthCare System, Inc., simplifies a complicated topic: networks. The network is fundamental to the success of a PACS, as the movement of data around the department directly effects all users. If there are network problems, technologists are unable to send images, radiologists are unable to interpret studies, and referring clinicians are unable to receive images.

The development of the Digital Imaging and Communication in Medicine (DICOM) standard further bolstered the integrity of digital imaging, ensuring that a standard existed for image generation, transfer, and storage. It also forced the development of a standard for hardware elements to communicate with each other, allowing easier integration of new computer tomographic (CT) scanners, magnetic reonance imaging (MRI) scanners, and other devices into the PACS. In Chapter 5, Dr. David Clunie, Director of Medical Imaging Research at ComView Corporation and Co-chair of the DICOM Committee, a well known leader in the field, and Dr. John Carrino, of Thomas Jefferson University Hospital, explain many of the features and elements of the DICOM standard. Again, this chapter may serve as a reference to many, but an understanding of the DICOM standard can help you to plan elements of the PACS, especially when purchasing new image acquisition devices that require DICOM compliance.

During PACS deployment, users quickly realize not all legacy devices are DICOM-compliant. In Chapter 6, Dr. Katherine Andriole, the PACS Clinical Coordinator at the University of California at San Francisco, reviews issues surrounding choice, integration, and use of imaging acquisition devices. This chapter marks the beginning of **Section III** of the text entitled Advanced Imaging Technologies. This section provides an understanding of the specific technologies within the digital department, beginning with image acquisition.

In Chapter 7, Drs. Eliot Siegel, Chairman of the Department of Radiology at the Baltimore VA Medical Center, and Bruce Reiner, Director of Radiology Research at the same institution, discuss issues surrounding workflow within the radiology department. A keen understanding of the pathway of patients, images, reports and other ancillary functions within the radiology department can greatly impact the selection of systems in all aspects of PACS. This is especially pertinent in choosing archives, brokers, web servers, and workstations. Radiologists interpret imaging studies on workstations. The use of workstations represents a radical shift for most radiologists, who have trained with and are used to interpreting film on alternators. The transition from reading "hard copy" to "soft copy" can have a great impact on diagnosis as well as efficiency.

In Chapter 8, Dr. Steven Horii, Professor of Radiology at the University of Pennsylvania, discusses the development of workstations—historical aspects, current offerings, and future trends. This affords the reader an appreciation for workstation issues that a radiology group should consider when purchasing a PACS. Workstations harvest their images from a storage device, generically named the archive.

The archive is a key component of the PACS, as indicated by the acronym itself. Once images are acquired and interpreted, they are stored on large disk drives, tape drives, and hard drives within the department. Along with issues surrounding the selection of archive devices, in Chapter 9, Dr. Douglas Tucker, a leader in the field of storage devices, discusses the role of archives in PACS as well as various trends surrounding image storage. He explains options a prospective PACS user should consider when purchasing storage solutions.

Digital images are large files.

In Chapter 10, Dr. Stephen Mann of Pegasus Imaging, a leader in the field of compression technologies, describes techniques to reduce the size of storage of such large image files. He provides both technical and non-technical descriptions of many complicated compression routines. Finally he touches upon the future of this technology, which will allow radiology departments to decrease the size and the costs associated with storing medical image data.

As radiologists, we are responsible not only for the interpretation of images, but for the generation of reports to convey findings to the referring physicians. Traditionally, we have employed dictation systems and transcriptionists to perform this task. With decreasing budgets and demand for improved service, however, alternate strategies are necessary. In Chapter 11, we describe issues and the technology behind voice recognition. The experience in the marketplace is limited; we describe our successes with the technology and our implementation strategies to help you make the transition if you choose it as a solution. With improved report turnaround times with voice recognition, referring physicians also demand the ability to view images associated with these reports rapidly.

In Chapter 12, we describe various solutions for distributing images. An understanding of options for providing images to referring clinicians is important once the commitment is made to install a PACS and reduce filming. The impact of a "filmless" enterprise affects all physicians in a healthcare organization, and an understanding of remote strategies is paramount prior to deployment. The ability to transfer digital data for referring physicians in remote locations can also enhance radiology services by using the technology in the field of teleradiology.

In Chapter 13, Dr. James Thrall and Dr. Giles Boland, the Director of Teleradiology at Massachusetts General Hospital, discuss issues surrounding teleradiology technology, opportunities, and workflow. By the completion of this chapter, you should understand the key concepts of incorporating a teleradiology solution as an adjunct to your PACS. Many of the nonmedical and nontechnological issues raised in using a teleradiology system include licensure in sending and receiving locations.

In Chapter 14, Drs. John Smith, Director of Regulatory Affairs of the Center for Integration of Medicine and Innovative Technology (CIMIT) at the Massachusetts General Hospital, and Harry Zibners, President of the Sacramento Radiology Medical Group, review the issues facing radiology departments using PACS and digital imaging. Chapter 14 represents the first chapter in Section IV: Future Opportunities. In this section, you should gain an understanding of nontechnological and nonclinical issues surrounding PACS.

In Chapter 15, Dr. David Avrin of the University of California, San Francisco, describes the various advances and changes PACS has made in the realm of research and education. As a developer of various elements of technologies that are currently employed by both vendors and academic medical centers, Dr. Avrin describes various tools and methods that will change the way research and education are implemented.

As a continuation of this theme, in Chapter 16, Dr. Robert Bramson, Vice-Chairman of the Children's Hospital, Boston, and CEO of Partners Radiology at Harvard Medical School, explains another benefit of computer-based adjunct technology—reviewing the field of medical utilization. Medical utilization technology allows the streamlined use of resources within the healthcare enterprise and along with PACS can lead to large savings in operational and utilization budgets. Medical utilization represents a good example of the adjunctive improvements PACS technology can make in the healthcare enterprise by ensuring that proper imaging studies are ordered and costs are maintained at a minimum.

In conclusion, this text should provide you with the language, understanding, and vision behind PACS technology. By the end of this book, you should be able to understand the key elements in an RFP, discuss with your vendors the appropriate needs of your department, and begin to explore many of the other added benefits PACS technology offers the healthcare enterprise.

I sincerely hope you find the book useful and stimulating and welcome your feedback, whether kudos or criticisms.

CHAPTER 2

FINANCIAL MODELING

SYRENE R. REILLY • DAVID AVRIN

This chapter provides an overview of the financial concepts and tools that are useful in the financial evaluation of PACS. Section I discusses various analysis methods and makes a case for using net present value (NPV) methodology. Section II looks at the major cost elements that should be considered and quantified. Section III explores the cost saving opportunities and nonfinancial benefits of implementing PACS. These three sections should help you on your path to justifying PACS financially.

ANALYSIS METHODS

There are numerous ways to evaluate a capital investment such as PACS. It is worthwhile to understand all of them, and to determine which methods are most widely used and respected at your organization, especially by those with decision rights. It is often helpful to use several methods, as each provides a different lens through which you can analyze your investment opportunity. Different methods appeal to different constituencies. The nonfinancial benefits need to be enumerated as clearly as the financial benefits if you are to fully evaluate any investment opportunity, especially in a health care environment. To add credibility and quality to the financial results, this analysis is best done by an impartial person who has business analysis skills.

It is important to define the objectives of the financial analyses at the outset. Objectives can be any or all of the following:

- Determining whether investing in PACS makes sense financially
- Obtaining organizational approval
- Negotiating discounts with PACS vendors
- Analyzing different scenarios/sensitivity analyses
- Developing budget estimates
- Tracking results

It is possible to incorporate all of the above features in one model. The best financial models are those that clearly lay out assumptions and sensitivities to those assumptions, and assign cost savings responsibilities to parties who control the use of film and the film library. Cost savings produced by eliminating conventional film systems are discussed in detail later.

CASH

Most investment analysis methods are based on cash flow. A major difference between accounting income and cash flows is the treatment of capital assets. For accounting income, the cost of a capital asset is allocated to the periods that benefit from the asset via depreciation expense. For cash, each year reflects cash spent on the capital asset. To evaluate a capital project, you'll want to weigh the capital outlays associated with the project against the benefits in terms of capital returned to the enterprise, all in the form of cash.

Example: A company purchases a $10M asset that produces $2M of annual income (cash) and has an expected life of ten years. Accounting income spreads the cost of an asset over the asset's useful life and matches the cost of the asset to the income it produces. This is the theory behind depreciation. If the asset continues to produce $2M in revenue in the eleventh year (as shown in Tables 2.1 and 2.2), there is no depreciation expense because the asset has been fully depreciated over the prior ten years.

TABLE 2.1
Cash Flow Method

Year	Cash Outlay	Cash Inflow	Annual Net Cash Flow
0	10		(10)
1		2	2
2		2	2
3		2	2
4		2	2
5		2	2
6		2	2
7		2	2
8		2	2
9		2	2

TABLE 2.2
Accounting Income Method

Year	Depreciation Expense	Revenue	Annual Income
0	1		(1)
1	1	2	1
2	1	2	1
3	1	2	1
4	1	2	1
5	1	2	1
6	1	2	1
7	1	2	1
8	1	2	1
9	1	2	1
10	1	2	1
11	—	2	2

SUNK COSTS

The purpose of all these techniques is to evaluate a possible capital invest-ment. A sunk cost is a cost that has already been incurred and cannot be changed. Sunk costs are irrelevant to the decision of whether to make an investment. Thus, the cost justification effort is less burdensome for those who have already made past investments in digital equipment, information systems, and hardware.

IRRELEVANT COSTS

Costs that would be incurred regardless of the implementation of PACS should be ignored. This is particularly appropriate for organizations that al-ready plan to implement computed radiography. Such costs are not relevant in the financial justification of PACS. Similarly, the decision to invest in voice recognition technology is separate from the PACS decision and should be analyzed separately.

PAYBACK PERIOD

Payback period represents the number of years it takes for an organization to recover its initial investment via the cash flows generated from the in-vestment, without adding the cost of capital (interest). This is also the point at which the project breaks even on a cumulative cash flow basis. Some or-ganizations establish required payback periods in addition to other financial hurdles (described later). The benefits of this method are the ease of use and simplicity of application, but it does not help determine the true value of the investment over its lifetime, or its value relative to other investment opportunities (see Table 2.3).

An example of analyzing the payback period concept is illustrated in Table 2.4. After the payback period of five years, the investment yields pos-itive cumulative cash flow to the organization.

NET PRESENT VALUE (NPV)

The net present value method assesses the worth of a project by bringing all cash inflows and outflows associated with the project into one value in

TABLE 2.3
Payback Analysis: Advantages and Disadvantages

Advantages:

1. East to do
2. Quick financial reality check
3. Helps identify capital costs
4. Helps identify sources and magnitudes of savings

Disadvantages:

1. Does not take account of the cost of capital (current market interest rules)
2. Does not account for risk of project
3. Does not quantify tghe investment value of the project

today's dollars. With a 10% interest rate, an investor with $1.00 today can generate a future value of $1.10 in one year. Alternatively, this investor would value a riskless payment of $1.10 in one year at $1.00 today, in "today's dollars." In this example, $1.00 is the present value, $1.10 is the future value, and the discount rate is 10%. Net present value is the current

TABLE 2.4
Payback Analysis Example

Year	Init Inv	Increm CF	Cum CF
0	10		(10)
1		2	(8)
2		2	(6)
3		2	(4)
4		2	(2)
5		2	—
6		2	2
7		2	4
8		2	6
9		2	8

value of the cash inflows less the current value of the cash outflows. For example, suppose this investor were offered an alternative project in which he would get $1.10 at the end of the year if he invested $.98 today. Since the $1.10 in the future is worth $1.00 to him today, and the cost of the investment is only $.98, he gains $.02 by accepting this project versus his first alternative. This $.02 return is the net present value of the project. An investment is worth making if it has a positive NPV; an investment is not worth making if it has a negative NPV. This is the most widely accepted and respected analysis method.

The underlying concept of net present value can best be understood by the following example: Assume that someone promises to pay you $100 one year from now. What would you be willing to give that person today? To someone you know and trust to pay you back, you would be willing to give them market rate, or approximately $93 at 8% (=$100.44) for one year. On the other hand, if you do not know the person, the risk rate is substantial, and you may be willing to give them only $80, or even $50, based on the higher risk of not being paid back.

Furthermore, if the term of the promise were longer, say five years instead of one, like a savings account in reverse, the interest would have to be compounded over the term of the investment, usually on an annual or a more accurate monthly basis. The formula for this process, net present value (NPV), is similar to the familiar interest compounding formula, but with the compounding portion in the denominator, as shown:

$$NPV = P/(1[+d)^n$$

where:
P = future value (being discounted)
d = discount rate per period
n = the number of periods

The discount rate has two components: (1) the underlying (riskless) market rate or cost of capital for the term (including inflation), and (2) an estimate of the risk premium, or interest rate related to the risk of the project. Risk of PACS project implementation is a complex topic that we do not discuss in detail, other than to consider that the risk factor should encompass all of the assumptions of the project: costs of implementation, timeliness of implementation, and realized cost savings. Some of the risks that should be considered are listed in Table 2.5.

There are many ways for a PACS project to get off track. Major obstacles, or risks with major or even disastrous consequences, are often referred to as "show-stoppers" by information technology professionals. Note that because the discount rate includes an inflation factor, the cash flows it

---

TABLE 2.5
Risks of PACS Implementation

Technology:

Integration/interoperability

   1. Modalities—DICOM compliance

   2. RIS/HIS

Software: stability/(robustness)

Scaling

Network infrastructure

   1. Institution

   2. Community

Disaster Protection

Organization:

Acceptance

   User interface

      Radiologists

      Clinicians

Realization of film and personnel savings

Lack of in-house expertise

---

is applied to should also include an inflation factor so the analysis compares "apples to apples."

RISKS OF PACS IMPLEMENTATION

Where an organization has more projects than capital, the discount rate should be set at the risk-adjusted return that the funds could generate on a competing project, as a hurdle rate (e.g., build an operating room suite vs. PACS). A certificate of deposit bearing 7% offered by a bank insured by the FDIC has a risk-adjusted return of 7% because there is no risk. A PACS implementation expected to generate 20% returns if the implementation is flawless may have a risk-adjusted return of 12% to 15% to reflect the risk that savings might not materialize or additional revenue might not be generated. In this case, enterprises generally set the discount rate or hurdle rate at the corporate level. That rate is usually 15% to 20%, depending on the risk profile of the enterprise. In health care, information technology projects are often assigned higher risk rates because they have a reputation of not being able to produce the desired return, and PACS falls into this category. For certain IT projects in health care, there are often other enterprise-wide strategic reasons to proceed, even if the expected returns do not overcome the hurdle rate.

If the investment and/or savings occur at different times (years) and/or in differing amounts, the NPV calculation is the sum of each value for the specific length of time from the time of investment into the future:

$$NPV = \Sigma \ P_i/(1 + \text{discount rate per period})^i$$
$$i = 1, n \text{ where } n = \text{number of periods}$$

The simplest way to calculate the NPV is to discount the annual *net cash flow*, or the sum of capital outlays (termed investment,) and cost savings (termed incremental cash flow), as demonstrated in Tables 2.6 and 2.7. At a discount rate of 15%, cash flows beyond 10 years have a marginal im-

TABLE 2.6
Net Present Value Example with Initial Investment of $10

Year	Investment	Incremental Cash Flow	Net Cash Flow	Discontinued Cash Flow
0	$10.00		−$10.00	−$10.00
1		$2.00	$2.00	$1.74
2		$2.00	$2.00	$1.51
3		$2.00	$2.00	$1.32
4		$2.00	$2.00	$1.14
5		$2.00	$2.00	$0.99
6		$2.00	$2.00	$0.86
7		$2.00	$2.00	$0.75
8		$2.00	$2.00	$0.65
9		$2.00	$2.00	$0.57
10		$2.00	$2.00	$0.49
			NPV	$0.02

TABLE 2.7

Net Present Value Example with Initial Staggered Investments of $6.00, $2.00, and $2.00

Year	Investment	Incremental Cash Flow	Net Cash Flow	Discontinued Cash Flow
0	6.00		(6.00)	(6.00)
1	2.00	2.00	0.00	0.00
2	2.00	2.00	0.00	0.00
3		2.00	2.00	1.32
4		2.00	2.00	1.14
5		2.00	2.00	0.99
6		2.00	2.00	0.86
7		2.00	2.00	0.75
8		2.00	2.00	0.65
9		2.00	2.00	0.57
10		2.00	2.00	0.49
				NPV: $0.77

pact, as evidenced in the table examples, in which the $2M in cash flow in year 10 has a present value of $490,000, or 25% of its future value.

It is useful to project out as many years as it takes to reach steady state cash flows or to the point at which no further benefits are expected from the investment. The capital outlay occurs in the first year(s). Operating costs will ramp up as the system reaches completion and should be adjusted each year for inflation. Savings ramp up as the enterprise discontinues its use of film. So if the organization plans to implement PACS over two years, and to take five years from implementation before achieving its film elimination targets, the analysis should be carried over for seven years (two years to implement plus five years to achieve full cost savings). The PACS life expectancy would serve as a time cap on this exercise.

In reality, enterprises may have more capital projects with positive NPVs than can be funded with the capital available. As a result projects with the highest return win in the battle for capital. Sometimes the political and nonfinancial considerations increase or decrease the financial value of a project. Those who prepare on all fronts increase the likelihood that the capital project will be approved.

INTERNAL RATE OF RETURN

The internal rate of return (IRR) is the discount rate at which the NPV of a project is 0. Instead of solving for a project's worth in dollars after applying a predetermined hurdle rate, the formula is solved for the discount rate itself, specifically the rate at which the NPV equals 0. This method offers one of the most common ways enterprises evaluate portfolios of opportunities, particularly if the decision is made on a financial basis only. This approach is somewhat shortsighted, since some of the costs (savings) are difficult to measure, particularly those that accrue outside the radiology department, and there are enterprise-wide strategic reasons to invest in PACS.

Tables 2.8 and 2.9 demonstrate the IRR method for the preceding example of a phased investment in PACS in years zero through two. The IRR calculation in a spreadsheet function such as the one in Excel solves for the unknown rate of return by using iterative or repeated calculations of the NPV formula. One actually has to make a guess or initial estimate of the rate, but usually any starting point between 0 and 10% will work. The NPV is calculated and driven to 0 by repeated adjustments to the rate, until the NPV is close to 0. This then yields the calculated internal rate of return for

TABLE 2.8
Internal Rate of Return at 7 Years

Year:	Investment:	Savings:	Discnt rate: Net CF:	11% Disc CF
0	$6.00	$0.00	−$6.00	−$6.00
1	$2.00	$2.00	$0.00	$0.00
2	$2.00	$2.00	$0.00	$0.00
3		$2.00	$2.00	$1.46
4		$2.00	$2.00	$1.32
5		$2.00	$2.00	$1.19
6		$2.00	$2.00	$1.07
7		$2.00	$2.00	$0.96
				NPV: ($0.00)
			IRR: 11.0%	

TABLE 2.9
Same Data as Table 2.9, but with Return Extended Out 10 Years

Year:	Investment:	Savings:	Discnt rate: Net CF:	17.5% Disc CF
0	$6.00	$0.00	−$6.00	−$6.00
1	$2.00	$2.00	$0.00	$0.00
2	$2.00	$2.00	$0.00	$0.00
3		$2.00	$2.00	$1.23
4		$2.00	$2.00	$1.05
5		$2.00	$2.00	$0.89
6		$2.00	$2.00	$0.76
7		$2.00	$2.00	$0.65
8		$2.00	$2.00	$0.55
9		$2.00	$2.00	$0.47
10		$2.00	$2.00	$0.40
				NPV: ($0.00)
			IRR: 17.5%	

the project, or the rate at which future discounted cash savings balance the initial and future discounted investments in the project.

For each year, a net cash flow is determined by subtracting the investment and other additional costs in that year from the savings. The net cash flow is then discounted by the IRR rate, as shown in Table 2.10 in the column labeled "Disc CF." That column is not actually produced by the IRR calculation in the spreadsheet, but is provided here for illustration, using the present value formula with the IRR rate.

BREAK-EVEN ANALYSIS AND FIXED AND VARIABLE COSTS

It is useful to compare the fixed and variable costs of the organization's film-based system to PACS to determine the volume level at which PACS produces lower *total* costs than conventional methods. Fixed costs are costs that

TABLE 2.10
Sensitivity of IRR to Magnitude of Capital Investment

NPV Example		IRR Example: $12.50 to $1000 investment			
Rate: 8%					
Year 1	250	Year 1	−1000	−1000	−750
Year 2	250	Year 2	250	250	250
	250	Year 3	250	250	250
	250	Year 4	250	250	250
Year 5	250	Year 5	250	250	250
		Year 6	0	250	0
NPV: $998.18		IRR: 0.0%	7.9%	12.6%	

do not change as volume changes. Variable costs vary directly with volume and are 0 if nothing is produced. Because the objective is to solve for the volume, it is best to do this as a one-year snapshot. To arrive at an annual cost, spread the capital costs over the useful life of the asset. Most of the capital costs are fixed, although one could argue that the cost of storage varies with volume. The personnel required to manage the PACS is also somewhat fixed. Variable costs are minimal. A conventional system's fixed costs are lower, since there is less capital equipment. The conventional system's variable costs consist mainly of film (and other disposables) and film library support activities (personnel). Although these are the major ingredients, you could try to capture numerous other costs that are more difficult to quantify. (We discuss those more fully later in this chapter.) These economic relationships are depicted in Figure 2.1.

In this diagram, the dashed line (traditional fee-for-service income) no longer exists as such, but is replaced by an underlying linear demand line for imaging services, to which a value can be assigned or ascribed. For example, in a managed care or capitated healthcare enterprise, a demand for imaging services is some function of the number of insured lives (linear), demographics (nonlinear), utilization profile of the referring physicians (complex), and possibly other factors. Some generalizations can be made, however. If the horizontal axis is labeled " insured lives," then the slope of the demand line is proportional to the diagnostic imaging utilization profile, and determines the volume of examinations. An institution still has to

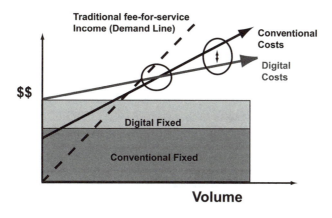

FIGURE 2.1

Break-even analysis.

provide this volume of services: however the important differential is not between the demand line and the cost line (digital or conventional), but between the conventional and digital, where the crossover occurs at some volume level. That's because the incremental or variable costs of a digital study are lower, particularly for the digital modalities.

COSTS

FACTORS DETERMINING COSTS

There is no boilerplate solution for how to determine the costs of implementing PACS. The costs depend on the sophistication of the enterprise's existing information system network and its imaging equipment inventory and needs. These capital costs, together with ongoing costs for operating the system, determine what levels of savings are required to justify PACS. Investing in PACS represents a trade-off: decreased operating costs (film and film personnel) versus increased capital costs together with PACS maintenance and personnel costs. To produce a credible financial analysis, it is best to err on the side of overstating costs and understating savings to the extent that the results allow.

Determining the cost to acquire, move, and store images is critical. An equipment inventory assessment must be done by a technician who understands how each radiology practice operates, what equipment exists, and what PACS equipment is needed. As the cost of software and maintenance

TABLE 2.11

Categories of Expenditures

Imaging Equipment: captures image in digital form

Workflow Managers/Servers: store retrieve, and distribute images

Archive: longer term storage of images

Display Stations: displays images to radiologists and clinicians throughout the enterprise

Facility Upgrades: temperature, humidity, and security controlled environment for equipment; furniture
and lighting changes for reading areas

Clinical distribution and viewing

is often in question and the discounts are flexible, the price to pay for the system could be calculated by using the number that generates a positive NPV. The required discount could be calculated by comparing this number to the list price offering. Equipment vendors can easily supply list prices and customary discounts. This discount, which can be substantial, is influenced by negotiation, size of purchase, and reputation value to the vendor of the enterprise. In addition, list prices are in a deflationary mode as technological advances and competition drive down prices.

CAPITAL EXPENDITURES

The initial capital outlay consists of the following categories of expenditure, listed in Table 2.11, the technical nature of which are discussed more fully in the following chapters. Archive capital costs will continue to decrease, and in spite of early skepticism, creative methods for management of hierarchical storage promise to decrease storage costs even further in the near future.

COST REDUCTION AND REVENUE ENHANCEMENT

Once the capital and operating costs are defined, determine the cost savings and revenue enhancements that will result from implementating PACS. There is a credibility continuum, with hard costs such as film and associated costs being the most credible, and soft ones such as improved patient outcomes being the least credible. An analysis that financially justifies PACS without including savings, which are more difficult to quantify and demonstrate, will be better received than one that shows an impressive financial impact but is built on extensive, unproven assumptions. In other words, proceed along the credibility continuum only until the cost is justified. Doing so also eases the follow-up analysis that may or may not be required to demonstrate postimplementation outcomes.

Partners HealthCare System, Inc. (*Partners*) in Boston provides an example of how one organization proceeded along the credibility continuum, using the financial techniques outlined earlier in this chapter, until PACS was justified. At *Partners*, founded in 1993, by the Massachusetts General Hospital and Brigham and Women's Hospital, PACS was financially justified based on savings from decreased film and film library costs alone, and no further analysis of cost savings or revenue opportunities was necessary. The *Partners* system is armed with a world-class information system infrastructure, consisting of the largest integrated Intel/Microsoft platform in the world connected to 30,000 desktop computers for almost the same number of employees. The two hospitals were also well on their way to converting to computed radiography when this analysis was conducted.

Partners arrived at an implementation cost of approximately $12.6M, along with operating costs of approximately $1.5M per year, together composing the cost to be justified. The analysis was based on an annual volume of 775,000 radiology examinations per year. This represented 2.7M films, at a film cost of $3.5M and a film library cost of $1.7M. An eight-year analysis was performed to cover three years of investment and implementation, three years to break even, and two years to reach steady state savings. All of these factors resulted in an NPV of 0 dollars, or break-even (using a discount rate of 10% required by its treasury department). Likely but difficult-to-quantify cost savings and revenue enhancement opportunities would clearly produce a positive financial return, not to mention all of the nonfinancial benefits such as improved clinical outcomes.

On a per unit (per exam) basis, *Partners* estimated that it would save $8 per exam for film and film library expenses on an annualized basis, for an additional PACS operating cost of $2 per exam, resulting in a net savings of $6 per exam. This however requires a one-time capital investment in PACS infrastructure of $16 per annualized exam but only $3.20 per exam, assuming a useful life of PACS investment of five year (see Table 2.12).

Mayo authors divided personnel costs associated with film into those occurring inside the radiology department and those outside. These costs

TABLE 2.12
Mayo Study: Total Estimate per Exam: $15.82!

Film	$6.25
Supplies	$1.46
Personnel	$5.91 (direct) and $2.20 (indirect)

are incurred by nursing and clerical staff when engaged in both the "film search game" and in traditional methods of requesting and managing exams needed in the clinic or operating rooms. The Mayo authors also made the comment that "Our estimated cost of film per exam per year is most likely an underestimation of real costs when compared to other institutions."

FILM COST

To capture film costs it is necessary to develop assumptions about the number of annual exams, films per exam, and cost per film over the life of the capital investment in PACS. Annual savings is the product of annual exams multiplied by number of films per exam multiplied by the expected film cost per sheet. For example, an enterprise that generally conducts 10,000 annual MRI exams using eight films per MRI at a cost of $1.50 per film would save $120,000 if it eliminated 100% of its film use. It is easiest to combine all associated film costs, including chemicals, processing, folder jackets, etc., with the film commodity cost for simplicity.

For most enterprises, it is necessary to ramp up film elimination from 0% to 90% or so over some number of years. It is difficult to eliminate film entirely (thus the 90%) because of the need to produce films for clinicians outside of the enterprise, for legal proceedings, and so on. Nevertheless, it is necessary to reach a fairly aggressive target quickly in order to justify PACS currently. The rapidity with which film use is eliminated is the *key* factor in cost savings. A long implementation perpetuates dual systems and processes, delays savings, and destroys value. A commitment must be made by the clinical enterprise that film use will be eliminated as soon as PACS is implemented. To make these assumptions real, keep in mind that a replacement for image distribution must be in place as well as a PACS prior to successful film elimination.

FILM LIBRARY COST

The film library cost consists mainly of personnel managing the contents of the film library. Like film costs, the savings here would ramp up and shadow film reduction. The analysis could also include costs saved by reducing the space required for film storage. For many institutions the space saved depends on legal requirements for film storage, which may take several years to develop, as the law generally follows practice, and these, from a legal perspective, are uncharted waters. For the analysis to capture space savings, the organization must have an alternate need for the space, and by gaining the film storage space, be able to avoid leasing additional space. It may be easier to treat such space savings as a wash when anticipating the increased space required for the PACS equipment and its staff, but this needs to be determined on a case-by-case basis.

The analysis can also phase in a reduction in warehouse costs for film storage that shadows the implementation phases. This reduction would also have to respect the film storage time required by law.

LOST EXAMS

The financial impact study could also include the elimination of incremental costs and lost revenue associated with misplaced films. Savings may materialize from a decrease in staffing required of practitioners and administrative personnel to serve existing volumes, or as increased throughput (revenue less incremental costs). This impact is difficult to quantify, and the inclusion of these costs depends on whether the institution tracks this information.

It is also difficult to quantify the cost to the enterprise of not producing a film for a legal proceeding, or the cost of the department's and institution's reputation in not being able to produce a film for a patient or physician who needs it. The nonquantifiable cost to the patient might be staggering if a previous study is needed for comparing with a present study before a clinician can make an informed diagnosis. These situations can be enumerated in the analysis as nonquantifiable benefits.

RE-DOS

PACS virtually eliminates the need for re-dos for two reasons. First, computed radiography imaging modality has a very wide range of latitude for exposure error, compared to film. Second, the rate of lost exams in a well-engineered PACS is very low compared to the estimated 10% to 15% temporary or permanent loss rate in a conventional film library. In order to calculate this savings, estimate the cost of re-dos to the organization in terms of time and materials. The savings in time depends on whether the clinician would be serving other patients instead of repeating the process whereas the savings in cost depends on whether a reduction in staffing would result. Such savings apply not only to radiologists but also to clinicians who are detained by re-dos. Savings on materials are calculated by the number of re-done exams multiplied by films per exam multiplied by the cost per film.

Again, it is difficult to quantify the cost to patients associated with the delay caused by a re-do. At the risk of being overly dramatic, we can say that a savings in time can make the difference between life and death for patients whose critical condition may depend on a rapid diagnosis.

SAVED TIME FOR PRACTITIONERS AND ADMINISTRATIVE STAFF

PACS makes image distribution faster, easier, and more reliable. This feature translates into a cost reduction if staff are eliminated or into an additional financial contribution (incremental revenue less incremental costs) if an unmet demand for services (additional volume) exists. This impact will not be felt until the PACS is fully implemented and all radiologists and clinicians are proficient in its use. This time saved is difficult to measure without comparing the task time today versus the task time in a carefully projected environment, but little data is available for such comparison.

Faster turnaround time will likely translate into shorter stays, which in turn can reduce costs of care or produce additional income if additional patients can be served. The potential impact on length of stay and increased admissions would be difficult to substantiate. It is difficult to know or measure how PACS contributes to shortening length of stay because there are so many complex factors that contribute to length of stay. It is difficult to segregate PACS as a single component.

SITE OPPORTUNITIES: REMOTE, CONSOLIDATION

Just as the electronic revolution makes it possible for millions of people to spend more time working from home, electronic imaging makes the locus of work far less important for radiology services. PACS enables diagnostic images to be available anytime, anywhere they are needed, with little or no human intervention. This eliminates the necessity and cost of having radiologist coverage in multiple sites within an entity and in many entities within a system. The mobility of images created by PACS facilitates peer or expert review of images inter- and intranetwork. This mobility reduces the potential number of radiologists required to serve a given population, and also the time in which those services can be provided. Enterprises that take advantage of these site opportunities will be able to serve existing patients with fewer resources (reduce costs) or serve additional patients with existing resources (increase revenue).

IMPROVED COHESION (MULTISITE OR MULTIENTITY ENTERPRISES)

This benefit refers to the ability to better manage the peaks and valleys of demand by diverting image reading to alternate sites. Diversion allows for more effective use of resources, faster turnaround times, and improved patient outcomes. It also lets any appropriate radiologist read images for a clinician anywhere within the defined network, thereby allowing patients to receive care in their own locales, and in some instances, allowing clinicians to receive radiology services with only a technician, rather than a radiologist, on their sites.

IMPROVED PATIENT OUTCOMES

Perhaps the most difficult benefit to quantify is improved patient outcomes, yet such benefits represent perhaps the most compelling argument. Improved outcomes are the product of many factors: image clarity, fewer lost exams and re-dos, multi-availability of digital images, and most importantly, turnaround time. The latter is especially true where distance is involved. There is no simple quantitative value that can be placed on improved detection of disease or image availability, nor is there a simple way to assess the value of a secure and fast repository of images. These factors will have a huge impact on the way medicine is practiced and the quality of care patients receive.

COMPETITIVE IMPACT

A financial analysis could attempt to capture whether implementing PACS would have an impact on the organization's overall revenue and admissions.

Many enterprises, especially integrated delivery networks, will see the decision to implement PACS simply as a necessary step in maintaining their market position. If PACS is financially justified and greatly improves patient outcomes, the entity or system that adopts it first will have a competitive advantage.

▶ REFERENCES

Avrin DE. *PACS Economic Issues and Justifications*. AAPM 1999 Summer School: Practical Digital Imaging and PACS. Sonoma State University, Rohnert Park, CA.

Avrin DE, Andriole KP, et al. *Hierarchical Storage Management (HSM) Solution for Cost-Effective On-Line Archival and Disaster Recovery Using On-Site Lossy Compression and Off-Site Tape Backup*. RSNA 1999, Chicago.

Excel integrated online help manual. Excel, Microsoft Corp. Redmond, WA.

King BF, Ward S, Bruesewitz RT, et al. *Cost of film: Purchasing, processing, packaging, storing and disposal over the lifetime of a film examination in a large radiology department*. SCAR Proceedings 1996, pp 152-156.

Pratt HM, Langlotz CP, Feingold ER, et al. *Incremental cost of department-wide implementation of a PACS and CR*. Radiology 1998; 206:245–252.

Spiro HT. *Finance for the Nonfinancial Manager, 2nd Ed*. John Wiley and Sons, NY, 1982.

COMPUTING
FUNDAMENTALS

CHAPTER 3

COMPUTING FUNDAMENTALS

KEITH J. DREYER

The personal computer revolution has dramatically changed all our lives forever. Over the past 20 years, with the decrease in hardware costs, increase in computational performance, and a seemingly endless supply of software products, computers have entered nearly every facet of our personal and professional lives. One of the best things about computers is that you don't have to know how they work to make them work. However, we find that if you can understand just the basics (which isn't too hard to do), you can better appreciate how computers can be applied to the field of radiology. With this in mind, the following pages review the basics of modern computers. We don't discuss mainframes or minicomputers. Instead, our goal is to define the fundamental components of a microcomputer—known today as a PC or personal computer—which could easily function as a primary interpretation workstation. We also discuss important software concepts such as operating systems and programming languages. Finally, we describe how these products can be used by us (or our computer engineers) to create the holy grail of computing—the software application program.

You can think of computers like humans in that they share four of the same basic functions—*input*, *output*, *memory*, and *processing* (or thought). And since all these functions occur at different locations, there needs to be a way for them to communicate with each other. Humans use the nervous system for this task and computers use a bus. As a human, there are certain things you know from birth (genetically acquired information), and certain things you learn. Computers are the same (they're just "born" a little differently). The set of preset functions or programs inherent to a computer, known as the operating system, has led to great debates throughout the industry as, like humans, computer's "genetic code" can be altered or reprogrammed by viruses. Finally, those tasks that are "learned" after "birth" (i.e., "installed" after "purchase") are known as application programs, and have made many of their "teachers" (i.e., "software manufactures") very wealthy. And, just as we need to use a language when teaching humans, computers need languages too.

The remainder of this chapter describes in detail these basic computer functions: *Input, Output, Memory, Processing, The Bus, Operating Systems, Computer Languages,* and *Application Programs.*

INPUT

Since our goal for computers is typically to have them communicate with their human owners, many of the input and output functions of computers are much like those of humans. For humans, input comes from the senses (vision, hearing, touch, smell, and taste). For computers, input comes from input devices (keyboard, mouse, microphone, and digital camera, for example) (see Figure 3.1). These devices provide a computer with a rudimentary

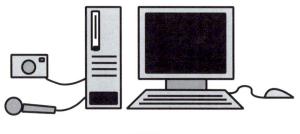

FIGURE 3.1

Modern personal computer with standard I/O devices.

form of three of the five human senses. (We still don't have input devices that provide a computer with smell or taste—probably because there hasn't been a big need for it.)

OUTPUT

Output for humans comes simply through the movement of muscles. This allows us to grasp and move other objects (such as a pencil or a musical instrument), which we can further use to communicate our output data (such as writing or playing music). We can also move certain muscles to generate sound (phonation) to further communicate our output (speech). So in summary, we humans write and draw, talk and sing, and move a variety of objects to generate output, or more properly stated, express our thoughts. With computers, we have tried to emulate several of these human outputs so our computer can communicate with us. Drawing and writing come in the form of computer monitors and printers (both the film and paper types) (see Figure 3.1). Talking and music generation come through a sound card and speaker connected to the computer, which have had limited use in business applications to date. Finally, the movement of objects through the use of computers (known as robotics) is well developed for specific applications (e.g., assembly line automation) but is not generally available to the public.

MEMORY

Human memory is poorly understood and quite variable. Its capacity is tremendous while its accuracy is anything but perfect (you can test this by trying to recite the last paragraph you've just read word-for-word). Computer memory, on the other hand, is well-defined, accurate, and available in large quantities, albeit expensive. Computer memory serves a variety of purposes and comes in a variety of forms. Memory is needed to store data (both input and output data, and recent and old data) (see Figure 3.2) and to store programs (that list of instructions that tell the computer what to do). To serve this variety of purposes best, a wide variety of memory types are available. In general, they come in three forms: integrated circuits, spinning media, and linear media, and these vary based on size, speed of access, volatility, and cost. For a complete description of computer memory options, refer to Chapter 9 on Archives.

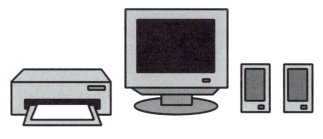

FIGURE 3.2

Removable (floppy) drive and media.

PROCESSING

At the core of the computer is the central processing unit or CPU ("processor," for short) (see Figure 3.3). It is the human brain analog. The CPU interprets a set of instructions (known as machine codes) and performs whatever tasks it is told to do. A list of these tasks, or instructions, is known as a computer program. Programs tell the CPU exactly what to do, and when to do it (but more on programs later).

Modern computers, at the time of this writing, execute instruction at the speed of nearly 1 GHz (that's nearly a billion instructions per second!). In 1979, computer processors were considered screamers if they ran at 1 MHz. Thus, modern CPUs are running a thousand times faster than they did just 20 years ago—and they keep getting faster.

A wide variety of CPUs are available today from a number of vendors. For instance, Intel makes the 80386 (a.k.a. 386), 80486 (a.k.a. 486), 80586 (a.k.a. Pentium), Pentium Pro (related to the 586), and Pentium IV (a Pen-

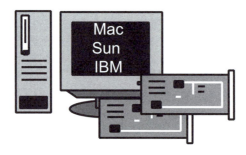

FIGURE 3.3

Various CPU boards.

tium Pro with MMX—Multi-Media eXtension—instruction set). Motorola makes a slew of different CPUs that power the Macintosh series. SUN Microsystems Inc. makes CPUs for its SUN Workstations and for Silicon Graphics for its SGI workstations. As long as manufacturers are able to place more and more transistors on a single integrated circuit, CPUs will continue to decrease in price while increasing in performance, thereby making all of our applications run faster.

THE BUS

Inside your computer is a "motherboard" (see Figure 3.4). Basically this board is the computer, to which is attached a power supply, a surrounding metal case, and all input/output devices (such as the keyboard, mouse, and monitor). On the motherboard sits the CPU, the RAM (random access memory, discussed in Chapter 9), and connections to the hard disk (also discussed in Chapter 9). The motherboard has connectors or slots for attaching other devices to your computer. The number of slots, which varies among computer motherboards, has a large impact on the expandability of a computer. You fill one slot with a video display board, which is how your computer tells the monitor what to display. Basically, if the information is an image, it is taken from the hard disk (and probably decompressed), written into the system's RAM, and then taken from system RAM and written to the video display card. The display card displays the information to the monitor through a cable connected to it from the back of your computer. (To make things more complicated, the video display card also has RAM, which is more expensive and less expandable than the "system" RAM. For

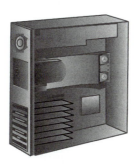

FIGURE 3.4

PC motherboard and power supply.

the most part, up to 64 MB of video card RAM is around what you can buy on a standard card.)

All this traffic must go back and forth quickly if your image is going to make it to the screen in the blink of an eye. Each time the information moves, it takes time. Additionally, the "pipe" through which it moves is known as the "bus," and it can be narrow or wide. There are many kinds of bus, but for the most part the combination of CPU and operating system function on a predetermined or specified bus. In other words, once you buy the computer, you can't change the bus. Because the bus is a bottleneck, a new bus is designed from time to time to speed performance. Since the original IBM PC made its debut, the ISA bus has been reworked a few times for just that purpose. First an extended ISA bus was designed (EISA), but it wasn't terribly popular because it increased the cost of the motherboard and improved performance to only a small share of the desktop market.

Then the VESA local video bus was designed to improve video performance—an improvement needed by many who were running video-intensive Windows applications. Recently, the PCI bus has made its appearance for similar purposes and seems to have succeeded as a standard. Also, AGP is evolving as a standard for high-speed graphic video cards and will probably play an important role in future workstation design.

OPERATING SYSTEMS

The operating system (OS) is the software at the heart of the computer. It is simply a program that performs a variety of basic functions for all other programs. (For example, the mouse pointer arrow is actually generated by the OS. Any program that needs a mouse pointer—like a radiology workstation—simply uses the OS to generate it.) Examples of some OSs that you might have heard of are: CP/M, DOS, LINUX, MacOS, MUMPS, OS/2, SOLARIS, UNIX, Windows 95, Windows 2000, Windows NT, and VMS. Without an OS your computer is merely a lump of silicon and metal. The operating system is what determines what software you can and can't run on the computer. If you have UNIX, forget about running Microsoft Word for Windows. If you have Windows 95, you can't run Macintosh OS-based software.

Historical Note: MUMPS was the first OS designed primarily for medical application programs. It was designed and developed in 1966 by G. Octo Barnett and Neil Pappalardo, respectively, to facilitate the management of text-based medical information through the use of a hierarchal storage array. It is still used in a number of modern radiology departments even today!

An operating system is usually designed to run on a specific CPU or series of CPUs. That is, you can run DOS on an Intel 286, 386, 486, or Pentium, but forget about running it on your Motorola-based Mac. As computers have become more powerful and compact, operating systems have been designed to take advantage of this power, and they have become graphical so that ordinary people can interact with the computer more intuitively. What facilitates their interactions are called GUIs (pronounced goo-eys) for Graphical User Interfaces. Because these GUI-based OSs expose many high-level functions to the end user (e.g., scrolling, drop and drag, wastebaskets), application programs running on them have a "common look and feel" regardless of who makes them. In 1984 Apple introduced the Macintosh. Its OS was probably the first widely accepted GUI. Shortly thereafter came the Microsoft GUI (a.k.a. Windows). Once the first GUI took hold, more GUIs followed in their footsteps, and programs started to take advantage of their advanced, yet common, functions and features. In fact, you can even find major medical equipment, including MR and CT scanners and virtually every kind of PACS component, running applications on GUI OSs on PCs.

COMPUTER LANGUAGES

At the lowest level, computers know of only ones and zeros. If you really want to communicate with a computer in its "native tongue" you would have to speak binary. Furthermore, the CPU of a computer knows very few, rudimentary instructions—what is known as machine language or machine code. Very few programmers can "talk" in this native tongue, and it is a very inefficient form of human-computer communication (kind of like getting your point across to someone by tapping on a table). Enter the high-level computer language.

Even though the computer can understand only this machine code, if it had an interpreter it could understand other languages as well. Therefore, if technicians could think of a logical way to communicate your commands to a computer, they would just have to write a program (known as an interpreter, a compiler, or an assembler) to convert that language to machine language and submit it to the computer. BASIC (Beginners All-purpose Symbolic Instruction Code) is an example of just that. It is high-level language that is much more intuitive for programmers to understand than machine code and therefore makes them much more efficient. A single line of BASIC might convert to thousands of lines of machine language, which the CPU can process in the blink of an eye. Visual BASIC is a specific version of the language from Microsoft Inc. that uses a GUI programming environment for RAD (Rapid Application Development). With Visual BASIC, major works can be developed in days. A limitation of Visual BASIC is that programs written in it currently run only on Microsoft OSs.

Other examples of popular, high-level languages include C, C++, and Java. Java, developed by SUN Microsystems, Inc., is the newest of these languages, and its popularity is growing rapidly because it can run on a variety of CPUs and OSs without altering any lines of code. This "write once, run anywhere" concept has been a dream of programmers since the beginning, and with Java, it may finally come true.

APPLICATION PROGRAMS

Application programs are those software packages that you purchase and install after you buy your computer. (Some are actually installed before you buy, but after the computer is manufactured, and are call "bundled" soft-

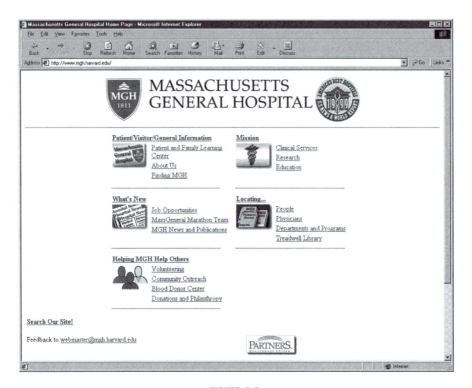

FIGURE 3.5

Sample Web site display using a Web browser.

ware.) Application programs are probably the reason you bought your computer in the first place. Examples include word processors, spreadsheets, and radiology primary interpretation workstations.

Sometimes application programs become so commonplace that they work their way into the OS. A good example of this is the browser application used to "surf the Web" (see Figure 3.5). Considerable debate has been underway recently as to whether "the browser" should reside in the OS or should be sold separately. This seemingly simple decision drastically changes the landscape of nearly every software vendor—thus the debate.

CONCLUSION

Computers are here to stay. In fact, we couldn't sustain civilization, as we currently know it, without them. They continue to improve in performance and usability and decrease in price and size. For them to become even more widely accepted, however, they will have to become better communicators. This is happening already (see Chapter 11, Voice Recognition). It is shortsighted to exclude anything from the possibilities of what computers may be able to do in the future. Compared to humans, they are evolving at unprecedented rates. One can only hope that before we make them too smart, we can teach them from whence they came.

CHAPTER 4

NETWORKING FUNDAMENTALS

SCOTT M. ROGALA

The world of networking and the world of PACS are two different environments that converge in such a way as to require a very special skill set. This chapter gives you the basics of computer networking and shows you how they apply to a PACS environment.

It is important to appreciate the role the network plays in a PACS implementation. Our goal is not to make you an expert network engineer, but rather to give you enough information so you can navigate the often confusing, cluttered world of computer networking. With the right kind of information you'll feel comfortable enough with the terminology to understand what your vendor(s) are providing, on both the PACS and network sides. We also want to impress upon you the importance of good network design and implementation; these are integral parts of the PACS system. Failure to create a strong, robust network infrastructure will result in unhappy users, finger-pointing, and loss of confidence in PACS. If the network is designed and implemented correctly, it can contribute immensely to a successful PACS implementation.

We'll start with some basic concepts, intended not for the veteran network engineer but for those who have had no exposure to computer networking. Through extensive use of analogies, most of you will grasp the concepts well enough to see how much thought is needed in the design of networks, and why the necessary investment of time and capital must be made to achieve a successful implementation. We hope that, by explaining in familiar terms what is considered wizardry and hocus-pocus will help bridge the gap between network engineers and radiologists.

FOR REFERENCE: THE OSI MODEL

The OSI model (see Figures 4.1 and 4.2) was set down by the International Organization for Standardization (OSI) as a framework to make it easier to construct computer networks from the application (as one views an image) all the way down to the physical layer (i.e., the wires). It defined how networks should interoperate. Note that the OSI model serves only as a guideline, and no network, to our knowledge, is set up exactly to the OSI definition.

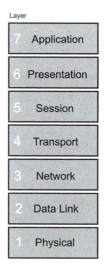

FIGURE 4.1

The OSI model.

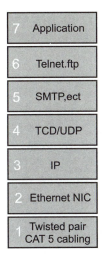

FIGURE 4.2

The OSI model with Ethernet and TCIP/IP.

A SIMPLE NETWORK

Let us start by setting up a very simple network of two computers, a server and a client, to illustrate many of the concepts.

In our example, the server machine is an image archive in a small PACS system and the client machine represents a primary interpretation worksta-tion. For the PACS to work, these two computers exchange data with one another, radiology images, for instance. It would look something like Figure 4.3.

What are the components of this architecture? First we'll work top down, and then explain in more detail from the bottom up.

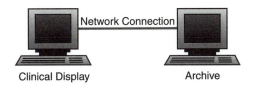

FIGURE 4.3

Two computers connected.

THE ARCHITECTURE AND COMPONENTS AND THE OSI MODEL

The archive machine hosts the images the clinical display needs. An application on the archive knows how to answer image requests from clinical displays. In the OSI model this portion of communication happens at the higher levels. The application needs to transfer this information from itself to the clinical display requesting the information. The overall picture would look something like Figure 4.4. Figure 4.4 is an extremely simplified way of looking at the OSI model. It is displayed in this way to emphasize the fundamental components that we will need to understand to effectively make PACS networking decisions.

Each layer is interested only in the exchange of information between the layer directly above and that directly below. (For example, the hardware layer generally does not care how the protocol layers pass information to the application: it is concerned only with passing the information up to the protocol layer.) In this way the application communicates with the protocol stack, which in turn hands the information over to the hardware layer (the Network Interface Card, or NIC). Next, the hardware layer puts the information out onto the network.

Each layer has a different and well-defined task. The application layer knows the data it wants to transmit, and it knows which machine it wants to transmit it to. The protocol stack knows how to find the computer in question (or to find a device that knows how to locate it). The network layer knows how to transmit the data over the network and the network knows how to transmit the data to its destination. On the other end, the informa-

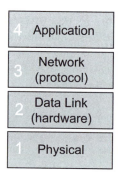

FIGURE 4.4

A simplified OSI model.

tion works its way back up until it ultimately reaches the application and the image is viewable.

In many ways, this is analogous to the way the U.S. Postal System works. In our scenario it would look something like Figure 4.5.

In this example it's easy to see how each layer is independent of each other. It is not important to the envelope what information is contained in it, only that the information fits. The same goes for the post office box, which doesn't care what size envelope or even small box is put in it, only that it's not a koala or something else that doesn't belong in post office boxes. Moreover the box could care less about the contents of the envelope. As we'll see later, the post office system uses the address on the envelope to move the envelope throughout the postal system.

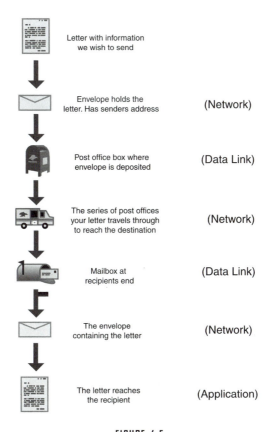

FIGURE 4.5

Postal system analogy.

Now we'll work our way back up through the layers, starting with the physical layer. The physical layer consists of the wires that make up the network. It may also include the NIC in the computers attached to it. In general, the physical layer can be thought of as the "plumbing" or highway of a network. The quality and width of the pipe can determine the speed at which the data can be transmitted, the reliability of the network, and the distance we can transmit data.

Most of you have probably seen the cable coming out of the wall plate and connecting to your computer's NIC. These are commonly known as unshielded twisted pair (UTP) copper cabling, also referred to as CAT5 or CAT3, depending on the exact quality. Networks can also be made up of telephone wires, coax cable (otherwise known as thinnet or 10Base5), and other types of wires. One advance that has changed networks dramatically in recent years has been the use of fiber optic cabling, which can transmit more data over longer distances than conventional cabling by using light or lasers instead of electrical signals. The relatively high cost of fiber cabling has relegated it generally to the core of networks where bandwidth is needed most. Of late, fiber cabling has become the only type of cabling that can support faster transmission rates, and it is finding its way to the desktop as it becomes more popular and less expensive. Later in this chapter, we will discuss which types of cabling are generally used where.

Returning to our example in Figure 4.3, our hypothetical network will use Category 5 cabling between the two workstations for now. They could be directly connected or, using a device discussed earlier, we could use a hub, to which both devices can be connected, as shown in Figure 4.6. Just

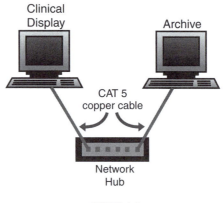

FIGURE 4.6

Two computers connected with a hub.

like the hub of a wheel, a hub in networking terms is a device connecting multiple computers. Hubs can have from as few as four to as many as 24 or 48 connections for computers.

Moving up a layer, the hardware (data link) layer consists of the Network Interface Card, as well as the software drivers installed on the computer that allow the computer to communicate with the hardware. The most common types of cards are Ethernet cards, which are designed to communicate on Ethernet networks. There are also ATM cards (Asynchronous Transfer Mode, discussed later), token ring cards, and a variety of others. As with all the other layers, direct communication occurs between cards of the same type (i.e., Ethernet to Ethernet, or ATM to ATM). As we get into more complicated network topologies, we'll see that networks can become very diverse, consisting of computers with Ethernet cards, ATM cards, and token ring cards, all communicating via the use of various internetworking devices.

For now, to keep it simple, let's say that both computers have Ethernet cards in them. Both computers also have the appropriate software drivers installed.

As we continue to move up our simplified OSI model, we need to discuss protocols. Loosely defined, protocols are a set of predetermined rules that two or more parties follow in communication or other interactions. In computer networks, protocols are the set of rules, or languages, that enable computers to communicate over the underlying network infrastructure. Protocols and how they are used are very much akin to languages in the real world: just as humans speak languages such as English, French, and Swahili, networks use languages such as TCP/IP, IPX, and Appletalk. For two computers to communicate they must be speaking the same language. In our scenario we'll say our two computers are speaking TCP/IP with one another, thus using a common language to communicate over an Ethernet network on CAT5 cabling.

Last, but not least, is the application that uses this language to communicate. In this example, that application is PACS.

COMMUNICATION AND CONVERSATIONS

It's time to delve more deeply into exactly how conversations occur. Once we establish that two computers want to exchange data, they must use their shared set of rules (protocols) to do so. Further, these protocols need to communicate over a network. So far we've talked about Ethernet, ATM, and token ring. These are sometimes called network topologies, and they all occur at the data link layer. Certain rules must be followed on these topologies for them to work correctly. We have also identified a few of the more common protocols (or languages) such as TCP/IP and IPX. These computer communication languages operate at the network layer. Any protocol that is routable is using layer three, the network layer, to make decisions. Protocols that aren't routable are called bridged protocols, and are only aware of the data link layer. We discuss this further when we discuss routing and bridging.

To better explain the relationship between a topology, such as Ethernet, and a protocol, such as TCP/IP, we again use the analogy of human communication. When we communicate, we can do so via a wide variety of media: the air (speech), paper (the written word), or hands (sign language). What language we use is completely independent of the medium we use. Similarly, computers can communicate via TCP/IP or IPX and do so over Ethernet or copper wire or token ring or fiber optic cabling. (Later we discuss devices that do the functional equivalent of taking written English and verbalizing it, or vice versa. You are much less likely to find a network device that does the functional equivalent of translating from English to French; however, such devices are commonly referred to as gateways.)

Since protocols are much like languages, it is useful to use the conversation model to explain how computers communicate. The primary obstacle in using this analogy is that communication for us is second nature; we talk and write without being aware that we are in fact following a set of rules. In the world of computers, where only logic exists and everything is taken literally, conversations are actually very complicated to carry out.

As an example, in human behavior, there are protocols for starting a conversation, such as saying "Hello, how are you?" and responses such as "Good, and yourself?" These sorts of things occur naturally (assuming everyone is civil!). Similarly, ending a conversation has sets of rules concerning good-byes, and so on. Even during the conversation, it's important not to interrupt the person speaking, and to acknowledge what they are saying with a nod. If you don't understand what they are saying, you ask them to repeat themselves. Very similar things happen on computer networks, as we will explain.

AN EXAMPLE OF A CLASSIC COMPUTER NETWORK—SHARED ETHERNET

To get a better understanding of how computers handle this, let's look at a conversation between our archive computer (server) and our clinical display (client) and postulate how they might communicate. The client knows it wants certain information from the server. Its request makes its way down through the protocol stack using a language that it knows the archive understands. This message makes its way out onto the wire, heading for the destination machine. The destination, in this case the archive, is listening for anybody looking to talk to it, and sees the packet (piece of data) on the network. The two machines begin with their "Hello, how are you?" routine and agree to communicate with certain rules.

They agree, for instance, on how much data the two will transmit at any given time, what to call their conversation, and a great number of other things. All the while, since there is a single shared network between the two devices, only one of the two computers can be speaking at any given time. If the client and archive attempt to send information at the same time, both of their transmissions are lost, and they need to start their sentences over. When such a situation arises it is termed a "collision," because the electrical signals effectively collide with one another on the network of shared cabling. In these instances, algorithms in the program determine when it is safe to start trying to repeat the message while decreasing the likelihood for another collision.

When only two computers are in the equation, the likelihood of a collision is smaller than you might imagine. However, as more and more computers compete for the same network, the likelihood of two or more computers trying to transmit at once increases greatly. At some point, when you are building networks with hundreds of computers on them or networks where computers are constantly trying to communicate, collisions become the norm rather than the exception, and the network can't bear the burden of all those sentences in the conversation. The sentences, in network terms, are called packets.

What we are describing is called shared Ethernet, where all of the computers share the same network. Even today it is probably the most popular type of network in the world, although newer technologies are becoming more prevalent. Only one computer can be transmitting its electrical impulses onto the network at any given time. We like to use the example of a conference room to make the idea of a shared medium a little easier to understand (see Figure 4.7).

Let's say that our conference room holds 200 people. First, we set up a simple rule: anybody can talk to anybody else, but only one person in the entire room can be talking at a time. If somebody tries to talk while somebody else is in mid-sentence, they both have to stop and start their sentences again. One can see very quickly how, in a room full of people operating under these rules, very little is going to get said, especially if a lot of conver-

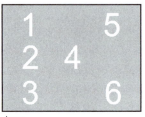

layer

4   PACS, baseball
3   English or TCP/IP
2   The people
1   The air the sound travels over

FIGURE 4.7

The conference room.

sations are in progress. In this example, the conference room is analogous to a network segment, the air is the medium (Ethernet), the people are the computers, and the information they are trying to transmit could be PACS knowledge, baseball news, or the latest juicy gossip. Some could be speaking English or French, but only those who understand French are able to communicate with others who understand French. Similarly, on our network, computers could be talking TCP/IP to one another while others are speaking IPX. They all share the same network segment, but they communicate only with those speaking the same language.

ENTER BRIDGING

You can see in this scenario how inefficient such communications can be. The same was true for early networks. The first attempt to tackle the problem of collision was with a concept called bridging. A bridge is a device that connects two or more networks together. (As we see later, a bridge understands only the two lower layers of our simplified OSI model. Next we talk about a device that understands the lower three layers, a router.)

To explain exactly what a bridge does, let's take the conference room and split it in two. We assign each person a unique number, known as his or her MAC address, or Media Access Control address. The MAC address is unique not only in the conference room, but also throughout the world. In computing, the MAC address is derived from the Network Interface Card. It is how each computer (or in our example, each person) is identified.

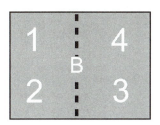

FIGURE 4.8

The conference room split by a bridge.

In Figure 4.8 you see that the conference room is split in two, with people numbered 1, 2, and 3 on the left side and 4, 5, and 6 on the right side. In the middle of the conference room is a dividing wall, which stops all noise unless the bridge, "B," allows it through. It's the bridge's job to keep track of who is where, and to bridge the traffic through the dividing wall as necessary.

For the bridge to do its job effectively, it listens to all network traffic. It does this by listening for broadcasts. In a network, a broadcast is a method a computer uses to locate another computer when it doesn't know exactly where to find that computer. It's almost like yelling out, "Joe, where are you?" In the case of a simple shared network segment, the client looking for the archive for the first time sends out a broadcast requesting the MAC

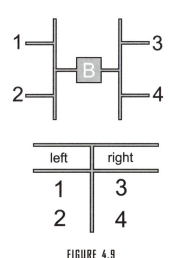

FIGURE 4.9

A segmented network with a bridge and the bridge's table.

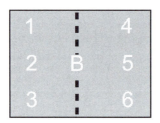

FIGURE 4.10

The equivalent conference room.

address of the archive. The archive answers this request, and the conversation between these two computers ensues. In the case of our conference room without the dividing wall, these broadcasts are just like any other packet—they can cause a collision.

A bridge sits between two network segments (i.e., in the middle of the conference room) and keeps track of who is on which half. Initially the bridge has no idea who is on which side, so it begins to listen to traffic and build a list. When device 1 makes a request to find device 2, the bridge records that 1 is on its left side and that 2 responded from the left side. This is illustrated in Figure 4.9, and the conference room analogy is carried forward in Figure 4.10.

From this point on, any traffic between 1 and 2 are isolated from the right half, effectively creating two different *collision domains*. Devices 1 and 2 can communicate directly with one another without affecting the right side. Similarly, devices 3 and 4 on the right side can function the same way. When the bridge sees device 4 broadcast to locate device 1, the bridge knows that device 1 is on its left side, and will pass the traffic. In performing this sort of task on what once had been one large, congested segment, the bridge can greatly decrease the number of collisions, provided that it is properly located (that is, that proper network design and traffic analysis have been performed). We look more closely at those functions as we design our PACS network.

ROUTING

Bridging solved some, but not all of the problems computer networks faced with respect to traffic. Devices still needed to broadcast in order to find their destinations, and in larger networks with many segments bridged together, networks could still collapse under the sheer weight. On networks that comprised hundreds and even thousands of computers, bridging just wasn't up to the task. Also, although we won't go into detail here, another problem was that bridging didn't scale particularly well, meaning that large, complex networks were susceptible to prolonged outages that could be very difficult to troubleshoot.

The challenge facing programmers was to create a more intelligent networking device that could limit broadcasts and more efficiently use the bandwidth. Routing is a technology developed in the mid 1980s to address these problems. Routing made use of protocols that had more intelligence built in to them so they could pass traffic more effectively throughout the network. Protocols that came along before routing existed had no concept of layer three of the OSI model; they simply made use of the MAC address and used broadcasts to find their destinations. Protocols like that are called *bridged protocols*, and examples are LAT and Netbeui. When routing was introduced, protocols came along such as TCP/IP and IPX, which sent out information in packets that routers could use to more intelligently handle the traffic. These are commonly referred to as *routable protocols*. Such protocols could limit broadcasts and make it much easier to find devices on a large network.

Again we'll use the conference room example, except this time we'll expand our world to include the hallway outside the conference room, and add other conference rooms off this hallway (see Figure 4.11).

In this example, each room has a letter assigned to it: A through D. There are folks in each room and now they can be addressed in two ways. MAC addresses still need to be unique, but the protocol address needs to be unique only within that conference room. Addressing at the routable protocol level would look something like Table 4.1.

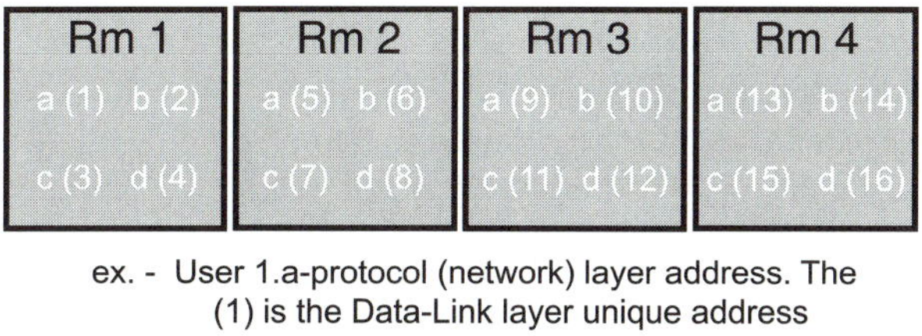

Rm 1	Rm 2	Rm 3	Rm 4
a (1) b (2)	a (5) b (6)	a (9) b (10)	a (13) b (14)
c (3) d (4)	c (7) d (8)	c (11) d (12)	c (15) d (16)

ex. - User 1.a-protocol (network) layer address. The
(1) is the Data-Link layer unique address

FIGURE 4.11

Four conference rooms (A–B) with devices in each.

TABLE 4.1
Conference Rooms and Addresses of Their Devices

Room	Devices addresses
A	A.a, A.b, A.c, A.d
B	B.a, B.b, B.c, B.d
C	C.a, C.b, C.c, C.d
D	D.a, D.b, D.c, D.d

The benefit is realized when we have many conference rooms, as in Table 4.1. When device A.a wants to communicate with device D.c, it knows that (1) device D.c is not in the same conference room as itself (otherwise it would have the same room letter) and (2) that the hallway knows how to find room D. So device A.a sends its information out into the hallway (the router, sometimes referred to as its "default gateway"), and the router relays the conversation to room D, where device D.c receives the information.

Earlier we mentioned that there are devices that can take the spoken word and convert it to written, and the reverse, as well. Both routers and bridges are capable of doing this, and commonly do. For instance, room C could be a room in which all of the devices are communicating via the written word, while A, B, and D are communicating via oral speech. The router would know how to verbalize everything coming out of room D and going into the other rooms, and know how to do the reverse for traffic going into room C.

Routing has been tremendously beneficial in large, complicated environments. Although it adds another layer of complexity and requires significantly more engineering to set up, it goes a long way towards simplifying, troubleshooting, and preventing a network from collapsing during heavy traffic. Unfortunately, routing can slow traffic down, because it has to perform some intensive tasks in order to determine exactly where the packet needs to travel. Keeping with our analogy, the time spent using the hallway to get to another conference room slows the conversation. In most cases the slowdown is negligible, but as we discuss in designing PACS networks, it can be detrimental to PACS performance.

A router is slow because it has to examine more of the packet in order to make routing decisions. Bridges work much more quickly because they have fewer decisions to make. The nature of networks is such that they are never set up as efficiently as possible—the server you need so you get your information inevitably has two or three routers in the way. Even still, as bandwidth demands increase, segments need to become smaller, which means more routers, which means slower response time to the server. When routing became too slow, another technology was introduced. Enter switching.

SWITCHING

Switching, as simple as it is, revolutionized the networking industry. Many networks were collapsing under the sheer weight of routers, and engineers were unable to break up their segments any more than they already had without creating hopelessly complex architectures. The idea of switching is to step back and look at only as much of the packet as a bridge looks at, the Data Link layer. This means that a switch is essentially a bridge. To a lot of people this is confusing, so let's look at it this way—a switch is basically a bridge with many, many interfaces, and sometimes each interface has only one device connected to it. Switches were developed because it became cost-effective to build bridges with numerous interfaces on them. They are essentially bridges that are applied in a different manner than original bridges because they are more powerful. As we begin to look at network design and talk about bandwidth, we'll see how the idea of switching (and the fact that it came about as higher-speed networks were being developed), when incorporated with routing, help make network bottlenecks easier to remove.

Switches are used in a variety of ways. Some switches are used in the core of the network (more on this later), whereas other switches are used to replace hubs. When they replace hubs, they have the same effect as changing the rules in the conference room. Recall our first rule of the conference room: *anybody can talk to anybody else, but only one person in the room can be talking at a time*. If more than one person speaks we have a collision. To help alleviate the problem we first installed a bridge in the conference room, then we added conference rooms with a router as the hallway. But that scheme can be applied only so far. At some point we can't take everybody out of the conference room, and 50 chatty people are going to have some serious collision problems. It doesn't seem productive to install 25 bridges in the conference room. But when switching came along, it greatly simplified the situation by doing just that. In effect switching looked at the rules we established concerning talking and changed one rule in the conference room—that which was the most inefficient. Switching allows us to say that anybody can talk to anybody else, as long as each person is talking to only one other person. Sometimes when a switch is used to separate everybody from everybody else in the conference room, it is referred to as a switching hub.

But what happens when the users in the conference room don't want to talk to each other, but instead want to talk to somebody in another room, i.e., through the router? Then we need to talk about bandwidth.

BANDWIDTH

Bandwidth, simply stated, is the rate at which information can be transmitted in a specific time interval, usually seconds. In computer networks the rate at which data can be transmitted is measured in bits per second. A bit, or binary digit, is either a 0 or a 1. A bit can be considered the atom of the computer world. Eight bits are called a byte. The reason eight bits are significant is that eight ones in binary form (11111111) are equivalent to 255 in decimal form, which is enough to represent all variations in the English alphabet of upper- and lower-case letters, numbers, and other characters.

One million bytes are commonly referred to as one megabyte, or 1 MB. This is how most computer users understand file sizes, hard drive sizes, etc. In the data networking world, however, transmission rates are measured in megabits, not megabytes. One megabit is denoted as 1 Mb to distinguish it from a megabyte (1 MB). In this way, data transmission rates can be deceiving because a network that can transmit data at 10 Mb per second is really transmitting 1.25 MB per second (one-eighth the speed). Why megabytes are used when referring to file sizes and megabits are used when referring to data transfer rates is a mystery. It could have been a marketing ploy by network vendors to make their networks sound faster than they really are.

To most people, megabits mean very little. It's like telling people your car has 282 HP when they haven't experienced 150 HP, 250 HP, or 300 HP. To put megabits into perspective, let's use the example shown in Table 4.2.

Many different types of common networks are available. Along with the shared Ethernet mentioned in our example network, others are listed in Table 4.3 in relative order of performance (though bear in mind that certain traffic conditions may alter the order somewhat, meaning that mileage may vary).

As data transmission rates increase, so does the quality of the cabling required to support those rates. For instance, there is no standard to transmit anything faster than 100 Mb/s Ethernet on copper cabling. All speeds

TABLE 4.2

Putting Megabits into Perspective

The typical individual reads at approximately 600 bits/second.

The image transmitted to your television screen represents about 3,000,000 bits/second.

Most modems connect to the Internet at 56,000 bits/second.

The most common type of network in existence today is shared Ethernet, which operates at 10,000,000 bits/second.

higher than 100 Mb/s require some type of fiber optic cabling. The industry continues to work on the standard for Gigabit Ethernet which will support copper, but the distance will likely be very short (25 meters).

Note that all network transmission rates are theoretical speeds. To say that 10 Mb/s Ethernet can transmit a 1.25 MB file in one second would be fallacious. It's important to make the distinction between theoretical and actual bandwidth and understand why the difference (sometimes called overhead) exists.

Many factors contribute to the difference. To understand overhead, consider how in shared Ethernet there is the possibility of a collision. This is one form of overhead. Any time there is a collision, the data that is being transmitted is discarded and must be retransmitted. In a shared Ether-

TABLE 4.3

Different Types of Networks Available and Their Speeds

4Mb/s token ring

10Mb/s Ethernet

16Mb/s token ring

100Mb/s Ethernet (also known as Fast Ethernet)

155Mb/s ATM (also known as OC3)

622Mb/s ATM (also known as OC12)

1000Mb/s Ethernet (also known as Gigabit Ethernet)

2488Mb/s ATM (also known as OC48)

net segment, this affects the actual bandwidth. Other network types, such as token ring, ATM, and to a lesser extent switched Ethernet, don't share the problems of collisions, but all network types must deal with some form of overhead that prevents them from reaching their theoretical bandwidth.

To understand some of the other factors, we need to examine conversations again, and realize just how little of the conversation in a data network has to do with the actual data being transmitted. Each half of spoken dialog is made of sentences. In a network, each of these sentences is called a *packet*. Packets are the elements composed of bits that carry data between the two computers on the network.

Let's look at the example of the letter and the envelope to see how a packet is formed.

In Figure 4.12, the letter represents the data that needs to be sent to the recipient. Realize that this letter is only a small part of what is actually getting sent through the postal system. The letter requires the envelope, the recipient's address, and the return address. All of this contributes to overhead. In some cases, the actual data could comprise as little as 33% of the packet. On top of that, each packet must be checked to make sure it made it to its destination without any errors (from electrical interference, for instance, which may cause a 0 to be interpreted as a 1 or vice versa). There is overhead in doing the checking, as well. As you might imagine, all of this extra information can quickly contribute to overhead on a network, gobbling up bandwidth you thought you had all to yourself. In some protocols, packets also have to be acknowledged by the receiver, or else the sender resends the packet. Imagine the overhead involved in sending a message that simply says, "Yes, I got your letter." There's very little data in that packet as compared to the actual bandwidth it consumes.

(Bear in mind that the packet in Figure 4.13 is an *example* of a packet, and not to be taken too literally. Each packet is actually made up of other information, depending on the exact protocol and data link layer for which it is designed. Our example packet has been simplified dramatically.)

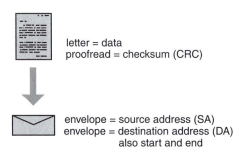

letter = data
proofread = checksum (CRC)

envelope = source address (SA)
envelope = destination address (DA)
also start and end

FIGURE 4.12

A letter and envelope with address is like a packet.

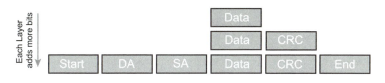

FIGURE 4.13

A simplified packet.

All of this goes a long way toward dragging the actual bandwidth of a network down. Most engineers agree that between collisions and overhead, actual bandwidth on a shared Ethernet segment is somewhere between 3 and 4 Mb/s. Any time you try to transmit more than that you will experience the law of diminishing returns in which collisions become the norm rather than the exception, and very little gets transmitted. The same holds true for 100 Mb/s shared Ethernet, which typically maximizes at somewhere between 30 and 40 Mb/s. Switching can go a long way toward bringing the theoretical and actual closer together by eliminating collisions on a segment. For example, on 100 Mb Ethernet segments (known as Fast Ethernet) that have implemented switching, the maximum bandwidths are closer to 75% or 75 Mb/s. For reasons we discuss later, ATM has different theoretical figures based upon a variety of assumptions and other factors.

FACTORS TO CONSIDER IN BUILDING A NETWORK

Up to this point we've discussed all of the various working parts of a network. We've discussed hubs, routers, bridges, and switches. We've examined different types of cabling used in building networks, and we've discussed how data actually is transmitted between computers. Given the vast array of protocols, hardware, and topologies at our disposal, how is one supposed to determine exactly how to go about building a network? Our original example network is quite simple: two computers, a server, and a client connected to a hub using Category 5 cabling to transmit image information. Depending on how important it is to get the information from the archive to the client, we could upgrade them to a faster network speed, such as 100 Mb/s Ethernet. What happens as we start to add workstations (see Figure 4.14).

If all of the devices are connected to the same hub, which means they share the same collision domain. Because all the devices are relatively close together (within 300 feet), we continue to use Category 5 cabling. Each device

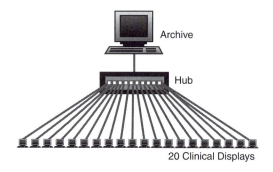

Archive

Hub

20 Clinical Displays

FIGURE 4.14

Adding workstations to our network.

is configured to communicate on the network at 10 Mb/s. In this scenario, each of the clinical displays is attempting to access information on the archive computer. The clinical display can theoretically access the information at 10 Mb/s, and the fastest the archive can respond with information *collectively* is 10 Mb/s. Even if we were to implement a switched architecture here, that would only make the situation worse, as the clinical displays currently don't have to compete with each other to send out their packets. They only have to compete for the archive's 10 Mb/s of bandwidth. Here we can see a bottleneck.

Another way to look at bottlenecks is to look at the example of a human conversation. Let's say that with speaking and listening you can process 200 words per minute in a dialogue hypothetically. This means that you can listen at the rate of 200 words per minute or you can speak at the rate of 200 words per minute. Any more than that and you might become confused and request the other person to slow down in speaking, or you have to slow yourself down in speaking. For argument's sake, let's say you are pretty good at multitasking and can actually be having two conversations at once; you can be discussing PACS networking with one individual and the Red Sox with another. Nevertheless, you can discuss these two subjects collectively at a total of 200 words per minute. If two more people try to talk to you, those 200 words need to be divided among all four parties. At some point you become the bottleneck, as each of the other four parties are capable of handling 200 words per minute but you are able to give them only 50 words a piece. They either have to get their information from another source, or you've got to find a way to speak and listen more rapidly. Similarly, we'll see how we can intelligently upgrade our network in the proper places to get the most for our investment. In our example, we could upgrade the server to "speak" at 100 Mb/s Ethernet, while keeping the clinical displays at 10 Mb/s Ethernet. Upgrading all of the clinical displays to 100 Mb/s Ethernet while the archive processes at 100 Mb/s will accomplish little except in an environment where only one or two clinical displays are requesting information at once, in which case optimum transmission rates can still be realized. If multiple workstations are operating at 100 Mb/s and requesting data from the archive, the archive could again become the bottleneck, at which time we could upgrade it to Gigabit Ethernet or ATM of one type or another.

It's clear there are multiple ways to handle this arms race. In the next example, we begin to integrate the various devices and architectures into a coherent PACS solution.

A REAL-WORLD EXAMPLE

It would be helpful to use a real-world example of how our institutions used to use switching and routing together to increase productivity for several thousand users on a network experiencing high utilization, collisions, and very poor performance. In one case, 1200 users in a particular building were using one 10 Mb/s Ethernet segment sharing the same collision and broadcast domain; that is to say, they were all in the same conference room. Each computer in the room was a client, all accessing servers off their network segment (outside the conference room). Simply installing a bridge would have accomplished little in this case, because all the traffic was attempting to use the same 10 Mb/s router interface. We couldn't take half the users and put them on a different routed segment, because that would have meant readdressing 600 computers by hand to tell them they were on a different network segment (in a different room). We needed to somehow keep all of the users on the same

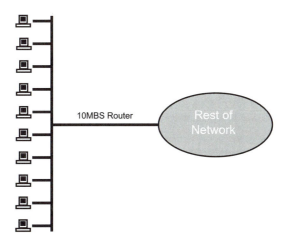

FIGURE 4.15

Network before upgrade.

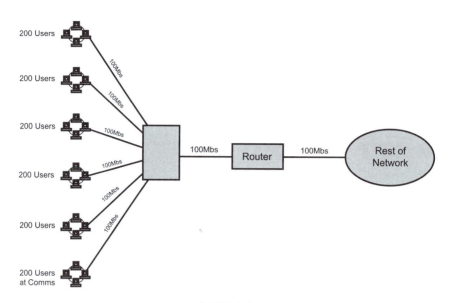

FIGURE 4.16

Network after upgrade.

segment, while decreasing the number of collisions. Installing a switch for all of these users would help some, as they would still be competing for the same 10 Mb/s interface on the router. We needed to do a combination that allowed faster access out of the conference room (the router interface) and use switching within the room so all 10 Mb/s users would suffer from fewer collisions. New equipment enabled us to install a switch and give the router a 100 Mb/s interface into the room, while allowing all users to communicate on the network at 10 Mb/s in a switched architecture. In doing so, we dramatically decreased the number of collisions and circumvented the bottleneck that would have resulted from upgrading to 100 Mb/s the router's interface onto the segment (see Figures 4.15 and 4.16).

PACS NETWORKS

As you probably see by now, networks can be incredibly diverse. There are a number of factors to take into consideration when building a network, and we have many tools available to us in the form of routers, switches, Ethernet, ATM, and copper and fiber cabling. How effectively we put this together depends on the amount of knowledge we have of the tools available to us, as well as an intimate understanding of exactly how traffic on the network flows. We also need to take cost into consideration. Among the many important factors, four stand out (Table 4.4).

TABLE 4.4

Four Important Factors in Building a Network

Performance—How quickly the network can transmit data.

Reliability—How reliable the network is. How easy is it to maintain?

Upgradability—How easy is it to upgrade?

Price—How much does the network cost?

The decision-making process is similar choosing a car. Potentially, one could purchase a high-performance car for a mid-range price, but in the long run there may be reliability issues with it, and maintenance may be expensive. On the other hand, a more reliable car might cost the same amount but lack the performance we might require on the highway. Getting both reliability and performance costs more money.

PACS networks are different than most networks. Typical networks are intended to transmit e-mail, share small files, share printers, and handle other processes. If it takes two minutes or three minutes to transmit an e-mail, does it really matter? If it takes 10 seconds to open that Word document rather than eight, who's going to notice? On the other hand, PACS networks are transmitting large amounts of data, and that data needs to get where it is going quickly and reliably. PACS networks require both performance, because of the sheer amount of data being transmitted, and reliability, because of its clinical nature. The reason PACS is becoming so popular is that only recently have fast, reliable technologies become available to make PACS implementations practical and cost-effective. In the following examples, you'll see networks on three different scales and learn the rationale behind their design.

ATM

First let's look at few technologies that we'll use in building this network. One such technology is ATM, or Asynchronous Transfer Mode. We'll explain the differences between ATM and Ethernet by explaining how they were derived.

Ethernet, in its purest form, is a "dumb" medium. It does not know what traffic is passing over it, nor does it need to. It operates under simple rules and principles that govern how traffic will be transported. Your e-mail about the Red Sox has no higher or lower priority than a PACS image or a telephone call. In this sense, Ethernet is said to have no concept of Quality of Service, or QoS.

ATM, on the other hand, was designed with the intent of allowing the network administrator to classify different types of traffic with different priorities. In this sense, an ATM network offers different levels of QoS depending on the application or workstation.

ATM is able to do this so well in large part because it is a much more predictive architecture. In an Ethernet network, packets can vary in size, reaching a maximum of 1500 bytes. However, some packets can be 300 bytes, some 50 bytes, and some 1500 bytes. Thus, it's very difficult for an Ethernet network to be able to predict traffic patterns. On the other hand, ATM packets are called "cells" and are always 53 bytes in length. Because of the constant size of the cells, ATM is predictive: a packet of streaming video won't get "stuck" behind a 1500 byte e-mail packet in a router while it tries to reach its destination.

ATM is often compared to a telephone network because of the high predictability it ensures. ATM networks can be built so that voice cells will have a high priority and always get through. ATM does this in much the same way the telephone system does. When you pick up the telephone and attempt to make a call, the ATM or telephone network checks to see if it can complete the call with the parameters you require. In the case of ATM and computer networks, you may request a certain amount of bandwidth. If the ATM network cannot guarantee that amount of bandwidth, the computer and the network can negotiate a lower bandwidth rate, or not start the conversation at all. This is very much like a telephone call, especially a cell phone call, where you occasionally get a "fast busy" because the voice network cannot guarantee enough bandwidth to complete the call.

That said, ATM has had a long, troubled journey toward universal acceptance. It has taken years from its inception to make it to a finished product. Along the way various vendors have released product based only loosely upon not-yet-agreed-upon standards that make vendor interoperability very unlikely. Because of this, when you choose an ATM vendor, understand the high probability of the product's not working with other ATM hardware.

Another consideration in choosing to use ATM in networks is the work a router or switch needs to perform in converting packets into cells and back. This conversion contributes a certain overhead, which is often viewed as detrimental. Strong consideration should be made when mixing ATM with other network types, such as Ethernet. However, those considerations go beyond the scope of this book.

There are other downsides to ATM. The number of ATM installations in most LAN environments is rather small when compared to those of Ethernet. Hence, it can be harder to find engineers who have expertise in the area. What is more, the price/port of ATM is significantly higher than Ethernet. Add to this the fact that Gigabit Ethernet is beginning to

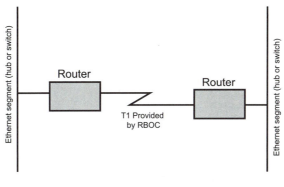

FIGURE 4.17

Illustration of how leased circuits from RBOCs can be integrated into LANs to allow connectivity between two LANs.

gain steam and provide high bandwidth at a smaller price, so an investment in ATM may not be a good one.

WAN NETWORKING

All of the technologies that we've talked about so far (ATM, Ethernet, token ring) have been designed for local campus settings; that is, for connections where we can run either fiber or copper cabling. When we leave the campus setting, however, we no longer have the luxury of being able to run our own cable. Whether trying to go across the street, across town, or across the world, we need an external provider to connect sites. Telephone companies (also known as Regional Bell Operating Companies, or RBOCs) such as Bell Atlantic or AT&T, have massive networks designed for handling telephone calls all over the world. They can use these networks to provide data transmission as well.

RBOCs lease "circuits" to companies over which to transmit data. These circuits are generally point-to-point connections between two sites. Generally speaking, the circuits they provide offer bandwidth from 56 Kbs all the way up to 155 Mb/s. Unfortunately, charges are recurring (usually monthly), and the price per megabit is much higher than on the LAN for a connection of the same speed. For instance, a standard type of circuit, a T1, operates at 1.554 Mb/s, and can cost several hundred dollars per month. The farther the circuit extends, the more the RBOC charges. Several factors in the industry have kept these costs fairly stable for many years, but technologies to get around these charges are becoming more popular, and competition is starting to drive down prices (see Figure 4.17). We discuss some of these technologies and the competition factors later in this chapter.

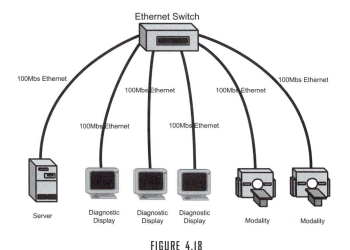

FIGURE 4.18

A simple PACS network.

A SIMPLE PACS NETWORK

Figure 4.18 shows a relatively simple PACS network. As you can see, there are two modalities, three clinical and diagnostic displays, and an archive server. All of these devices are connected to a central Ethernet switch, probably using CAT5 cabling. This network assumes that all devices connecting to the central switch are within cable spec for connecting at speeds of 100 Mb/s.

In this diagram the archive server is connected at 100 Mb/s, as are the diagnostic/clinical displays. The modalities are connected at 10 Mb/s. As most traffic is being sent to the archive server and retrieved from the archive server, we see our first potential bottleneck, but in a network of this size, it is very unlikely that the 100 Mb/s connection will be swamped. In some cases, a 1000 Mb/s (Gigabit Ethernet) connection could be substituted for the 100 Mb/s connection to the server, but the likelihood that it would enhance performance is minimal.

MAKING LIFE MORE COMPLICATED

Now we'll complicate our PACS network somewhat. First, we'll add some modalities and displays. Let's say these additions are located at the other end of the building and thus the distance exceeds our maximum cable re-

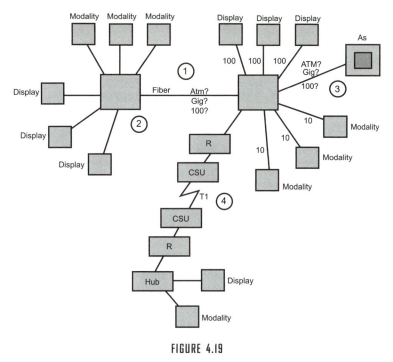

FIGURE 4.19

A more complicated network.

quirements. We'll need to connect them to a second Ethernet switch, and then connect the Ethernet switches together, probably with fiber optic cabling because the two switches are 750 feet apart.

Adding this additional closet (switch) causes us to look at our network in a whole new light. Now we have to consider how much bandwidth we need between the two closets (1, in Figure 4.19). This second switch has three modalities and three display stations and could conceivably saturate 330 Mb/s of bandwidth if all are transmitting at the same time. This is very unlikely, and Fast Ethernet is likely to be enough bandwidth for quite some time.

Still, just as in the simple PACS network, all of the traffic is going to the archive. So it is even more conceivable that the connection between the archive and the switch will be the most likely bottleneck. Given the technologies available these days, both links (2, in Figure 4.19) and (3, in Figure 4.19) could be either 155 Mb/s ATM, although that is not much of an improvement over 100 Mb/s Ethernet. We also need to consider the cell con-

TABLE 4.5

RBOC Circuit Types and Bandwidth

Circuit Type	Speed
Fractional T1	56Kbs—1.554Mbs
T1	1.554Mbs
T3/DS3	45Mbs
OC3	155Mbs
OC12	622Mbs

version if the rest of the devices are still Ethernet and if we want to add ATM to an all-Ethernet environment. Another option is 622 Mb/s (OC-12) ATM, which offers significantly better performance than 155 Mb/s ATM. Gigabit Ethernet is yet another option, and would probably come in at the same price point or better than 622 Mb/s ATM. These options offer a perfect example of how you must work with your PACS vendor and network vendor to determine which connection type best fits your situation.

In our network example let's say we decide to add a remote site across town. We have routers on each end (one at our local site and one at the remote site). Our RBOC is providing a T1 (1.554 Mb/s), a relatively slow connection speed for PACS. With the modality at the remote site, images could still be stored on the archive at a reasonable rate, meaning that compressed images could be read at the remote site. If we need to view uncompressed images in a more timely manner we probably need a faster connection type, perhaps multiple T1s or a T3 (which an RBOC offers at 45 Mb/s) (Table 4.5).

COMPLEX PACS NETWORK

Our complex network incorporates an very large number of devices. Including what is shown in Figure 4.20, 50 or so modalities could be spread around our hypothetical hospital, as well as 50 or more displays for reading the images. We will need a fast, robust network to address bandwidth and reliability concerns. Although the scale has changed dramatically, many of the same technologies are at our disposal. It's a question of how we use them.

We have chosen what is commonly referred to as a "star topology" for this network. In this architecture each switch "B" in Figure 4.20 connects via fiber to the core switch "A" in Figure 4.20. Modalities and displays can be connected to either the closet switch closest to them or to the core switch, if it is closer. We chose this design in our example because the archive server was centrally located to all of them, thus cutting down on wiring costs.

As for the actual connections between the core switch "A" and the closet switches "B," we have a number of technologies. Again, your PACS vendor may have preferences. In this case, we chose Gigabit Ethernet for the connections (uplinks) between the core and closet switches ("2" in Figure 4.20). You may notice that we include two fiber optic uplinks from the closets to the core switch. This allows greater reliability in the event that one of the pairs of fiberoptic connections experiences a failure, or if the fiberoptic connection on either the core switch or the closet fails.

Although not illustrated here, an even more resilient design would include two core switches "A," with the archive server having a connection to both core switches, and each closet switch having a connection to both core switches. This type of connection would create a somewhat more complicated design to troubleshoot in the event of a failure, and it would certainly

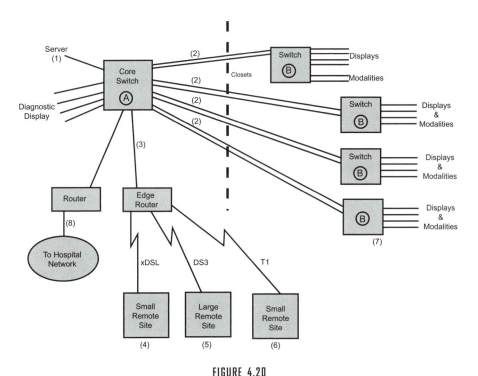

FIGURE 4.20

Complex PACS network.

cost more, but it provides a high level of redundancy (meaning cable failures and hardware failures have less of an impact on our network) and ensures a high degree of availability of the archive server.

You also should notice a connection "3" in Figure 4.20 to an edge router. This router acts just the same as the router in our previous PACS design, except that multiple sites of varying speed connect to it. In the current example (Figure 4.20), we are connecting to a remote site ("4") using xDSL at 144 Kb/s. This speed is too slow for sending or retrieving compressed images, but fast enough for a remote site that needs only to view compressed images ("6"). The site connected with the DS3 ("5") acts just like the site in the previous network example (Figure 4.19).

The site with the DS3 connection can communicate back to our main network at 45 Mb/s. This allows ample bandwidth for the large remote site to host a few modalities and display computers, although at a premium in terms of price. If bandwidth becomes an issue over this link we could upgrade to an OC3 connection providing 155 Mb/s, but the cost would be great.

Finally, "8" in Figure 4.20 shows a router that is providing connectivity to the rest of the hospital network, including its clinical systems. Note that this is the only router we are using on the LAN, and that in none of our previous examples did we include a router, as it can slow down performance in moving large images. However, in interfacing with the rest of a hospital network, a router should provide an efficient way of allowing us to move patient information between the two networks, as well as allowing clinicians to view compressed images throughout the hospital on lower-priced workstations.

FUTURE TRENDS

The networking industry as a whole experiences changes at an extremely rapid pace. The rate of change is dizzying. There are several changes in the industry that will affect how PACS is implemented in the near future.

GIGABIT ETHERNET

Gigabit Ethernet has gained acceptance. Now, Gigabit Ethernet is offered by nearly all vendors at reasonable prices. For the first time on the LAN, the ability for the network to provide cheap bandwidth has outpaced the computer's ability to transmit data. This means that since it is difficult for a Sparc workstation to transmit much more than 200 Mb/s, a Gigabit Ethernet connection offers plenty of bandwidth. Before Gigabit Ethernet, only expensive OC-12 ATM could make such a promise, while most workstations could saturate a 100 Mb/s Ethernet pipe. Of course, as computers get faster, their ability to transmit data will also increase. At this point, however, Gigabit Ethernet provides a lot of room for growth. Even so, it is possible for computers to collectively saturate Gigabit Ethernet backbones and connections, so careful network design is still required. Further, there are groups currently working on terabit Ethernet speed solutions.

RSVP

Earlier when explaining the advantages of ATM we said that ATM had the ability to distinguish between different traffic types, thus allowing it to efficiently pass video and voice traffic while still moving e-mail along at a reasonable rate. Ethernet vendors, not wanting to be left in the dust, recognized this distinguishing capability as an important feature, and have been working toward implementing some of those features into the Ethernet architecture. Called RSVP (Resource reserVation Protocol), this feature will give Ethernet some ATM-like capabilities by allowing it to offer a lesser degree of QoS (almost a poor-man's QoS). When combined with the brute force of Gigabit Ethernet, it offers a challenge to the future of the more elegant ATM in the LAN environment.

LAYER THREE SWITCHING

As detailed at length earlier in this chapter, switching occurs at the OSI model layer 2 and routing occurs at layer 3. The lines are becoming blurred, however, as vendors seek to offer the speed and flexibility of switching and the intelligence and efficiency of routing. Vendors are calling this layer three switching, although different vendors have widely varying ideas of how to implement it and what it means. In effect, layer three switching should combine the best of both worlds to such an extent that the idea of using the corridor in the conference room model will no longer be seen as an impediment to fast, efficient communication between different segments. In a large network, where PACS seeks to peacefully coexist with any number of applications, layer three switching offers potentially dramatic benefits by getting large images and studies out to a vast clientele.

VPN

VPNs, or Virtual Private Networks, have constituted a major buzzword in the industry. The goal of this technology is to make the Internet a safe medium for the secure transfer of private information, such as clinical data or images. It does this by encrypting the information at the source and decrypting it at the destination. In doing so a "private virtual network" is set up over the public, unsecure Internet. There is hope that the companies can use this technology to decrease costs by using the Internet to exchange information that they normally would be able to share only over private circuits leased from RBOCs, thus saving money. This is also an ideal technology to use for remote access to the corporate network for home users or in virtual office environments. In the near future, as this technology matures and vendors are able to produce scaleable solutions, VPNs will make a great impact on how the Internet is used.

LOWER COSTS

Competitiveness among vendors also means lower costs in the networking industry, just as in the computer industry. In the first year that Gigabit Ethernet became available, prices dropped nearly in half. The price of NICs continues to drop, as well as the price of routers and switches. On the WAN front, RBOCs are seeing increasing competition from each other, from cable providers, and from other third-party providers who are seeking to take advantage of the tremendous hunger for bandwidth on the WAN. The cost and speed of the connection to the home or remote office, often called the "last mile," is quickly reaching attractive price points for many applications, especially PACS. RBOCs will be forced to lower prices of T1s and T3s as new technologies such as cable modems, xDSL, and wireless become more common. Similarly, use of the Internet and technologies such as Virtual Private Networking will also allow for significant price reductions for remote access.

CHAPTER 5

DICOM

DAVID A. CLUNIE • JOHN A. CARRINO

OPEN STANDARDS FOR PACS

In a 1992 book on "second generation" PACS, Michel Osteaux writes:

> The absence of recognized standards such as image format and transfer protocol and physical interface has been identified as one major problem with the first PACS realizations. Substantial efforts have been made and significant results achieved. . . . However, the level of real implementation by the manufacturers upon the acquisition modalities is still rather low." (Osteaux, 1992)

By 2001, this situation improved; there has been a revolution in open standards for information technology. A universally adopted standard for medical image interchange has been developed, the DICOM (Digital Imaging and Communications in Medicine) standard. Today it is unusual to purchase an acquisition modality that does not provide a standard DICOM interface for the storage of images across the network. All modern PACS provide a standard DICOM interface to allow the reception of images. Although one cannot always "plug-and-play" modalities and PACS to achieve full functionality and an efficient workflow, considerable progress has occurred.

　　This chapter explains the scope and applicability of the DICOM standard and its relationship to other standards, and describes how to obtain the most benefit from the standard when implementing a PACS.

HISTORY OF DICOM

The interchange of digital images beyond closed proprietary architectures became a desirable feature in the early 1980s, largely as a result of the increasing popularity of digital modalities such as computed tomography (CT), magnetic resonance (MR), and computed radiography (CR). A joint committee was formed consisting of users, who were represented by the American College of Radiology (ACR), and medical imaging equipment vendors, represented by the National Electrical Manufacturers Association (NEMA). This committee produced a series of standards beginning with ACR-NEMA 1.0 in 1985, which was later revised to the ACR-NEMA 2.0 standard in 1989 (ACR-NEMA, 1989). The older standards never proved popular among vendors. These standards did form the basis for subsequent proprietary PACS standards. Standard Product Interconnect (SPI) was developed jointly by Siemens and Philips, and the Papyrus file format was developed at the University of Geneva. The earlier ACR-NEMA standards ultimately formed the basis for the DICOM 3.0 standard, which is now ubiquitous (DICOM, 1998). The scope of DICOM now extends well beyond radiology, having been embraced by vendors and professional societies from other medical specialties such as cardiology, dentistry, pathology, gastrointestinal endoscopy, and ophthalmology.

　　Why has DICOM been so successful where earlier standards failed? Some reasons include:

▶ the specification of a network protocol that runs on top of the Internet standard protocol TCP/IP, allowing DICOM devices to make use of commercial off-the-shelf (COTS) hardware and software,

▶ the specification of strict requirements on the contents of the image "header" and the form of the pixel data itself for each type of modality, thereby improving interoperability,

▶ the specification of a conformance mechanism, so that a user can decide whether or not devices are likely to interoperate, and

▶ an open standard development process that encourages the involvement and consensus of both vendors and users.

DICOM SERVICES FOR PACS—I

The DICOM standard is a large one, and not all of its features are used in a PACS environment. The standard consists of 15 parts, each of which addresses a functional aspect of DICOM (see Table 5.1). It defines services for communication across a network and on removable media. The standard is maintained and extended by the publication of supplements, which add features, and correction items, which fix errors. The standard is republished on a regular basis to incorporate these supplements and correction items.

The most relevant DICOM services apply to the following PACS functions:

- storage (transfer) of images across a network,
- query and retrieval (Q/R) of images, and
- scheduling of acquisition and notification of completion.

TABLE 5.1
Parts of the DICOM Standard

Part	Description
Part 1	Introduction and Overview
Part 2	Conformance
Part 3	Information Object Definitions
Part 4	Service Class Specifications
Part 5	Data Structures & Semantics
Part 6	Data Dictionary
Part 7	Message Exchange
Part 8	Network Communication Support for Message Exchange
Part 9	Point-to-Point Support Communication Support for Message Exchange
Part 10	Media Storage & File Format for Media Interchange
Part 11	Media Storage Application Profiles
Part 12	Media Formats & Physical Media for Media Interchange
Part 13	Print Management Point-to-Point Communication Support
Part 14	Grayscale Standard Display Function
Part 15	Security Profiles

Also relevant are DICOM services for printing images, storing images on media for interchange outside the PACS, and transferring reports.
DICOM services are useful for any application that involves the transfer of medical images between devices. For example, they may be used in:

- a simple configuration where one modality prints images or sends images to a workstation (Figure 5.1),
- a cluster of modalities, printers and workstations (Figure 5.2),
- a small PACS with multiple modalities and workstations and a single archive (Figure 5.3),
- a large centralized PACS with a proprietary internal architecture but DICOM modalities, special purpose workstations (e.g., for three-dimensional imaging) and printers (Figure 5.4), and
- a large distributed PACS with multiple DICOM modalities, general-purpose workstations, and archives, which uses DICOM services for communication between components (Figure 5.5).

It is important to realize that DICOM does not define or depend upon any particular PACS architecture. Rather, the standard specifies services that apply at the boundaries between PACS and imaging components. In different PACS, the use of DICOM may be confined to the periphery of the PACS, and used solely for acquisition of images from modalities, or DICOM services may be used internally within the PACS between PACS subsystems such as archives and display workstations. In addition, the

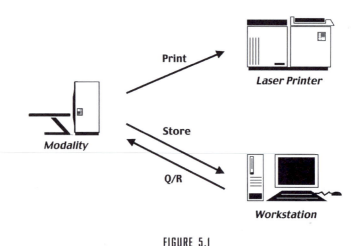

FIGURE 5.1

Single modality, workstation, and printer.

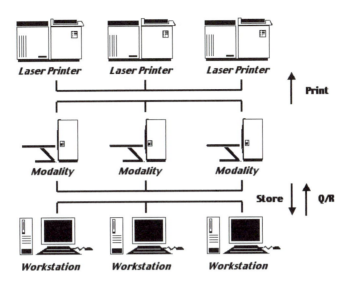

FIGURE 5.2

Cluster of modalities, workstations, and printers.

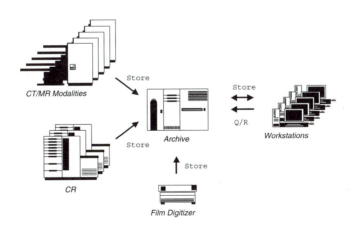

FIGURE 5.3

Small PACS.

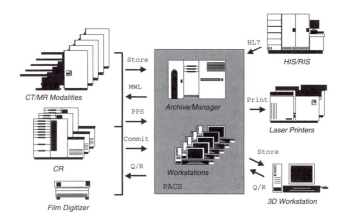

FIGURE 5.4

Centralized, proprietary PACS.

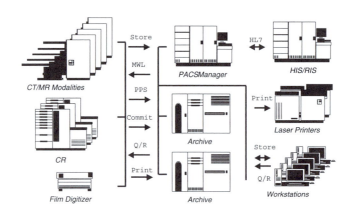

FIGURE 5.5

PACS using DICOM internally.

DICOM file format may be used internally on short-term storage or long-term archive media (although this is outside the scope of the standard conformance mechanisms), or images may be stored internally in a proprietary form and transformed to and from DICOM data sets as required.

Relevant DICOM services, and a brief description of their application to PACS, are listed in Table 5.2. From this table, one can see that the range of DICOM services does not cover every aspect of PACS operation (for example, there are no services for image deletion or migration or for prefetching), and not all devices can or should support all available DICOM services.

The key to the successful use of DICOM services in a heterogeneous (multivendor) environment is the correct matching of DICOM services and

TABLE 5.2
DICOM Services

DICOM Service	Typical PACS Uses
Image Storage	▶ Transfer images from modality to PACS archive
	▶ Transfer images from PACS archive to workstations
Query/Retrieve	▶ Browse/search archive from workstation
	▶ Retrieve images from archive to workstation
Print	▶ Print images from modalities
	▶ Print images from workstations
Modality Worklist	▶ Supply scheduling information to modalities
	▶ Provide modalities with demographics for image header
	▶ Facilitate matching received images with requests, old studies
Modality Performed Procedure Step	▶ Update schedule when procedure step commenced
	▶ Notify PACS when procedure step complete
	▶ Advise PACS of list of images comprising procedure step
Storage Commitment	▶ Allow modality to delete local images when PACS has confirmed they are stored
Interchange Media Storage	▶ Record images on media for transfer to another institution, physician or PACS
	▶ Receive images from outside sources (modalities or PACS)
	▶ Internal long-term archive format to reduce risk of obsolescence of storage media

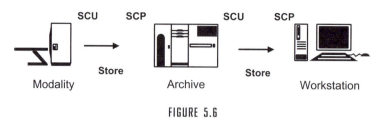

FIGURE 5.6

Service Class User and Provider roles.

roles. In DICOM terminology, the term "role" means that a device is either a "user" of a particular service (Service Class User or SCU) or a "provider" of a service (Service Class Provider or SCP). For example, when transferring an image across a network from a modality to a PACS archive, the modality acts as the SCU of an image storage service class, and the archive acts as the SCP. In the other direction, when the archive is transferring an image to a workstation, the archive acts as the SCU and the workstation acts as the SCP. This is illustrated in Figure 5.6.

DICOM STORAGE INFORMATION OBJECTS FOR PACS

To achieve interoperability between applications, it is not sufficient to specify generic image storage services. Rather it is necessary to define in detail the contents of images for each modality. Accordingly, the DICOM standard specifies Information Object Definitions (IODs), which describe the data structures that contain image data and associated information. Table 5.3 lists the IODs for the modalities currently defined or proposed. Not all of these definitions are for images, because DICOM can also be used to exchange other information such as reports, presentation states, radiotherapy plans, waveforms, and so on.

Differentiating information objects per modality is useful for the following reasons:

1. The form of the pixel data differs between modalities. For example: CT images are often represented as signed 12-bit grayscale values in Hounsfield Units, whereas ultrasound images are often 24-bit true color images containing a grayscale structural image with color Doppler velocity information.

TABLE 5.3
DICOM Information Object Definitions

IOD	Contains
Secondary Capture (SC) (scanned film, frame grabs, screen saves)	Single frame images
Computed Radiography (CR)	Single frame images
Digital X-Ray (DX)	Single frame images
Digital Mammography (MG)	Single frame images
Intra-oral Radiography (IO)	Single frame images
Computed Tomography (CT)	Single frame images
Magnetic Resonance (MR)	Single frame images
Ultrasound (US)	Single and multiframe images
Nuclear Medicine (NM)	Multiframe images
X-Ray Angiography (XA)	Multiframe images
X-Ray Fluoroscopy (XRF)	Multiframe images
Positron Emission Tomography (PET)	Single frame images
Radiotherapy (RT) Image, Dose, Plan, Structure Set, Record	Single frame images (RT Image)
Hardcopy Image (HC)	Single frame images
Visible Light (VL) Endoscopy, Microscopy, Photography	Single frame images
Waveforms (WV), including ECG, Hemodynamic and Audio	Time-based waveforms
Grayscale Softcopy Presentation State Storage (PR)	Rendering instructions
Structured Reporting (SR)	Reports, measurements, and annotations

2. The technique information differs between modalities, but can be standardized within a modality type, allowing the use of common attributes between vendors for display annotation and queries. For example, CT and MR images would normally be annotated with the slice thickness, whereas CR images would not, and MR images would be annotated with pulse sequence parameters like echo and repetition time, whereas CT and CR images would be annotated with peak kilovoltage and exposure.

3. The processing applied to images prior to display on a PACS workstation may be modality dependent. For example, a CR image might

have a nonlinear grayscale contrast lookup table applied, chosen on the basis of image statistics and anatomic location, whereas CT and MR images would normally be displayed with a linear window center and width.

In DICOM, the combination of a Service Class and an IOD is referred to as a Service-Object Pair (SOP) Class. A device may support the user (SCU) or provider (SCP) role for one or more SOP Classes. For example, a CT modality would typically adopt the SCU role for the CT Image Storage SOP Class to transfer images to an archive that supported the same SOP Class in the SCP role. The same archive acting in the SCU role of the CT Image Storage SOP Class could then transfer images to a workstation acting in the SCP role.

Typically an archive supports many different image storage SOP Classes, if not all of those defined in the standard. A workstation is specialized for a particular application and supports only a few Image Storage SOP Classes. For example, a 3D workstation typically supports only the CT, MR, and Secondary Capture Image Storage SOP Classes, and a projection radiography workstation typically supports only the CR, DX, and Secondary Capture Image Storage SOP Classes. A modality usually only supports its own specific SOP Class (as well as the Secondary Capture Image Storage SOP Class, if it supports a "screen save" operation).

DICOM CONFORMANCE STATEMENTS

Specifying and implementing a PACS using DICOM components requires an understanding of the DICOM Conformance Statement. The standard specifies that the manufacturer of any device claiming conformance shall provide a conformance statement that describes the capabilities of the device. To facilitate comparison, each conformance statement has a standard structure. Conformance statements can be obtained directly from the vendor and are often made available over the Internet on vendors' web sites.

DICOM conformance is voluntary. No official body has authority to enforce conformance with the standard. There is no certification or testing authority to verify claims of conformance.

Conformance to the standard does not guarantee interoperability between devices, but allows one to assess the feasibility of interoperability between devices. The purpose of the conformance statement is to allow the user to determine which features of the standard are supported by a particular implementation, and what extensions or specialization that implementation adds. By comparing the conformance statements of two implementations, a knowledgeable reader should be able to determine whether interoperability is possible.

SOP CLASSES AND ROLES

The conformance statement specifies which SOP classes the device supports and in which roles. One can determine from the conformance statement whether a device supports the services necessary to meet the user's requirements, and if two devices are compatible, in that they support the necessary SOP Classes in complementary roles.

For example, if a CT scanner's conformance statement specifies support for the CT Image Storage SOP Class in the SCU role, and, the image acquisition gateway for a proprietary PACS supports the CT Image Storage SOP Class in the SCP role, then the CT scanner should be able to transfer images to the PACS through the gateway.

Alternatively, if an ultrasound (US) machine's conformance statement specifies support for the US Image Storage SOP Class in the SCU role, but the PACS gateway does not support this SOP Class, then images cannot be transferred.

Closer inspection of the conformance statement of the ultrasound machine might reveal, however, that it can be configured to send grayscale ultrasound images as an SCU of the Secondary Capture SOP Class instead of the US Image Storage SOP Class, and that the PACS gateway supports this SOP Class as an SCP, so that images may be able to be transferred after all.

A more complex example illustrates the importance of careful comparison of the tables of SOP Class support for SCU and SCP roles in the conformance statements. Table 5.4 illustrates some typical modality, workstation, and PACS capabilities that might be found in a conformance statement.

How might these devices match potential PACS image transfer requirements (see Figure 5.7)?

1. Can the modality push CT images to the PACS?

   Yes—the modality and the PACS support the CT Image Storage SOP Class in complementary roles, with the modality as the sender (SCU) and the PACS as the receiver (SCP).

2. Can the modality push screen-saved images to the PACS?

   Yes—the modality and the PACS support the Secondary Capture Image Storage SOP Class in complementary roles, with the modality as the sender (SCU) and the PACS as the receiver (SCP).

TABLE 5.4
DICOM Conformance Statement Matching Example

Modality	PACS	Workstation
CT Image Storage—SCU	CT Image Storage—SCU & SCP	CT Image Storage—SCP
	MR Image Storage—SCU & SCP	MR Image Storage—SCP
SC Image Storage—SCU	SC Image Storage—SCU & SCP	
Study Root Q/R Find, Move—SCP	Study Root Q/R Find, Move—SCP	
Patient Root Q/R Find, Move—SCP		Patient Root Q/R Find, Move—SCU
Storage Commitment Push—SCU	Storage Commitment Push—SCP	
	Storage Commitment Pull—SCP	
Modality Worklist—SCU	Modality Worklist—SCP	
Performed Procedure Step—SCU		

3. Can the PACS push CT images to the workstation?

Yes—the PACS and the workstation support the CT Image Storage SOP Class in complementary roles, with the PACS as the sender (SCU) and the workstation as the receiver (SCP).

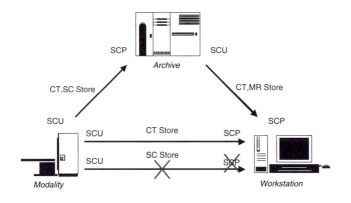

FIGURE 5.7

Conformance statement example—Storage.

4. Can the PACS push screen-saved images to the workstation?

No—even though the PACS supports the Secondary Capture Image Storage SOP Class in the sender (SCU) role, the workstation does not support the SOP Class as a receiver (SCP).

5. Can the workstation push CT and screen-saved images to the PACS?

No—the workstation does not support any Image Storage SOP Classes in the role of sender (SCU).

This example also illustrates the use of some DICOM SOP Classes that we have yet discussed in detail, such as query/retrieve (Q/R) and storage commitment. For now it is sufficient to assume that if the SOP Classes do not match exactly, they are not compatible.

Figure 5.8 illustrates some requirements for the interpretation of the DICOM Query/Retrieve SOP Classes specified in the conformance statement.

1. Can the workstation query the PACS about what images are available and retrieve them?

No—though the workstation supports Query/Retrieve Find and Move as an SCU and the PACS supports Query/Retrieve as an SCP, they support different models as specified by the Patient Root and Study Root SOP Classes and hence are incompatible.

2. Can the workstation query the modality about what images are available?

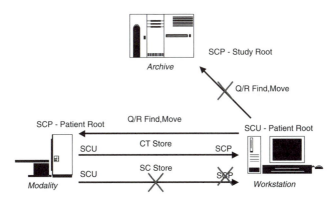

FIGURE 5.8

Conformance statement example—Query/Retrieve.

Yes—the modality and the workstation support the Patient Root Query/Retrieve Find SOP Class in complementary roles, with the workstation making the query (SCU) and the modality responding (SCP).

3. Can the workstation query the modality and have it send CT images?

Yes—the modality and the workstation support the Patient Root Query/Retrieve Move SOP Class in complementary roles, with the workstation making the query (SCU) and the modality responding (SCP) by initiating a transfer of the requested images using the CT Image Storage SOP Class with the modality as the sender (SCU) and the workstation as the receiver (SCP).

4. Can the workstation query the modality and have it send screen-saved images?

No—even though the modality and the workstation support the Patient Root Query/Retrieve Move SOP Class in complementary roles, with the workstation making the query (SCU) and the modality responding (SCP), the transfer of the requested images cannot occur because the workstation is not an SCP of the SC Image Storage SOP Class and cannot receive the images, even though the modality can act as the sender (SCU).

Figure 5.9 shows further requirements that illustrate the interpretation of some of the more advanced DICOM SOP Classes for modality/PACS integration that may be specified in the conformance statement.

1. Can the modality ask the PACS if images have been stored so they can be deleted from the modality's own local storage?

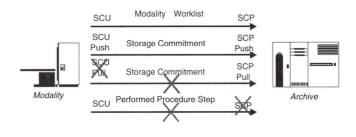

FIGURE 5.9

Conformance statement example—Integration services.

Yes—the modality and the PACS both support the Storage Commitment Push Model SOP Class in complementary roles, with the modality requesting the commitment (SCU) and the PACS responding (SCP); the PACS also supports the Storage Commitment Pull Model SOP Class as an SCP, but the modality doesn't support it as an SCU.

2. Can the modality query the PACS for a list of work to be performed?

Yes—the modality and the PACS support the Modality Worklist SOP Class in complementary roles, with the modality making the query (SCU) and the PACS responding (SCP).

3. Can the modality inform the PACS about what work it has performed and completed?

No—although the modality supports the Modality Performed Procedure Step SOP Class in the sender (SCU) role, the PACS does not support the SOP Class as a receiver (SCP).

One can see from the foregoing how important it is to match the SCU/SCP SOP Class tables in the conformance statements to determine whether devices are compatible and whether they meet the requirements of the PACS.

OTHER INFORMATION (IMAGE IODS, ANNOTATION, REAL-WORLD ACTIVITIES)

An actual conformance statement contains more than a list of supported SOP Classes in SCU and SCP roles. Matching the SOP Classes and roles is one important step towards determining interoperability, but a match is not a guarantee of interoperability. Other information in the conformance statement defines in greater detail precisely how, for example, an image transfer will take place, using what encoding or compression, over what kind of network connection, and with what associated attributes.

Most of this detail is not necessary for analyzing the compatibility of devices, since there are baseline requirements for such things as encoding. If one device supports some form of compression and the other does not, these capabilities will be negotiated when a connection is established, and a baseline of uncompressed encoding will be used to complete the transfer, if necessary. It is rarely important to dwell on the precise network hardware capabilities specified in the conformance statement, because these are usually inherited from the host computer. TCP/IP over some form of Ethernet is almost always supported. A few devices support TCP/IP over ATM instead of Ethernet, using either Local Area Network Emulation (LANE) or Classical IP.

The image IODs of the supported Image Storage SOP Classes specify sufficient mandatory attribute values for most routine PACS applications, such as image display, annotation, and 3D reconstruction.

When highly specific annotation or complex postprocessing is envisaged, the detailed list of attributes sent by a modality or stored by a PACS, as described in the conformance statement, may be helpful. The conformance statements should also specify what identifying attributes are sent by an SCU with the images and how the SCP uses them. For example, a modality may specify that it does or does not copy all relevant identifying attributes and codes from a worklist into the images, and a PACS may specify in what ways it "coerces" identifying attributes to match its (presumably greater) knowledge of the state of patients, studies, and requests. In particular it should be possible to determine from the conformance statement what is done with patient's names that are misspelled, whether accession numbers are supported, and what is done with temporary "trauma identifiers" once the patient's real name and identifier are known.

Also specified in the conformance statement are the real-world activities associated with invoking or responding to DICOM services. For example, one might read in a conformance statement for a modality that "pushing the send button at the study level will invoke transfer of images." One might deduce from this that images can be sent only as an entire study, not as individual series or images, and that there is no mechanism to configure the device to automatically send images as they are acquired and reconstructed. A conformance statement for a PACS might state that "after a delay of ten minutes, if no more images are received from the modality, the study is assumed to be complete and scheduled for reporting," which may or may not be compatible with the workflow of the institution or the modalities.

Close reading of the description of associated real-world activities in a conformance statement may reveal subtle but important assumptions, restrictions, dependencies, and configuration parameters that may cause interoperability problems.

For other than simple image storage services, the conformance statements contain additional information, such as definitions of query keys and models, and extended negotiation. It is necessary to understand each of the relevant services and its features in detail to interpret these conformance statements. Even for the more complex services, however, a simple matching of SOP Classes and roles often suffices for determining whether or not the devices have any chance of interoperating and meeting the requirements.

DICOM SERVICES FOR PACS—II

The Storage Service Class for the transfer of images has been described in previous sections. Some other DICOM services relevant to PACS have been mentioned and their role in matching conformance statements illustrated. In this section, further detail of some of these other services is provided.

QUERY AND RETRIEVAL

It is often not sufficient just to "push" images across the network to where they are needed. A useful facility is the ability to query a device for a list of available images, and then either to retrieve them or have them sent somewhere else. The DICOM standard provides the Query/Retrieve Service Class for this purpose. This service class supports the ability to ask for a list of patients, studies, series, or instances (the FIND operation), and to initiate the transfer of instances by patient, study, series, or instance list (the MOVE operation).

    The term "instance" is used in this context rather than "image", because the Query/Retrieve Service Class may be used to find and move objects that are not images, such as reports, waveforms, overlays, and curves. In addition, the term "MOVE" is something of a misnomer, because there is no implied deletion at the source (i.e., it is really a copy rather than a move). The MOVE operation transfers the selected instances on a separate "association" (the DICOM term for a network connection). This may be to a different device from that which requested the move. An operation called GET returns the instances on the same association as the request, but it is not widely supported and its use is deprecated.

    Not all systems support the concept of a patient. In many databases, the patient's details are considered attributes of a study. Accordingly, there are two Query/Retrieve Information Models (illustrated in Figure 5.10): Patient Root and Study Root.

    The following SOP Classes are defined:

▶ Patient Root Query/Retrieve Information Model—FIND,
▶ Patient Root Query/Retrieve Information Model—MOVE,

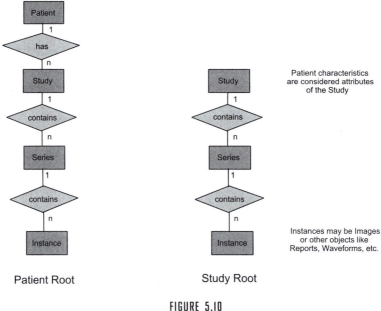

FIGURE 5.10

Query/Retrieve information models.

▶ Study Root Query/Retrieve Information Model—FIND, and

▶ Study Root Query/Retrieve Information Model—MOVE.

Some systems support both models; others support only one or the other. In general, the Study Root SOP Classes are more widely available, but many workstations support the ability to use either to initiate a query. A minority of modality vendors supports the Patient Root SOP Classes but not the Study Root SOP Classes.

The selection of what to query for or retrieve is specified by choosing a query "level," then selecting appropriate values for "keys" at that level. The baseline behavior is to support a strictly hierarchical model, such that a single entity (patient, study, or series) is selected at levels above the query level by specifying a value for designated "unique keys." Then, more flexible matching (by wildcards and ranges) is allowed at the query level itself. For example, to query for a list of the Instance Numbers (also known as Image Numbers) in a single series of a single study, one could use an instance level query using the Study Root Model Find SOP Class, by specifying the following keys:

▶ match a single study by using the Study Instance UID (Unique Identifier) as the unique key,

- match a single series by using the Series Instance UID as the unique key, and
- return all the Instance Numbers by specifying an empty (zero length) Instance Number key.

If one does not know a unique key value (which is always a UID except for patient level queries), one can determine it by performing a higher level query first. Alternatively, some systems support a fully relational (rather than hierarchical) model of query, for which unique keys are not required. This capability can be negotiated when the association is established, and the availability of this feature is documented in the conformance statement. Because relational queries are not widely supported, however, systems should be capable of meeting the user's requirements using the baseline hierarchical query mechanism whenever possible.

From the point of view of retrieving objects, it is not always necessary to perform a query (FIND) before retrieval (MOVE) if one already has enough information to specify the appropriate keys at the level of retrieval. For example, if one knows the Study Instance UID of a particular study and wants to transfer its entire contents (i.e., all its series and instances), one can initiate a study level MOVE using the value of Study Instance UID as the unique key.

MODALITY WORKLIST

In most PACS, modalities passively push images to the PACS as they are acquired. These images contain patient demographic details and study identification information that has been entered manually by the operator. Much of this information is already available to the PACS or the information system (HIS or RIS) in its database. Repeated manual entry of the same identifying data is reported to have an error rate of 15 to 20%. Therefore there is often a mismatching between identifiers entered at the modality and identifiers stored in the PACS or RIS/HIS. This leads to a "lost study" problem in the PACS, which cannot automatically match new images with requests or old studies, or route images to appropriate worklists or stations for reporting. If such a discrepancy occurs, the PACS must either reject the images or route them to a special list for manual intervention.

Furthermore, modality operators have traditionally received information about what work that is scheduled from printed or handwritten lists, or from a RIS/HIS terminal. The use of "paperless" scheduling mechanisms is desirable to enhance workflow efficiency.

The DICOM Modality Worklist service was created to facilitate more accurate identification of images and to provide scheduling information. It allows a modality to query a worklist SCP for information about Scheduled Procedure Steps. The query can be made based on modality, station, date, and time or by individual request, study, or patient identifiers. The modality can use the result of the query either to build a list of work to be performed, from which the operator can select scheduled procedure steps, or accurately and automatically to fill in the identification and demographic information for a scheduled step that is already known to the operator (e.g., based on a known accession number used as a query key).

An effective modality implementation of the Modality Worklist service as an SCU can considerably improve the efficiency of the modality operator by reducing reentry of data, and improve the efficiency of the PACS by filling out the DICOM image "header" information more completely and accurately. A popular strategy is to combine the use of bar code readers with DICOM Modality Worklist to automatically select worklist entries by scanning bar-coded patient wristbands or identification cards, request forms, or charts.

The provider of the worklist information (the SCP) need not necessarily be the PACS or the RIS/HIS. A common configuration uses a stand-alone "box" that monitors RIS/HIS transactions and builds an internal database of request information, then acts as a Modality Worklist SCP to provide the information to modalities on demand. Gateway devices like this act as an effective interface between the "event-based" model upon which many RIS/HIS systems are built, and the "query-based" model favored by modality implementers.

After the network Image Storage Service Class, the Modality Worklist Service Class is the most important DICOM tool for improving the productivity of a PACS. Whenever possible, avoid buying modalities or PACS that do not support Modality Worklist, and retrofit older equipment with additional hardware or software to support the service. In some cases, a "gateway" or "broker" can be interposed between older PACS and acquisition devices that do not directly support the Modality Worklist facility.

MODALITY PERFORMED PROCEDURE STEP

The modality worklist service provides a means for a PACS or Information System (IS) to keep the modality informed. The Modality Performed Procedure Step service "closes the loop" in the other direction by informing the PACS or IS:

- when a procedure step has started,
- when a procedure step has been completed (or aborted),
- what images were generated by the procedure step, and
- what other potentially useful information exists for billing and quality control, such as use of consumables, radiation dose delivered, and so on.

One of the important objectives of this service is to help the PACS and IS to know when to trigger further actions in the workflow. Specifically, the PACS and the IS need to know when to remove a scheduled step from their scheduling worklists, and when to add a study to a reporting worklist (i.e., to indicate that it is "ready" for reporting).

The latter event is especially difficult to determine and often requires human intervention, either at a separate IS or PACS terminal or a Quality Control (QC) workstation. Even when a procedure step at the modality has been completed, it may not be possible to determine whether that procedure step completely satisfies what was requested. A request that generates a complete study may involve multiple procedure steps performed on multiple devices at different times. For example, a barium procedure may include "spot" or "cine" images (XRF) obtained on one device during fluoroscopy as well as static projection radiography (CR or DX) images obtained on a different device later in the study.

The best that DICOM can do under these circumstances is to provide notification that a particular procedure step has been performed, link it to what was scheduled, and let the PACS know what images it should have. If the PACS does not yet have all those images, then the procedure step is definitely not ready for reporting. In the past, determining what images it should have has been a difficult problem for the PACS. Numerous heuristic approaches to determining this have been devised. They are based on the assumption that:

- all the images for one procedure step are sent on a single association, which is then closed,
- when an image from another procedure step is received, there are no more images for the earlier one, and
- when a configurable time has elapsed since an image has been received, the procedure step is finished.

These approaches are fraught with difficulty. They need to be configured per device and software release. They do not cope well with transient device or network failures. It may be necessary to cope with older installed devices to achieve, but whenever possible, new modalities should implement the Modality Performed Procedure Step SOP Class as an SCU.

STORAGE COMMITMENT

Although a modality may have sent its images to the PACS for storage using the DICOM network image storage service, it has no guarantee that the PACS has successfully stored them. It needs to know this before it can safely delete the images locally. In many cases, a manual check has to be performed by a human operator to be sure that it is safe to delete images on the modality. Sometimes such a decision needs to be made in "the heat of the moment" when there is suddenly no more disk space during the course of an examination.

DICOM provides the Storage Commitment service class to solve this problem. It allows the modality to ask the PACS if it commits to storing a list of images. In the "push" model of Storage Commitment, the PACS should have received the images transmitted to it by the modality. The PACS does not make the commitment until after it has received and stored all the images. Once a commitment is received, the modality may safely flag the images as "archived" and delete them, immediately or later, manually or automatically, according to local policy.

Note that the PACS should not try to imply more semantics from a request from the modality for storage commitment. There is no implication that the list of images is a complete procedure step or study; the modality may well make commitment requests before it has finished acquiring all the images in a procedure step.

There is also a "pull" model of Storage Commitment, in which the SCP is expected to query for the images on the list and retrieve them before making the commitment (i.e., the modality does not automatically send them). The pull model is not widely supported and its use is deprecated. Regardless, all SCUs and SCPs of the pull model are required by the standard to also support the push model.

PRINT

As much as a goal of installing a PACS is to avoid the use of film whenever possible, film is still required for some applications, including referral or transfer of patients to outside institutions, and display of images in areas where soft copy does not work well, including brightly lit areas such as operating rooms.

Historically, medical quality laser printers using transmitted media (i.e., "film") were connected to single devices by point-to-point proprietary interfaces. Over time, multiple printers were connected to multiple source devices by proprietary print networks, often through "spoolers."

The details of the DICOM Print service class for grayscale and color printing are beyond the scope of this chapter. However, some of the advantages of using DICOM rather than proprietary print services include the ability to:

- mix printers and sources from different vendors,
- expand or contract the pool of available printers on demand or in the event of failure,
- print to a device that is conveniently located,
- print directly from workstations and modalities without involving the PACS (e.g., in the event of failure),
- incorporate the use of cheaper, lower quality printers (such as plain paper or dye sublimation printers) that support DICOM print, without requiring special effort by the source device, and
- provide a consistent approach to achieve consistent grayscale contrast (i.e., the film looks "the same" regardless of the display or print medium).

The trend over recent years among modality and workstation vendors has definitely been to support DICOM print in preference to proprietary point-to-point links. All modern medical printers support DICOM. Additional attention has been directed to the issue of consistent grayscale appearance, and the DICOM Basic Print services have been expanded to support the use of the DICOM Grayscale Display Function Standard.

The DICOM Print service class includes several different approaches to printing, including:

- the Basic Print SOP Classes, which send preformatted images to the printer,
- the Referenced Print SOP Classes, which specify images that are to be retrieved and how they are to be formatted for printing, and
- the Stored Print SOP Classes, which allow preformatted print sessions to be archived.

In practice, almost all printers and print service users support only the Basic Print mechanism. The Referenced Print mechanism was not widely supported and has been retired from the standard.

INTERCHANGE MEDIA

Traditionally, physicians, institutions, and remote sites have exchanged medical images using some form of printed film. Despite the increased bandwidth and reduced cost of wide area networks for teleradiology, the size of some image sets and the image quality required dictate that some form of physical medium be used.

It is not technically difficult to record images in DICOM data sets on physical media such as floppy disks, recordable CDs (CD-R), and magneto-optical disks (MODs). There are challenges, however, if one expects the recipient to be able to read and display the images. Accordingly, the DICOM standard supports the concept of Media Application Profiles that specify in advance:

- what media to use (e.g., CD-R or 90 mm or 130 mm MOD of a particular capacity),
- what format to write on the media (e.g., DOS FAT16 or ISO 9660 file system),
- how to encode the images (e.g., with or without compression), and
- what objects are written on the media (e.g., cardiac angiography, CT, etc.).

When all these capabilities are defined in advance and agreed upon by both parties, interoperability can be achieved. Which Media Application Profiles are supported by a device is specified in the conformance statement.

The "Basic Cardiac Angiography" profile is the most widely implemented. It specifies the use of ISO 9660 CD-R to encode, using lossless JPEG compression, 512 matrix 8-bit multiframe cardiac X-ray angiography images. This profile is intended to replace the use of 35 mm cine film as an interchange medium, and has largely achieved this goal. All modern digital cardiac angiography modalities support this profile. The CD-R can be used either in place of a PACS for interchange within an institution, or as an input and output medium for a cardiology PACS.

Currently specified in the DICOM standard are profiles for:

- general purpose exchange of any uncompressed images on CD-R,
- basic and 1K angiography images compressed with lossless JPEG on CD-R,
- CT and MR images compressed with lossless JPEG on CD-R and 130 mm MOD, and
- ultrasound images uncompressed or compressed on CD-R, 90 mm and 130 mm MOD.

More profiles are added to the standard as new applications and media types become available. For example, some form of recordable DVD is likely to be added.

UNIQUE IDENTIFIERS

To keep track of objects in a PACS, it is necessary to identify them unambiguously and to avoid the possibility of operator entry error. DICOM defines a mechanism of identification using Unique Identifiers (UIDs). Each study is identified by a Study Instance UID, each series by a Series Instance UID, and each image by a SOP Instance UID.

Since a PACS may expand or merge with other PACS as enterprises grow, it is important that these identifiers be globally unique. This is achieved by specifying a string of numeric values separated by periods that begins with a "root" and is extended with additional values by whomever is assigned authority to delegate that root.

For example, International Standards Organization (ISO) is responsible for the top-level root "1.2" and delegates below that to national ISO member bodies. American National Standards Institute (ANSI) in the U.S. is assigned the root of "1.2.840." A hypothetical vendor might apply to ANSI for its own root and be assigned "1.2.840.9999." All of that vendor's devices might further disambiguate this root using a serial number, "1.2.840.9999.serial-number". A device with serial number 1234 might assign all its SOP Instance UIDs with a root of "1.2.840.9999.1234.1," distinguishing them by using the date, time, and process number, creating UIDs such as "1.2.840.9999.1234.1.19990520125930.4321."

UIDs are used for other purposes than identifying instances. They are also used to designate SOP Classes and Transfer Syntaxes that are defined in the standard. For example, the CT Image Storage SOP Class is identified (during negotiation and in conformance statements) by the UID "1.2.840.10008.5.1.4.1.1.2." The root "1.2.840.10008" is assigned by ANSI to NEMA for DICOM.

DICOM COMPOSITE INFORMATION OBJECTS

DICOM Information Object Definitions (IODs) are constructed from Modules that contain Attributes. Modules describe characteristics of real-world entities that are defined by the DICOM information model. For example, certain modules describe characteristics of the *Patient* entity, the *Study* entity, the *Series* entity, the *Image* or *Instance* entity, etc. Other entities describe the *Equipment* on which the image was acquired, and spatial or temporal *Frames of Reference* that may be used to relate images in space or time.

When information about more than one entity is present in an IOD it is referred to as a *Composite* IOD, as opposed to a *Normalized* IOD, which contains information about only one entity. All of the image objects in DICOM are composite IODs, and each DICOM image contains in a single data set a comprehensive description of the patient, study, and series, as well as the image itself. Individual modules may be mandatory (M), user optional (U), or conditionally present (C) if a specified condition is satisfied. Image objects typically share a common set of modules. They may define additional modules to provide modality-specific attributes, such as those related to acquisition technique. They may specialize the content of more general modules, for example, to restrict the type or bit depth of the image pixel data. Figure 5.11 illustrates some of the general and modality-specific modules from which IODs are constructed. Table 5.5 illustrates a typical image IOD, in this case the CT Image IOD.

A Module is described as a list of Attributes, with descriptions of their meaning, and requirements on their usage. Type 1 Attributes are required, Type 2 Attributes are required but may be sent empty if their value is unknown, and Type 3 Attributes are optional. Table 5.6 illustrates a typical Module, in this case part of the Image Pixel Module.

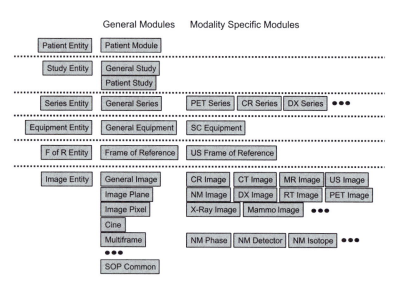

FIGURE 5.11

Example of Composite Image Modules.

TABLE 5.5
CT Image IOD

Information Entity	Module	Usage
Patient	Patient	M
Study	General Study	M
	Patient Study	U
Series	General Series	M
Frame of Reference	Frame of Reference	M
Equipment	General Equipment	M
Image	General Image	M
	Image Plane	M
	Image Pixel	M
	Contrast/bolus	C—Required if contrast media was used in this image
	CT Image	M
	Overlay Plane	U
	VOI LUT	U
	SOP Common	M

As an example of how Attributes in a general Module like the Image Pixel Module may be specialized, consider the list of the Attributes extracted from the CT Image Module illustrated in Table 5.7. In this example, the CT Image Module specializes some Attributes from the Image Pixel Module by restricting the range of allowed values, although it does not change the requirements on their presence or absence. For example, the Image Pixel Module allows RGB photometric interpretation, whereas the CT Image Module restricts the photometric interpretation to grayscale.

As an example of how additional Attributes specific to a modality may be added, consider the list in Table 5.8, also extracted from the CT Image Module. This is not an exhaustive list of all the CT-specific Attributes in the CT Image Module, but it illustrates some typical Attributes. The example shows that some modality-specific Attributes are always required, such as the rescale values necessary to convert stored pixel values into Hounsfield Units. Others are optional.

TABLE 5.6
Attributes from Image Pixel Module

Attribute Name	Tag	Type	Attribute Description
Samples per Pixel	(0028,0002)	1	Number of samples (planes) in this image.
Photometric Interpretation	(0028,0004)	1	Specifies the intended interpretation of the pixel data.
Rows	(0028,0010)	1	Number of rows in the image.
Columns	(0028,0011)	1	Number of columns in the image.
Bits Allocated	(0028,0100)	1	Number of bits allocated for each pixel sample. Each sample shall have the same number of bits allocated.
Bits Stored	(0028,0101)	1	Number of bits stored for each pixel sample. Each sample shall have the same number of bits stored.
High Bit	(0028,0102)	1	Most significant bit for pixel sample data. Each sample shall have the same high bit.
Pixel Representation	(0028,0103)	1	Data representation of the pixel samples. Each sample shall have the same pixel representation. Enumerated Values: 0000H = unsigned integer. 0001H = 2's complement.
Pixel Data	(7FE0,0010)	1	A data stream of the pixel samples which comprise the Image.

PACS-FRIENDLY IMAGE OBJECTS

Experience with the use of DICOM image objects in PACS suggests that efficiency can be improved if more information were made available by the acquisition modalities. In particular, PACS routing algorithms and worklists, as well as default display (hanging) protocols, have become more sophisticated. Although ad hoc site-specific mechanisms and conventions have been devised, often using information entered in comment fields, it is desirable that such mechanisms be standardized. Still, it is often not possible to determine from a DICOM Computed Radiography (CR) or Secondary Capture (SC) image

TABLE 5.7
Image Pixel Attributes Specialized in CT Image Module

Attribute Name	Tag	Type	Attribute Description
Samples per Pixel	(0028,0002)	1	Number of samples (planes) in this image. For CT Images, shall have an Enumerated Value of 1.
Photometric Interpretation	(0028,0004)	1	Specifies the intended interpretation of the pixel data. For CT Images, shall have one of the following Enumerated Values: MONOCHROME1 MONOCHROME2
Bits Allocated	(0028,0100)	1	Number of bits allocated for each pixel sample. Each sample shall have the same number of bits allocated. For CT Images, shall have the Enumerated Value of 16.
Bits Stored	(0028,0101)	1	Number of bits stored for each pixel sample. Each sample shall have the same number of bits stored. For CT Images, shall have the Enumerated Values of 12 to 16.
High Bit	(0028,0102)	1	Most significant bit for pixel sample data. Each sample shall have the same high bit. For CT Images, shall have only the Enumerated Value of one less than the value sent in Bits Stored.

which side of the body an image represents, or even how the image should be oriented for display. Checking and correcting orientation manually reduces productivity. In addition, there has been increasing emphasis on consistency of grayscale image contrast, leading to the development of the DICOM Grayscale Standard Display Function. Softcopy display systems can be calibrated to this function to achieve similarity of image appearance.

Accordingly, when the opportunity arose to define new DICOM image objects for use with flat panel digital sensors, an effort was made to incorporate these additional PACS requirements. The Digital X-Ray (DX)

TABLE 5.8
Additional CT Image Module Attributes

Rescale Intercept	(0028, 1052)	1	The value b in relationship between stored values (SV) and Hounsfield (HU). $HU = m*SV + b$
Rescale Slope	(0028,1053)	1	m in the equation specified in Rescale Intercept (0028,1052).
KVP	(0018,0060)	2	Peak kilovoltage output of the X-Ray generator used.
Reconstruction Diameter	(0018,1100)	3	Diameter in mm of the region from within which data were used in creating the reconstruction of the image. Data may exist outside this region and portions of the patient may exist outside this region.
Gantry/Detector Tilt	(0018,1120)	3	Nominal angle of tilt in degrees of the scanning gantry. Not intended for mathematical computations.
Exposure Time	(0018,1150)	3	Time of X-Ray exposure in msec.
Convolution Kernel	(0018,1210)	3	A label describing the convolution kernel or algorithm used to reconstruct the data.

family of objects was added to the standard. This family includes application-specific objects for Digital Mammography and Digital Intra-Oral Radiography. The DX objects can also be used for photo-stimulable phosphor plate and optically scanned film acquisition devices, in place of the existing CR and SC image objects, if the additional mandatory requirements are met.

The DX objects add the following requirements for improving PACS productivity:

▶ more extensive use of coded terms to describe anatomy, projection, and technique in a consistent manner among vendors,

▶ increased mandatory requirements for describing laterality, orientation, anatomy, and projection,

- restriction to a single exposure per image object,
- distinction between images intended for presentation (i.e., those that already have a grayscale lookup table or window information) and those intended for further processing, and
- encoding of the image output using the P-Value units of the Grayscale Standard Display Function, which are output-device independent.

Some of this information is already available to existing acquisition devices (e.g., the body part and view are often entered into a generator protocol selector). Before now, manufacturers might have opted not to encode this information in earlier DICOM objects because it was not mandatory, or they might have had no standard place to encode it.

An example of the use of some of the required attributes is illustrated in Figure 5.12.

ASSOCIATIONS

The DICOM standard defines not only the form in which images may be stored and what they contain, but also protocols and services used to exchange images and other messages. When a DICOM device or application wishes to connect to another device in order to send images or perform some other service, it attempts to establish an Association with the other device.

To make the connection, the *initiator* of the Association needs to be configured with sufficient information, including:

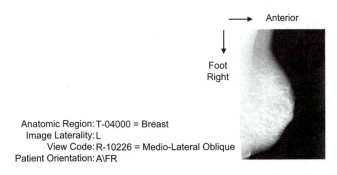

FIGURE 5.13

Digital mammography required Attributes for PAS productivity.

▶ the IP address of the other device (or host name if a name service is available),

▶ the TCP port number to connect to (usually 104),

▶ the Called Application Entity (AE) Title of the other device, and

▶ the Calling AE Title to use as the initiator's own name.

The *acceptor* of an Association needs to be configured with:

▶ the TCP port number to listen on (usually 104),

▶ the AE Title by which to identify itself, and

▶ the IP addresses and Calling AE Titles from which Associations are accepted.

The Calling and Called AE Title of a device is sometimes, but not always, the same as its host name. Many devices do not care what AE Title they are "called" by when accepting an Association, and many do not care who is calling them either. Such "promiscuous" devices are easy to configure. However, many devices are finicky and need to be specifically configured to allow other devices to connect to them. Some devices also allow or require a list of which SOP Classes and which Transfer Syntaxes to offer to, or accept from, other devices.

The process of establishing an Association involves:

▶ the initiator opening a TCP/IP network connection to the acceptor,

▶ the initiator proposing a list of SOP Classes to use, and Transfer Syntaxes to encode them, as well as a list of optional extended negotiation items, and

▶ the acceptor returning a list that is the subset of the proposed SOP Classes and Transfer Syntaxes that it agrees to support.

At this point, an Association is established and the exchange of messages can begin. In the simplest case, an SCU of an Image Storage SOP Class, which has acted as initiator of an Association, can begin transmitting images.

For example, consider an ultrasound machine transferring images to an archive. It attempts to initiate an Association with the archive, with the intention of acting in the role of an SCU of the US Single-frame, US Multi-frame, and SC Image Storage SOP Classes. This device is also capable of performing lossless JPEG compression of the images in order to reduce transmission time. It therefore offers the following SOP Classes and Transfer Syntaxes (which are referred to as Presentation Contexts):

- US Image Storage SOP Classes with Implicit VR Little Endian Transfer Syntax (the default),
- US Image Storage SOP Classes with Lossless JPEG Compression Process 14 Selection Value 1,
- US MF Image Storage SOP Classes with Implicit VR Little Endian Transfer Syntax (the default),
- US MF Image Storage SOP Classes with Lossless JPEG Compression Process 14 Selection Value 1,
- SC Image Storage SOP Classes with Implicit VR Little Endian Transfer Syntax (the default), and
- SC Image Storage SOP Classes with Lossless JPEG Compression Process 14 Selection Value 1.

The Association acceptor (the archive), which acts in the role of SCP in this example, responds that it accepts:

- US Image Storage SOP Classes with Implicit VR Little Endian Transfer Syntax (the default), and
- SC Image Storage SOP Classes with Implicit VR Little Endian Transfer Syntax (the default).

It rejects all other Presentation Contexts offered. In other words, the archive does not accept lossless JPEG compression and does not support the US Multi-frame Image Storage SOP Class. If the ultrasound device has cine loops to be transferred in addition to single frame images, it needs to split them into individual frames before sending them to the archive.

Once established, an Association persists until it is explicitly closed from either end or until some implementation-dependent timeout occurs. Usually, an association initiator opens an Association, performs a certain discrete task (such as transmitting all the images in a study), and then closes the Association. For most services, however, no particular semantics are defined in the standard for the persistence of an Association. Images from one study may be transmitted across multiple Associations, or multiple studies over one Association, or even on a separate Association for each image.

In the real world, because failures occur, both devices need to be capable of recovering and re-establishing Associations to perform outstanding operations that were interrupted.

ENCODING AND TRANSFER SYNTAX

DICOM objects are encoded in binary form as lists of Attributes. Each Attribute (or Data Element when one is speaking of encoding) is identified by
a Tag consisting of a 16-bit group and 16-bit element number, which together uniquely identify the Data Element. The Data Elements in the data
set are sorted sequentially by ascending Tag number, and each Data Element is sent only once. In other words, the data set is not encoded in the
structure or order that is described in the IODs. When an IOD contains
modules that define the same Tag more than once (e.g., to specialize its requirements or behavior), it is actually encoded only once. Those Data Elements in even-numbered groups are standard DICOM elements. Those with
odd group numbers are Private Data Elements, whose requirements and behavior are implementation-dependent.

The meaning of the value of a Data Element is defined by the IOD
in which it is used. The form or Value Representation (VR) (i.e., whether
it is a date or time or binary value or string or name, etc.) is defined by
the Data Dictionary. The Data Dictionary is the part of the DICOM
standard that defines the VR for all the standard Data Elements, as well
as their Value Multiplicity (VM). The Data Dictionary itself is not transmitted with the data set. One has to know from the standard that Data
Element (0010,0010) is Patient Name; there is nothing contained in the
encoded data set to indicate this. Explicitly encoded in the Data Element
is a field describing the length of the value in bytes called the Value
Length (VL). See Figure 5.13.

The VR may or may not be encoded in the data set. In the ACR-
NEMA standards, prior to DICOM 3.0, it was not: hence, the baseline or
default encoding or Transfer Syntax is referred to as an Implicit VR Transfer Syntax. All network implementations of DICOM must support this default Transfer Syntax. All other Transfer Syntaxes explicitly encode a two-
character field that identifies the VR of the Data Element. The available
Value Representations are shown in Table 5.9.

DICOM provides several different Transfer Syntaxes for transferring
images across the network or for storing them in files. There are three broad
classes of Transfer Syntaxes, which include:

- ▶ the default Implicit Value Representation Little Endian Transfer
  Syntax,

- ▶ the Little and Big Endian Explicit Value Representation Transfer
  Syntaxes, and

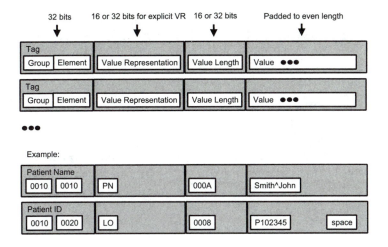

FIGURE 5.12

Data Element encoding.

▶ the compression Transfer Syntaxes (which are all Explicit Value Representation).

The Little and Big Endian choices are provided because some implementers believe there are performance advantages to using the native

TABLE 5.9
Value Representations

AE	Application Entity	AS	Age String	AT	Attribute Tag
CS	Code String	DA	Date	DS	Decimal String
DT	Date Time	FL	Float Single	FD	Float Double
IS	Integer String	LO	Long String	LT	Long Text
OB	Other Byte	OW	Other Word	PN	Person Name
SH	Short String	SL	Signed Long	SQ	Sequence
SS	Signed Short	ST	Short Text	TM	Time
UI	Unique Identifier	UL	Unsigned Long	UN	Unknown
US	Unsigned Short	UT	Unlimited Text		

byte ordering of the host computers. In practice, few implementations support other than Little Endian. The currently available compression Transfer Syntaxes include lossless and lossy JPEG compression, as well as a Run-Length Encoding (RLE) scheme popular with ultrasound vendors.

Which transfer syntax is used is either negotiated when the Association is established in the case of network transfers, or defined a priori in Media Application Profiles in the case of storage on interchange media.

In the case of interchange media, the stored file also contains a Meta Information Header, always in Explicit VR Little Endian Transfer Syntax, which specifies what Transfer Syntax has been used to encode the data set that follows.

COMPRESSION

The DICOM standard takes no position on what is an appropriate compression algorithm or compression ratio to use for any particular application, nor will it ever do so. Such decisions are the responsibility of professional practice standards, and are derived from the body of evidence in the scientific literature.

DICOM does provide a framework for the use of compression technology. Where standards in common use for medical image compression are available, they are specified as standard Transfer Syntaxes. For example, the full range of lossless and lossy JPEG processes defined in ISO 10918-1 are specified in DICOM (ISO 10918-1/ITU T.81, 1993). This does not mean that the use of lossy compression using JPEG is recommended, or that any particular compression ratio is recommended.

Additional standard transfer syntaxes will likely be added to DICOM as new compression standards become available, such as JPEG-LS (ISO 14495-1/ITU T.87, 1999), a new form of lossless compression, and JPEG 2000 (ISO 15444-1/ITU T.800, 2000), a wavelet-based progressive lossless and lossy compression scheme.

At any time, subject to successful negotiation at Association establishment, a Private Transfer Syntax specifying a proprietary compression scheme may be used. This mechanism is widely used to allow proprietary wavelet-based lossy compression schemes to be used with DICOM for teleradiology applications.

COMMON PACS DICOM PROBLEMS

The majority of PACS installations using DICOM services perform as expected, even when relatively complex services and workflow are involved. Difficulties, however, range from minor annoyances (like having to reset the window center and width on every image), to potential disasters (such as having images displayed out of anatomical order), through the occasional catastrophe (such as "losing" images or entire studies on an intermittent basis).

Sometimes such difficulties are a consequence of the flexibility in the DICOM standard that is necessary to reach consensus amongst vendors. Some examples include:

▶ alternative ways of representing image pixel data for the same modality (e.g., CT and MR data may be signed or unsigned, may not always be 12 bits, and may have padding values outside the expected range of valid pixel values).

▶ window center and width values may or may not be supplied by the modality, or may be relatively unhelpful statistically generated defaults, depending on whether images are intended to be transmitted before or after an operator checks them.

▶ different Query/Retrieve models (Patient or Study Root) may be supported depending on internal database architecture.

▶ all the images for a single series or study may not be transmitted in any particular sequence (such as ordered by anatomical location from caudal to cranial) nor even over a single association; this may confuse any receiving application that depends on such behavior.

▶ Attributes that are optional in the standard, or that may be sent empty if their value is unknown, may not be sent at all, leading to reduced functionality, or confusion on the part of a receiver that depends on the presence of a valid value (typical examples are accession number and laterality of body part, neither of which are present in the user interface of many older modalities).

▶ different ways of organizing images into series, confusing devices that apply display protocols or perform 3D reconstruction (e.g., some CT scanners put localizers in the same series as the axial images, others in a different series; some put images acquired at the same time and location but with different reconstruction kernels in the same series).

❱ different ways of annotating images and specifying relationships (e.g., some CT and MR scanners allow operators to save localizer images marked with lines portraying the location of orthogonal images burned in or overlaid; others specify the relationship by reference; many display workstations ignore any convention other than that of their own vendor's scanners—the standard is essentially silent on this issue).

From the perspective of the DICOM device manufacturer, some design strategies reduce the risk of incompatibility:

❱ write only perfect DICOM objects,

❱ read anything vaguely resembling a DICOM object,

❱ assume nothing about the contents of objects or the sequencing of messages, and

❱ make everything configurable.

For example, as an image creator, one should always fill all mandatory Attributes with appropriate values, use standard defined terms for values, fill as many optional Attributes as possible, and where possible, design the user interface and internal database architecture using the DICOM Patient/Study/Procedure Step/Series/Image model.

As an image user one should be prepared to accept almost any image that can possibly be interpreted and displayed, regardless of how much information is missing or malformed, and how strangely the images are organized. A particularly common problem occurs with an image-viewing application that does not take into account "unusual" but legal forms of image pixel data, to the point that some images cannot be displayed or windowed at all.

The more complex an application, the more difficult it becomes to avoid making assumptions about the content or sequence of transactions. However, many applications can be implemented without resorting to private services or private Attributes, and without depending on the presence of specific values in standard optional Attributes. Most problems arise in practice because the implementer is limited by the capabilities of an existing application that is being extended, or because image senders and receivers from the same vendor are built to use DICOM only as a tool for communication between them, without considering interoperability with devices from other vendors.

Most importantly, one should avoid "creatively" interpreting or applying the standard. In particular, it is inappropriate to use services for applications other than as intended, or in combinations beyond those intended. Otherwise, such applications will not work with those of other implementers who do not make the same assumptions.

The purchaser or integrator of a PACS rarely has the luxury of being able to make changes in the implementation of devices that are not working together. Under these circumstances one can:

▶ request one of the vendors to fix the problem once the cause has been clearly established,

▶ choose different equipment (in which case it is important to detect these problems during acceptance testing rather than clinical use), or

▶ interpose some sort of "box" that performs translation or mapping of objects and services into a form that is acceptable and usable; this is an expensive solution but sometimes expedient.

TESTING

Having matched conformance statements for likely candidates to build or extend a PACS configuration, the next step is to test whether or not they work. Few organizations have the luxury of being able to try entire scanners or PACS before buying them, but some vendors can provide "modality simulators" that run the same software and simulate the user interface of a real device. These can be used to exercise the necessary functions using a stored set of images and a simulation of the real workflow. Even if a vendor can or will not test before installation, at the very least the vendor should be able to confirm that testing between involved vendors has occurred (using similar hardware and software configurations and versions), or that the same configuration is in production at another site (which you may want to visit). Furthermore, the contract with the vendor(s) should clearly specify what functionality is required before the installation is accepted, and who is responsible for achieving that functionality.

It should come as no surprise that when two or more parties are responsible for a complex installation, a certain amount of "finger pointing" is inevitable if things do not work as planned. Not infrequently, one hears claims from both sides that their equipment is "DICOM compliant." Indeed conformance statements, other documents, results of stand-alone testing, and testimonies from satisfied customers may be produced to prove it.

It should be clear, however, that no such simple claim as "DICOM compliant" is valid: the DICOM standard contains tools to achieve interoperability, but adherence to the standard cannot guarantee it. End-users are not interested in conformance to standards per se, only in installations that actually work.

As a user or integrator it is necessary to:

▶ have realistic expectations—do not expect "plug-and-play" results without serious analysis and thorough testing,

▶ define responsibility in advance—do not be left with responsibility for integration unless you have the necessary expertise, and

▶ be reasonable—vendors' engineering and marketing lifecycles do not allow for rapid fixes to minor or even major defects (unless they are safety-related).

An extreme example of specification and testing of DICOM-based PACS equipment can be found in the US Department of Defense's DIN-PACS contract (Defense Supply Center) and benchmark testing strategy (Richardson et al., 1999).

▶ REFERENCES

ACR-NEMA. *Standard PS 300—Digital Imaging and Communications.* NEMA, Washington DC 1989.

Defense Supply Center, Philadelphia. *Digital Imaging Network—Picture Archive and Communications System Contract.* Contract Number SP 020097-R-8002 DINPACS. URL: http://www.dpsc.dla.mil/medical/medequip/what.htm

DICOM. *Digital Imaging and Communications in Medicine—Version 3.0.* NEMA, Rosslyn VA 2000. URL: http://medical.nema.org/dicom/2000/

ISO 10918-1/ITU T.81. *Digital Compression and Coding of Continuous-Tone Still Images.* Geneva. 1993.

ISO 14495-1/ITU T.87. *Lossless and Near-Lossless Coding of Continuous Tone Still Images (JPEG-LS).* Geneva. 1999.

ISO/15444-1/ITU T.800. *JPEG 2000 Image Coding System.* Geneva, 2000.

Osteaux M et al. *Second Generation PACS Concept: A Global View. In A Second Generation PACS Concept.* Osteaux M (Ed.) Springer-Verlag. Berlin 1992. Page 314.

Richardson NE et al. *The philosophy of benchmark testing a standards-based PACS.* Journal of Digital Imaging 12:87–93, 1999.

▶ GLOSSARY AND ABBREVIATIONS

ACR   American College of Radiology.

AE   See Application Entity.

AET   See Application Entity Title.

APPLICATION ENTITY   The network representation of an application process, which is the element of a system that performs processing for a particular application. A single physical device may support more than one Application Entity.

APPLICATION ENTITY TITLE   The name by which an Application Entity is known to other Application Entities, and which is used in DICOM to map to a Presentation Address, to identify calling and called Application Entities during establishment of an Association, and to indicate where objects are located or should be sent.

APPLICATION PROFILE   A Media Storage Application Profile defines a selection of choices at the various layers of the DICOM Media Storage Model that are applicable to a specific need or context in which the media interchange is intended to be performed.

ASSOCIATION   A network connection between two Application Entities. The establishment of an Association in DICOM implies that the Application Entities have successfully negotiated a set of SOP Classes that are supported in complementary roles, as well as one or more Transfer Syntaxes to use to encode messages.

ATTRIBUTE   A property of an Information Object. An Attribute has a name and a value, which are independent of any encoding scheme.

ATTRIBUTE TAG   A unique identifier for an attribute of an information object composed of an ordered pair of numbers (a group number followed by an element number).

BIG ENDIAN   A form of byte ordering, where multiple binary values are encoded with the most significant byte encoded first and the remaining bytes encoded in decreasing order of significance.

CALLED APPLICATION ENTITY TITLE   The Application Entity Title of the (potential) acceptor of an Association.

CALLING APPLICATION ENTITY TITLE   The Application Entity Title of the initiator of an Association.

COMPOSITE IOD   An Information Object Definition, which represents parts of several entities in the DICOM application model. Such an IOD includes attributes that are not inherent in the real-world object that the IOD represents but rather are inherent in related real-world objects.

CONFORMANCE STATEMENT   A formal statement associated with a specific implementation of the DICOM Standard. It specifies the Service Classes, Information Objects, and Communication Protocols supported by the implementation.

DATA DICTIONARY   A registry of DICOM Data Elements that assigns a unique tag, a name, value characteristics, and semantics to each Data Element.

DATA ELEMENT   A unit of information as defined by a single entry in the Data Dictionary. An encoded Information Object Definition (IOD) Attribute that is composed of, at a minimum, three fields: a Data Element Tag, a Value Length, and a Value Field. For some specific Transfer Syntaxes, a Data Element also may contain a VR Field, where the Value Representation of that Data Element is specified explicitly.

DATA ELEMENT TAG   A unique identifier for an element of information composed of an ordered pair of numbers (a Group Number followed by an Element Number), which is used to identify Attributes and corresponding Data Elements.

DATA ELEMENT TYPE   Used to specify whether an Attribute of an Information Object Definition or an Attribute of a SOP Class Definition is mandatory, mandatory only under certain conditions, or optional. This translates to whether a Data Element of a Data Set is mandatory, mandatory only under certain conditions, or optional.

DATA SET   Exchanged information consisting of a structured set of Attribute values directly or indirectly related to Information Objects. The value of each Attribute in a Data Set is expressed as a Data Element. A collection of Data Elements—in order of increasing Data Element Tag number—which is an encoding of the values of Attributes of a real-world object.

DATA STREAM   The result of encoding a Data Set using the DICOM encoding scheme (Data Element Numbers and representations as specified by the Data Dictionary).

DEFINED TERM   The value of a Data Element is a Defined Term when the Value of the element may be one of an explicitly specified set of standard values; implementers may extend these values.

DICOM   Digital Imaging and Communications in Medicine.

DICOM FILE   A DICOM File has content formatted according to the requirements of Part 10 of the DICOM Standard. In particular, such files contain the File Meta Information and a properly formatted Data Set.

DICOM FILE FORMAT   The DICOM File Format provides a means to encapsulate the Data Set representing a SOP Instance related to a DICOM Information Object.

DICOM INFORMATION MODEL   An entity-relationship diagram used to model the relationships between the Information Object Definitions, representing classes of real-world objects defined by the DICOM Application Model.

ELEMENT NUMBER   The second number in the ordered pair of numbers that makes up a Data Element Tag.

ENUMERATED VALUE   The value of a Data Element is an Enumerated Value when the Value of the element may be one of an explicitly specified set of standard values; implementers may not extend these values.

EXPLICIT VR   A method of encoding Data Elements in which the Value Representation (VR) of the Data Element is explicitly encoded in the Data Element itself.

FILE META INFORMATION   The File Meta Information includes identifying information on the encapsulated Data Set. It is a mandatory header at the beginning of every DICOM File.

GROUP NUMBER   The first number in the ordered pair of numbers that makes up a Data Element Tag.

HL7   Health Level 7.

IE   See Information Entity.

IOD   See Information Object Definition.

IMPLICIT VR   A method of encoding Data Elements in which the Value Representation (VR) of the Data Element is not explicitly encoded in the Data Element itself, but rather is obtained from the Data Dictionary.

INFORMATION ENTITY   That portion of information defined by a Composite IOD that is related to one specific class of real-world object. There is a one-to-one correspondence between information entities and entities in the DICOM Application Model.

INFORMATION OBJECT   An abstraction of a real information entity (e.g., CT Image, Study, etc.), which is acted upon by one or more DICOM Commands.

INFORMATION OBJECT DEFINITION   A data abstraction of a class of similar real-world objects, which defines the nature and Attributes relevant to the class of real-world objects represented.

INFORMATION OBJECT INSTANCE   A representation of an occurrence of a real-world entity, which includes values for the Attributes of the Information Object Class to which the entity belongs.

ISO (INTERNATIONAL STANDARDS ORGANIZATION)   An international organization of national standards' bodies from approximately 100 countries, established in 1947 to promote standardization of intellectual, scientific, technological, and economical information worldwide. It produces international agreements, which are published, and international standards.

LITTLE ENDIAN   A form of byte ordering where multiple binary values are encoded, with the least significant byte encoded first and the remaining bytes encoded in increasing order of significance.

META SERVICE-OBJECT PAIR CLASS   A predefined set of SOP Classes that may be associated under a single SOP instance for the purpose of negotiating the use of the set with a single item.

MODULE   A set of Attributes within an information entity or Normalized IOD that are logically related to each other.

MULTI-FRAME IMAGE   Image that contains multiple two-dimensional pixel planes.

NEMA   National Electrical Manufacturers Association.

NORMALIZED IOD   An Information Object Definition that represents a single entity in the DICOM application model. Such an IOD includes Attributes that are only inherent in the real-world object that the IOD represents.

OSI (OPEN SYSTEMS INTERCONNECTION)   An ISO standard for network communication that serves as a framework for defining the structure of DICOM, although TCP/IP is used rather than OSI for actual exchange of DICOM messages.

PIXEL DATA   Graphical data (e.g., images or overlays) of variable pixel-depth encoded in the Pixel Data Element, with Value Representation OW or OB. Additional descriptor Data Elements is often used to describe the contents of the Pixel Data Element.

PRESENTATION ADDRESS   The network address of an Application Entity, usually the IP address and TCP port number.

PRIVATE DATA ELEMENT   Additional Data Element, defined by an implementer, to communicate information that is not contained in Standard Data Elements. Private Data Elements have odd Group Numbers.

REAL-WORLD ACTIVITY   That which exists in the real world that pertains to a specific area of information processing within the area of interest of the DICOM standard. Such a Real-World Activity may be represented by one or more computer information metaphors called SOP Classes.

REAL-WORLD OBJECT   That which exists in the real world upon which operations may be performed that are within the area of interest of the DICOM standard. Such a Real-World Object may be represented by one or more computer information metaphors called a SOP Instance.

SCP   See Service Class Provider.

SCU   See Service Class User.

SERVICE CLASS   A structured description of a service that is supported by co-operating DICOM Application Entities using specific DICOM Commands acting on a specific class of Information Object. Also, a collection of SOP Classes and/or Meta SOP Classes, which are related in that they are described together to accomplish a single application.

SERVICE CLASS PROVIDER   The role played by a DICOM Application Entity that performs operations and invokes notifications on a specific Association.

SERVICE CLASS USER   The role played by a DICOM Application Entity that invokes operations and performs notifications on a specific Association.

SERVICE-OBJECT PAIR CLASS   The union of a specific set of DIMSE Services and one related Information Object Definition (as specified by a Ser-vice Class Definition) that completely defines a precise context for communication.

SERVICE-OBJECT PAIR INSTANCE   A concrete occurrence of an Information Object and a communication context.

SOP CLASS   See Service-Object Pair Class.

SOP INSTANCE   See Service-Object Pair Instance.

STANDARD DATA ELEMENT   A Data Element defined in the DICOM Standard, and therefore listed in the DICOM Data Element Dictionary in PS 3.6.

TAG   See Data Element Tag.

TRANSFER SYNTAX   A set of encoding rules that allow Application Entities to unambiguously negotiate the encoding techniques (e.g., Data Element structure, byte ordering, compression) they are able to support, thereby allowing these Application Entities to communicate.

UID   See Unique Identifier.

UNIQUE IDENTIFIER   A string of characters that uniquely identifies a variety of items, guaranteeing uniqueness across multiple countries, sites, vendors, and equipment. In addition, the scheme used to provide global unique identification for objects. It uses the structure defined by ISO 8824 for OSI Object Identifiers.

VALUE   A component of a Value Field. A Value Field may consist of one or more of these components.

VALUE FIELD   The field within a Data Element that contains the Value(s) of that Data Element.

VALUE LENGTH   The field within a Data Element that contains the length of the Value Field of the Data Element.

VALUE MULTIPLICITY   Specifies the number of Values contained in the value Field of a Data Element.

VALUE REPRESENTATION   Specifies the data type and format of the Value(s) contained in the Value Field of a Data Element.

VALUE REPRESENTATION FIELD   The field where the Value Representation of a Data Element is stored in the encoding of a Data Element structure with explicit VR.

VR   See Value Representation.

VM   See Value Multiplicity.

ADVANCED IMAGING TECHNOLOGIES

CHAPTER 6

IMAGE ACQUISITION

KATHERINE P. ANDRIOLE

This chapter discusses in detail the digital acquisition of data from the various imaging modalities for input to a picture archiving and communication system (PACS). This includes essential features for successful clinical implementation, including conformance with the digital imaging and communications in medicine (DICOM) standard, radiology information system-hospital information system (RIS-HIS) interfacing, and workflow integration. Image acquisition from the inherently digital cross-sectional modalities, such as computed tomography (CT) and magnetic resonance imaging (MRI), are reviewed, as well as digital acquisition of the conventional projection X-ray utilizing computed radiography (CR), digital radiography (DR), and film digitizers for digital acquisition of images already on film.

Quality assurance (QA) and quality control (QC) for a PACS are described, with emphasis given to QA-QC procedures and troubleshooting problems occurring specifically at image acquisition. Future trends in image acquisition for digital radiology and PACS are introduced, including anticipated changes in image data sets (such as increased matrix size, increased spatial resolution, increased slice number and study size, and improved image quality); changes in the imaging devices themselves (such as smaller foot-prints and more portability); and image processing capabilities for softcopy display.

INTRODUCTION

INTEGRATION INTO PACS

Image acquisition is the first point of data entry into a picture archiving and communications system (PACS), and as such, errors generated here can propagate throughout the system, adversely affecting clinical operations. General predictors for successful incorporation of image acquisition devices into a digital imaging department include: ease of device integration into the established daily workflow routine of the clinical environment, high reliability and fault tolerance of the device, simplicity and intuitiveness of the user interface, and device speed (Andriole 1999a).

DICOM

Imaging modality conformance with the digital imaging and communications in medicine (DICOM) standard is critical. DICOM consists of a standard image format as well as a network communications protocol. Compliance with this standard enables an open architecture for imaging systems, which bridges hardware and software entities and allows interoperability for the transfer of medical images and associated information between disparate systems.

    The push by the radiological community for a standard format across imaging devices of different models and makes began in 1982. Collaboration between the American College of Radiology (ACR) and the National Electronic Manufacturers Association (NEMA) produced a standard format (ACR-NEMA 2.0) with which to store an image digitally. It consisted of a file header followed by the image data. The file header contained information relevant to the image, such as matrix size or number of rows and columns, pixel size, and grayscale bit depth, as well as information about the imaging device and technique (e.g., Brand X CT scanner, acquired with contrast). Patient demographic data such as name and date of birth were also included in the image header. The ACR-NEMA 2.0 standard specified exactly where in the header each bit of information was to be stored, so that the standard required image information could be read by any device simply by going to the designated location in the header. This standard unified the format of imaging data but functioned only as a point-to-point procedure.

In 1994, at the Radiological Society of North America (RSNA) Meeting, a variety of imaging vendors participated in an impressive demonstration of the new and evolving imaging standard (ACR-NEMA 3.0) or what is currently known as the DICOM standard. Participants attached their devices to a common network and shipped their images to one another. In addition to the standard image format of ACR-NEMA 2.0, the DICOM standard included a network communications protocol or a common language for sending and receiving images and relevant data over a network. The DICOM standard is covered in greater detail in Chapter 5 of this volume, so only a basic summary is included here.

The DICOM standard language structure is built on Information Objects (IO), Application Entities (AE), and Service Class Users (SCU) and Providers (SCP). Information Objects include, for example, the image types, such as CT, MRI, and CR. The Application Entities include the devices, such as a scanner, workstation, or printer. The Service Classes (SC*) define an operation on the Information Object via Service Object Pairs (SOP) of IO and SCU and SCP. The types of operations performed by an SCU-SCP on an IO include Storage, Query/Retrieve, Verification, Print, Patient, Study and Results Management, and Study Content Notification.

An example of a use of the DICOM standard would be the negotiation of a transaction between a compliant imaging modality and a compliant PACS workstation. The scanner would notify the workstation, in a language both understand, that it has an image study to send to it. The workstation would reply to the modality when it is ready to receive the data. The data would be sent in a format known to all, the workstation would acknowledge receipt of the image, and the devices would end their negotiation. Figure 6.1 shows the results of a sample PACS tool for reading the DICOM header. Shown are elements in Groups 8 and 10, pertaining to image identification parameters (such as study, series, and image number) and patient demographics (such as patient name, medical record number, and date of birth), respectively.

Prior to DICOM, the acquisition of digital image data and relevant information was extremely difficult, often requiring separate hardware devices and software programs for different vendors products, and even for different models of devices made by the same manufacturer. Most of the major manufacturers of imaging devices currently comply with the DICOM standard, thus facilitating an open systems architecture using multiple vendor's devices. For many legacy devices purchased prior to the establishment of DICOM, an upgrade path to compliance can be performed. For those few

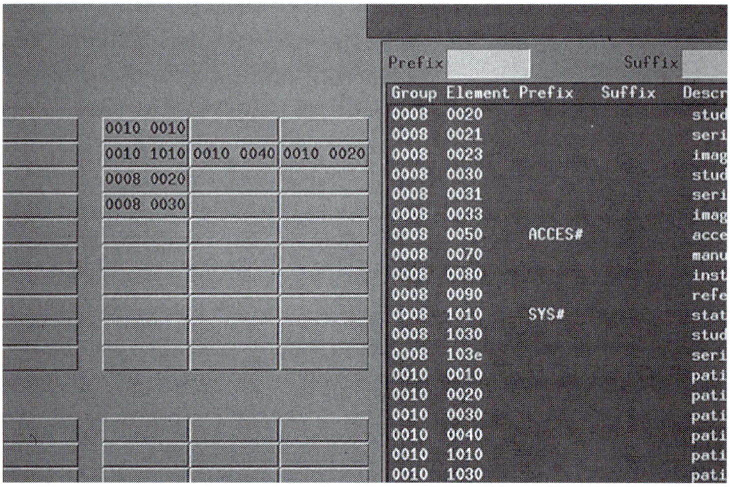

FIGURE 6.1

The output of an example PACS tool for reading the DICOM header. Shown are elements in Groups 8 and 10, pertaining to image identification parameters (such as study, series, image number) and patient demographics (such as patient name, medical record number, date of birth) respectively.

devices that do not yet meet the standard, interface boxes consisting of hardware equipment and software programs that convert the image data from the manufacturer's proprietary format to the standard form are available.

RIS-HIS INTERFACING FOR DATA VERIFICATION

Equally essential, particularly at acquisition, is integrating the radiology information system (RIS) and/or hospital information system (HIS) with the PACS. This facilitates input of patient demographics—name, date, time, medical record number (MRN) to uniquely identify a patient, and accession number (AccNum), to uniquely identify an imaging examination, exam type, imaging parameters—and enables automatic PACS data verification, correlation, and error correction with the data recorded in the RIS-HIS. Several imaging modalities are tightly coupled with the RIS (i.e., some CR manufacturers) and provide automatic downloading of demographic information from the RIS by barcode readers to the modality and hence to the DICOM header. This eliminates the highly error-prone manual entry of data at acquisition.

Health Language 7 (HL7), also called Health Link 7, is the RIS-HIS standard and compliance with it is desirable. RIS-HIS databases are typically patient-centric, enabling query and retrieval of information by the patient, study, series, or image data hierarchy. Integration of RIS-HIS data with the PACS adds intelligence to the system, helping to move data around the system based on "*how, what* data should be delivered *where* and *when*," thereby automating the functions performed traditionally by the film librarian.

Figure 6.2 diagrams an example of how RIS, HIS, and PACS systems might interact upon scheduling an examination for image acquisition into a PACS (Andriole 1999b). For more information on RIS-HIS-PACS integration, see Chapter 7 of this volume.

MODALITY WORKLIST

Some vendors also provide the capability to download RIS-HIS schedules and worklists directly to the imaging modality, such as many computed tomography (CT), magnetic resonance imaging (MRI), and digital fluoroscopy (DF) scanners. In these circumstances, the imaging technologist need only choose the appropriate patient s name from a list on the scanner console monitor (i.e., pointing to it on a touch-screen pad), and the information

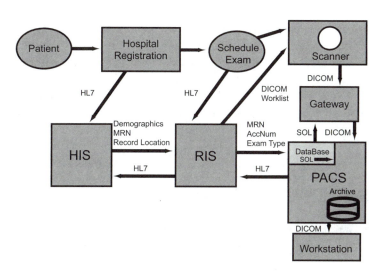

FIGURE 6.2

Diagram of how RIS, HIS, and PACS systems might interact upon scheduling an examination for image acquisition into a PACS.

consistent with the RIS-HIS database is downloaded into the PACS header for that patient examination.

The general DICOM model for acquisition of image and relevant data from the imaging modality involves the modality device acting as an SCU and storing it to an SCP device such as a PACS acquisition gateway or an image display workstation. In the Modality Worklist function, however, the image device receives the pertinent patient demographics and image study information from a worklist server, such as a PACS, RIS, or RIS-HIS interfaced device.

There are two modes for accomplishing the RIS-HIS data transfer to the imaging modality. The first involves data being transferred automatically to the modality based on the occurrence of an event trigger, such as examination scheduled or patient arrived. The second method involves a query from the modality to the RIS-HIS. This may be initiated by entry of some identifier at the modality. For example, bar coding the study accession number or the patient medical record number from the scheduling card may be used at the point of study to initiate a request for the associated RIS-HIS information (patient name, date of birth, etc.) to be sent from the worklist server on demand.

The benefits of the DICOM Modality Worklist cannot be understated. Incorrect manually entered patient demographic data, such as all the permutations of patient name, can result in errors such as mislabeled image files and incomplete study information, which is critical to maintaining the integrity of the PACS database. Furthermore, the improvements in departmental workflow efficiency and device usability are greatly facilitated by Modality Worklist capabilities. A number of vendors currently offer DICOM Modality Worklist for their imaging modality devices; alternatively, several interface or broker boxes are available that interconnect PACS to RIS-HIS databases translating DICOM to HL7 and vice versa.

ACQUISITION OF THE NATIVE DIGITAL CROSS-SECTIONAL MODALITIES

DIGITAL ACQUISITION VERSUS ANALOG ACQUISITION

Digital image acquisition from the inherently digital modalities such as computed tomography (CT) and magnetic resonance imaging (MRI) just makes sense. There are two methods for accomplishing this: direct capture and frame grabbing. Direct digital interfaces allow capture and transmission of image data from the modality at the full spatial resolution and bit depth or grayscale inherent in the modality, while analog (video) frame grabbers digitize the video signal voltage output going to an image display, such as a scanner console monitor. In the frame-grabbing method, as in printing an image to film, the image quality is limited by the process to only 8 bits (or 256 gray values). This may not allow viewing in all the appropriate clinical windows and levels or contrast and brightness settings.

For example, when viewing a CT of the chest, one may wish to view in lung window and level settings and in mediastinal and bone windows and levels. Direct capture of the digital data will allow the viewer to dynamically window and level through each of these settings on-the-fly (in real time) at the softcopy display station. To view all appropriate window and level settings on film, several copies of the study would have to be printed, one at each window and level setting. If one performs the analog acquisition or frame grabbing of the digital data, the viewer can only window and level through the 8 bits captured, which may not be sufficient. Thus, direct capture of digital data from the inherently digital modalities is the preferred method of acquisition. Table 6.1 lists commonly PACS-interfaced cross-sectional modalities and their inherent file sizes.

TABLE 6.1
The Commonly PACS-Interfaced Cross-Sectional Modalities and their Inherent File Sizes

Modality	Image Matrix Size	Grayscale Bit Depth
Computed Tomography (CT)	512 × 512 pixels	12–16 bits
Digital Angiography (RA) &	512 × 512 pixels or	8–12 bits
Digital Fluoroscopy (DF)	1024 × 1024 pixels or	
	2048 × 2048 pixels	
Magnetic Resonance Imaging (MRI)	256 × 256 pixels	12–16 bits
Nuclear Medicine Images (NUC)	64 × 64 pixels or	8–16 bits
	128 × 128 pixels or	
	256 × 256 pixels	
Ultrasound (US)	64 × 64 pixels or	16–32 bits
	128 × 128 pixels	

ACQUISITION OF PROJECTION RADIOGRAPHY

Methods for digital image acquisition of the conventional projection X-ray include devices such as computed radiography (CR) or imaging with photostimulable or storage phosphors and digitization of existing analog film, as well as direct digital detectors falling under the general heading of digital radiography (DR), which are beginning to be used clinically. Digital acquisition of images already on film can be accomplished using a variety of image digitization devices or film scanners. These include the infrequently used analog video cameras with analog-to-digital converters (ADC), digital cameras, charge-coupled devices (CCD), and laser scanners.

FILM DIGITIZERS

Film digitizers will still be necessary even in the all digital or filmless imaging department, so that film images from outside referrals without digital capabilities can be input into the system and viewed digitally. Film digitizers convert the continuous optical density values on film into a digital image by sampling at discrete, evenly spaced locations and quantizing the transmitted light from a scan of the film into digital numbers. Several types of film digitizers exist today, with some used more frequently than others in PACS and teleradiology applications.

The analog video camera with ADC, or camera on a stick, has been used in low-cost, entry-level teleradiology applications but is infrequently used in PACS applications today because of its manual operation. The analog video camera requires an illumination source and careful attention to lens settings, focus, f-stop, etc. In addition, it has a maximum resolution of $1024 \times 1024 \times 8$ bits (256 grays), thus limiting the range of window and level or contrast and brightness values the resultant digital image can be displayed in. Digital cameras produce a digital signal output directly from the camera at a maximum resolution of $2048 \times 2048 \times 12$ bits (4096 grays), but are still used infrequently in PACS due to their high cost.

A more commonly used film scanner for PACS is the charge-coupled device (CCD) or flat-bed scanner, which uses a row of photocells and uniformly bright light illumination to capture the image. A lens focuses the transmitted light from the collimated, diffuse light source onto a linear CCD detector, and the signal is collected and converted to a digital electronic signal by an analog-to-digital (ADC) converter. CCD scanners have a maximum resolution of $4096 \times 4096 \times 8$ to 12 bits, but have a narrow film optical density range to which they can respond. CCD scanners have been used in high-end teleradiology or entry-level in-house film distribution systems, such as image transmission to the intensive care units (ICUs). CCD scanners are cheaper than laser scanners, the other commonly used PACS film digitizer.

The laser scanner or laser film digitizer uses either a helium-neon (HeNe) gas laser or a solid-state diode laser source. The laser beam is focused by lenses and directed by mirror deflection components, and the light transmitted through the film is collected by a light guide, its intensity detected by a photomultiplier tube, converted to a proportional electronic signal, and digitized in an ADC. Laser scanners use a fine laser beam of generally variable or adjustable spot sizes down to 50 μm (producing an image sharpness of approximately 10 line pairs/mm). They have maximum resolution of 4096 $\times$ 5120 $\times$ 12 bits and can accommodate the full optical density range of film. They are semi- or fully-automatic in operation and are currently the scanner of choice for PACS applications.

COMPUTED RADIOGRAPHY (CR)

Computed Radiography (CR) refers to projection X-ray imaging using photostimulable or storage phosphors. In this modality, X-rays incident upon a photostimulable phosphor-based image sensor or imaging plate, produce a latent image that is stored in the imaging plate until stimulated to luminesce by laser light. This released light energy can be captured and converted to a digital electronic signal for transmission of images to display and archival devices. Unlike conventional screen-film radiography in which the film functions as the imaging sensor, or recording medium, as well as the display and storage media, computed radiography eliminates film from the image recording step, resulting in a separation of image capture from image display and image storage. This separation of functions potentiates optimization of each of these steps individually. In addition, CR can capitalize on features common to all digital images, namely, electronic transmission, manipulation, display, and storage of radiographs (Andriole 1999c).

Recent technologic advances in CR have made this modality more prevalent in the clinical arena. Hardware and software improvements in the photostimulable phosphor plate, in image reading-scanning devices, in image processing algorithms, and in the cost and utility of image display devices have contributed to the increased acceptance of CR as the digital counterpart to conventional screen-film projection radiography. This section provides an overview of state-of-the-art computed radiography systems, including a basic description of the data acquisition process, a review of system specifications, image quality and performance, and advantages and disadvantages inherent in CR.

An explanation of the image processing algorithms that convert the raw CR image data into useful clinical images is provided. The image processing algorithms discussed include image segmentation or exposure data recognition and background removal; contrast enhancement; spatial frequency processing, including edge enhancement and noise smoothing; dynamic range control (DRC); and multiscale image contrast amplification (MUSICA). Note that the same types of image processing algorithms utilized for CR may be applied to DR images as well. Examples of several types of artifacts potentially encountered with CR are given, along with their causes and methods for correction or minimization.

REVIEW OF THE FUNDAMENTALS

PROCESS DESCRIPTION

A computed radiography system consists of a screen or plate of a stimulable phosphor material that is usually contained in a cassette and is exposed in a manner similar to traditional screen-film cassettes. The photostimulable phosphor in the imaging plate (IP) absorbs X-rays that have passed through the patient, thus "recording" the X-ray image. Like the conventional intensifying screen, CR plates produce light in response to X-rays, at the time of exposure. However, storage phosphor plates are also capable of storing some of the absorbed X-ray energy as a latent image. Plates are typically made of an europium-doped barium-fluoro-halide-halide crystallized matrix. Electrons from the dopant ion are trapped just below the conduction band when exposed to X-rays. Irradiating the imaging plate after the X-ray exposure with red or near-infrared laser light liberates the electrons into the conduction band, stimulating the phosphor to release some of its stored energy in the form of green, blue, or ultraviolet light—the phenomenon of photostimulable luminescence. The intensity of light emitted is proportional to the amount of X-rays absorbed by the storage phosphor (Bogucki 1995).

The readout process uses a precision laser spot scanning mechanism in which the laser beam traverses the imaging plate surface in a raster pattern. The stimulated light emitted from the IP is collected and converted into an electrical signal, with optics coupled to a photomultiplier tube (PMT). The PMT converts the collected light from the IP into an electrical signal, which is then amplified, sampled to produce discrete pixels of the digital image and sent through an analog-to-digital converter (ADC) to quantize the value of each pixel (i.e., a value between 0 and 1023 for a 10-bit ADC or between 0 and 4095 for a 12-bit ADC).

Not all of the stored energy in the IP is released during the readout process. Thus, to prepare the imaging plate for reuse and another exposure, the IP is briefly flooded with high intensity (typically fluorescent) light. This erasure step ensures removal of any residual latent image.

The steps involved in a CR system are diagrammed in Figure 6.3. In principle, CR inserts a digital computer between the imaging plate receptor (photostimulable phosphor screen) and the output film. This digital processor can perform a number of image processing tasks, including compensating for exposure errors, applying appropriate contrast characteristics, enhancing image detail, and storing and distributing image information in digital form.

SYSTEM CHARACTERISTICS

One of the most important differences between CR and screen-film systems is in exposure latitude. The exposure response of a digital imaging system relates the incident X-ray exposure to the resulting pixel value output. System sensitivity is the lowest exposure that will produce a useful pixel value, and the dynamic range is the ratio of the exposures of the highest and lowest useful pixel values (Barnes 1993). Storage phosphor systems have ex-

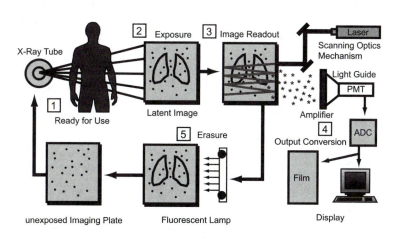

FIGURE 6.3

The image production steps involved in CR. The imaging plate is exposed to X-ray, read out by a laser scanning mechanism, and erased for reuse. A light guide collects the photostimulated luminescence and feeds it to a photomultiplier tube (PMT), which converts the light signal to an electrical signal. Amplification, logarithmic conversion, and analog-to-digital conversion produce the final digital signal, which can be displayed on a cathode ray tube monitor or sent to a laser printer for image reproduction on film.

tremely wide exposure latitude. The wide latitude of storage phosphor systems, and their effectively linear detector characteristic curve, allows them to capture a wider range of exposure information in a single image than is possible with any screen-film system. In addition, the wide dynamic range of CR allows it to be used under a broad range of exposure conditions without the need for changing the basic detector. This also makes CR an ideal choice for applications in which exposures are highly variable or difficult to control, as in portable or bedside radiography. The digital image processing in CR systems can usually create a diagnostic image out of under- or overexposures by appropriate lookup table corrections. In the screen-film environment, such under- or overexposures might necessitate retakes and additional exposure to the patient.

Dose requirements of a medical imaging system depend on the system's ability to detect and convert the incoming signal into a usable output signal. It is important to stress that CR systems are *not* inherently lower dose systems than screen-film. In fact, several studies have demonstrated a higher required exposure for CR to achieve optical density equivalent to screen-film (Andriole 1994, Wilson 1993). However, the wider latitude of storage phosphor systems makes them much more forgiving of under- or overexposure. As in any digital radiography system, when dose is decreased, the noise due to quantum mottle increases (Kodak 1992). Reader tolerance of this noise tends to be the limiting factor on the lowest acceptable dose.

In some clinical situations, the radiologist may feel comfortable lowering the exposure factor to reduce dose to the patient, as in pediatric extremity X-ray exams. When imaging the chest of the newborn, however, one may wish to raise the dose to avoid mistaking the more visible mottle (at lower doses) over the lungs for pulmonary interstitial emphysema, for example.

IMAGE QUALITY

DQE   Objective descriptors of digital image quality include the detective quantum efficiency (DQE), which is a measure of the fidelity with which a resultant digital image represents the transmitted X-ray fluence pattern (i.e., how efficiently a system converts the X-ray input signal into a useful output image) and includes a measure of the noise added (Barnes 1993). Also taken into account are the input/output characteristics of the system and the resolution response of unsharpness or blur added during the image capture process. The linear, wide-latitude input/output characteristic of CR systems relative to screen-film systems leads to a wider DQE latitude for CR, which implies that CR has the ability to convert incoming X-ray quanta into "useful" output over a much wider range of exposures than can be accommodated with screen-film systems (Kodak 1992).

Spatial Resolution   The spatial resolution response or sharpness of an image capture process can be expressed in terms of its modulation transfer function (MTF), which in practice, is determined by taking the Fourier Transform of the line spread function (LSF), and relates *input* subject contrast to *imaged* subject contrast as a function of spatial frequency (Barnes 1993). The ideal image receptor adds no blur or broadening to the input LSF, resulting in an MTF response of one at all spatial frequencies. A real image receptor adds blur, typically resulting in a loss of MTF at higher spatial frequencies.

The main factor limiting the spatial resolution in CR, similar to screen-film systems, is X-ray scattering within the phosphor layer. However, it is the scattering of the stimulating beam in CR, rather than the emitted light as in screen-film, that determines system sharpness (Kodak 1992, Matsuda 1993). Broadening of the laser light spot within the IP phosphor layer spreads with the depth of the plate. Thus, the spatial resolution response of CR depends largely on the initial laser beam diameter and the thickness of the IP detector. The reproducible spatial frequency of CR is also limited by the sampling used in the digital readout process. The spatial resolution of CR is less than that of screen-film, with CR ranging from 2.5 to 5 line pairs per millimeter (lp/mm) vs. the 10 lp/mm or higher spatial resolution of screen-film.

Contrast Resolution   The contrast or grayscale resolution for CR is much greater than that for screen-film. Because overall image quality resolution is a combination of spatial and grayscale resolution, the superior contrast resolution of CR can often compensate for its lack of inherent spatial resolution. By manipulating the image contrast and brightness, or the window and level values respectively, small features often become more readily apparent in the image. This is analogous to "bright-lighting" a bone film, for example, when looking for a small fracture. The overall impression is that the spatial resolution of the image has been improved, when in fact it has not changed—only the contrast resolution has been manipulated. More work needs to be done to determine the most appropriate window and level settings with which to initially display a CR image. Lacking optimal default settings, it is often useful to view CR softcopy images "dynamically" with a variety of window and level settings.

Noise   The types of noise affecting CR images include X-ray dose-dependent noise and fixed noise (independent of X-ray dose). The dose-dependent noise components can be classified into X-ray quantum noise, or mottle, and light photon noise (Matsuda 1993). The quantum mottle inherent in the input X-ray beam is the limiting noise factor, and it arises in the process of absorption by the imaging plate, with noise being inversely proportional to the detector X-ray dose absorption. Light photon noise arises in the process of photoelectric transmission of the photostimulable luminescence light at the surface of the photomultiplier tube (PMT).

Fixed noise sources in CR systems include IP structural noise (the predominant factor), noise in the electronics chain, laser power fluctuations, quantization noise in the analog-to-digital conversion process (Kodak 1992, Matsuda 1993). IP structural noise arises from the nonuniformity of phosphor particle distribution, with finer particles providing noise improvement. Note that for CR systems, it is the *noise* sources that limits the DQE system latitude, whereas in conventional X-ray systems, the DQE latitude is limited by the narrower *exposure response* of screen-film.

Comparison with Screen-Film   The extremely large latitude of CR systems makes CR more forgiving in difficult imaging situations, such as portable examinations, and decreases retake rates, as compared to screen-film, for improper exposure technique. The superior contrast resolution of CR can compensate in many cases for its lesser spatial resolution. Cost savings and improved departmental workflow can be realized with CR and the elimination of film.

AVAILABLE CR SYSTEMS

HISTORICAL PERSPECTIVE   Most of the progress in storage phosphor imaging has been made after World War II (Berg 1947). In 1975, Eastman Kodak Company (Rochester, NY) patented an apparatus using infrared-stimulable phosphors or thermoluminescent materials to store an image (Luckey 1975). In 1980, Fuji Photo Film (Tokyo, Japan) patented a process in which photostimulable phosphors were used to record and reproduce an image by absorbing radiation, and then releasing the stored energy as light when stimulated by a helium-neon laser (Kotera 1980). The emitted phosphor luminescence was detected by a photomultiplier tube (PMT) and an electronic signal produced, which reconstructed the image.

Fuji was the first to commercialize a storage phosphor-based computed radiography system in 1983 (as the FCR 101) and published the first technical paper (in *Radiology*) describing CR for acquiring clinical digital X-ray images (Sonoda 1983). The central processing type second-generation scanners (FCR 201) were marketed in 1985 (Matsuda 1993). Third-generation

Fuji systems marketed in 1989 included distributed processing (FCR 7000) and stand-alone (AC-1) types (Matsuda 1993). Fuji systems in the FCR 9000 series are improved, faster, higher performance third-generation scanners. Current Fuji systems in the 5000 series include an upright chest unit (5501) and a multi-plate autoloader.

In 1992, Kodak installed its first commercial storage phosphor reader, Model 3110 (Bogucki 1995). Their current model, the KESPR (Kodak Ektascan Storage Phosphor Reader) Model 400 or CR 400 Plus includes an autoloader device. In 1994, Agfa-Gevaert N.V. (Belgium) debuted its own CR system design (the ADC 70) (Agfa 1994). In 1997, Agfa showed its ADC Compact with greatly reduced footprint. This product is now sold exclusively. In 1998, Lumisys presented its low-cost, desktop CR unit (the ACR 2000) with manual-feed, single plate reading. Agfa also introduced a low-cost, entry-level single plate reader (the ADC Solo) in 1998, appropriate for distributed CR environments such as clinics, trauma centers, and intensive care units (ICUs).

Many companies have been involved in CR research and development, including: N.A. Philips Corp., Konica Corp., E.I. DuPont de Nemours & Co., 3M Co., Hitachi, Ltd., Seimens AG, Toshiba Corp., General Electric Corp., Kasei Optonix, Ltd., Mitsubishi Chemical Industries, Ltd., Nichia Corp., GTE Products Co., and DigiRad Corp. (Kodak 1992). However, the four distinct state-of-the-art commercially available computed radiography systems include devices by Agfa, Fuji, Kodak, and Lumisys.

RECENT TECHNOLOGIC ADVANCES Major improvements in the overall CR system design and performance characteristics include a reduction in the physical size of the reading/scanning units, increased plate reading capacity per unit time, and better image quality. These advances have been achieved through a combination of changes in the imaging plates themselves, in the image reader or scanning devices, and in the application of image processing algorithms to effect image output.

The newer imaging plates developed for the latest CR devices have better image quality (increased sharpness) and improved fading and residual image characteristics. Better image quality has resulted from modifications in the imaging plate (IP) phosphor and layer thickness. Smaller phosphor grain size in the IP (down to approximately 4 μm) diminishes fixed noise of the imaging plate, while increased packing density of phosphor particles counteracts a concomitant decrease in photostimulable luminescence (Matsuda 1993). A thinner protective layer is used in the plates, which tends to reduce X-ray quantum noise; in and of itself, this would improve the spatial resolution response characteristics of the plates as a result of diminished beam scattering. However, in the newest IPs, the quantity of phosphor coated onto the plate has been increased for durability purposes, resulting in the same response characteristic of previous imaging plates (Ogawa 1995).

An historical review of CR scanning units chronicles improved compactness and increased processing speed. The first Fuji unit (FCR 101) from 1983 required roughly 6 m^2 of floor space to house the reader and could only process about 45 plates per hour, while today's Fuji models (i.e., FCR 9000s) occupy less than 1 m^2 and can process approximately 110 plates per hour (Matsuda 1993). Thus, apparatus size decreased by approximately one sixth and processing capacity increased roughly 2.5 times. Desktop models reduce the physical device footprint even further.

CR imaging plate sizes, pixel resolutions, and their associated digital file sizes are roughly the same across manufacturers for the various cassette sizes offered. For example, the 14 in × 17 in (or 35 cm × 43 cm) plates are read with a sampling rate of 5 to 5.81 pixels/mm, at a digital image matrix size of roughly 2k × 2k pixels (1760 × 2140 pixels for Fuji [Matsuda 1993] and 2048 × 2508 pixels for Agfa and Kodak [Bogucki 1995]). Fuji images are quantized to 10 bits (for 1024 gray levels), and Agfa and Kodak images have a 12-bit logarithmic quantization (for 4096 gray levels). Thus, total image file sizes range from roughly 8 MB to 11.5 MB. The smaller plates are scanned at the same laser spot size (100 μm) and the digitization rate does not change, therefore, the pixel size is smaller (Bogucki 1995). The 10 in × 12 in (24 cm × 30 cm) plates are typically read at a sampling rate of 6.7 to 9 pixels/mm and the 8 in × 10 in (18 cm × 24 cm) plates are read at 10 pixels/mm (Bogucki 1995, Matsuda 1993).

IMAGE PROCESSING ALGORITHMS

Image processing optimizes the radiograph for output display. Each manufacturer has its own set of proprietary algorithms that can be applied to the image for printing on laser film or display on its own proprietary workstations. Prior to the DICOM standard, only the raw data could be directly acquired digitally. Therefore, to attain the same image appearance on other display stations, the appropriate image processing algorithms (if known) had to be implemented somewhere along the chain from acquisition to display. Now image processing parameters are passed in the DICOM header, and algorithms applied to CR images are displayed on generic workstations. In general, the digital image processing applied to computed radiography consists of a recognition or analysis phase, followed by contrast enhancement and/or frequency processing. Note that the same types of image processing applied to CR can also be used for processing DR images.

IMAGE SEGMENTATION   In the image recognition stage, the region of exposure (i.e., the collimation edges) is detected, a histogram analysis of the pixel gray values in the image is performed to assess the actual exposure to the plate, and the appropriate lookup table specific to the anatomic region is selected by the X-ray technologist when patient demographic information is input. Proper recognition of the exposed region is extremely important, as it affects future processing of the image data. For example, if the bright white area of the image caused by collimation at the time of exposure is not detected properly, its high gray values will be taken into account during histogram analysis, thereby increasing the "window" of values to be accommodated by a given display device (softcopy or hardcopy). The overall effect would be decreased contrast in the image.

Some segmentation algorithms, in addition to detecting collimation edges in the image, permit users to blacken the region outside these edges (Bogucki 1995, Kodak 1994). This tends to improve image contrast appearance by removing bright white backgrounds in images of small body parts or in pediatric patients. Figure 6.4B demonstrates this feature of "blackened surround," as applied to the image in Figure 6.4A.

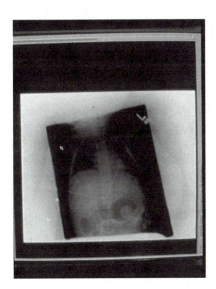
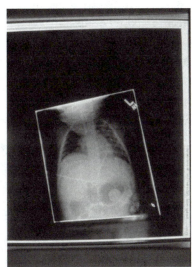

A   B

FIGURE 6.4

Example image segmentation algorithm detection of (white) collimation edges of image in image A, with "blackened surround" applied in image B, note the improved overall contrast in the image in B.

CONTRAST ENHANCEMENT Conventional contrast enhancement, also called gradation processing, tone scaling, and latitude reduction, is performed next. This processing amounts to choosing the best characteristic curve (usually a nonlinear transformation of X-ray exposure to image density) to apply to the image data. These algorithms are quite flexible and can be tuned to satisfy a particular user's preferences for a given "look" of the image (Gringold 1994). Lookup tables are specific to the region of anatomy imaged. Figure 6.5 shows an example of the default adult chest lookup table (A) applied to an image and the same image with high contrast processing (B). A reverse contrast scale or "black bone" technique—in which what was originally black in the image becomes white and what was originally white in the image becomes black—is sometimes considered beneficial for identifying and locating tubes and lines. An example is shown in Figure 6.6, where the contrast reversal algorithm has been applied to the image in Figure 6.6A, resulting in the image in Figure 6.6B.

SPATIAL FREQUENCY PROCESSING After contrast enhancement, spatial frequency processing, sometimes called edge enhancement, is usually performed. These algorithms adjust the frequency response characteristics of the CR systems, essentially implementing a high or band-pass filter operation to enhance the high spatial frequency content in edge information. Unfortunately, noise also contains high spatial frequency information and can be exacerbated by edge-enhancement techniques. To lessen this problem, a nonlinear unsharp masking technique is typically implemented, which suppresses noise via a smoothing process. (Unsharp masking is an averaging

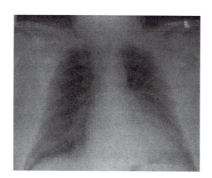
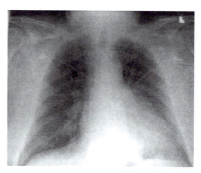

A   B

FIGURE 6.5

Chest image processed with A, default mode, and B, high-contrast algorithm applied.

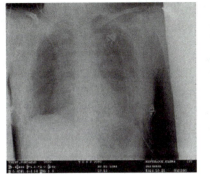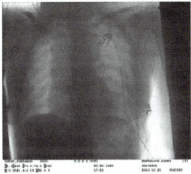

A   B

FIGURE 6.6

Chest image processed with **A**, default mode, and **B**, blackbone or contrast reversal algorithm applied.

technique that, via summation, tends to blur the image. When this is subtracted from the original image data, the effect is noise suppression.) Specific spatial frequencies can be preferentially selected and emphasized by changing the mask size and weighting parameters. For example, low frequency information in the image can be augmented by using a relatively large mask, while high frequency or edge information can be enhanced by using a small mask (Matsuda 1993).

DRC   Dynamic range control (DRC) processing is an advanced algorithm by Fuji for selective compression or emphasis of low-density regions in an image independent of contrast and spatial frequency (Ishida 1993). DRC performs an unsharp mask to suppress high spatial frequency information, then applies a specific lookup table that maps to selected regions (i.e., low-density areas). This mask is then added back to the original data, with the overall result being improved contrast in poorly penetrated regions without loss of high frequency and contrast emphasis. In a clinical evaluation of the algorithm for processing adult portable chest exams, five thoracic radiologists preferred DRC in a side-by-side comparison because it improved visibility of mediastinal details and enhanced subdiaphragmatic regions (Storto 1995).

MUSICA   Multiscale image contrast amplification (MUSICA) is a flexible advanced image processing algorithm developed by Agfa (Agfa 1994, Vuylsteke 1997). MUSICA is a local contrast enhancement technique based on the principle of detail amplitude or detail strength, and the notion that image features can be striking or subtle, large or small. The method is carried out by decomposing the original image into a set of detail images, where each detail image represents an image feature of a specific scale. This set of detail images, or basis functions, completely describes the original image. Each detail image representation and the image background are contrast-equalized separately; some details can be enhanced and others attenuated as desired. All the separate detail images are recombined into a single image, so that differences in contrast between features are diminished regardless of size—all features are more visible.

IMAGE ARTIFACTS

Artifacts can arise from a variety of sources, including the imaging plates themselves, image readers, and image processing. Several types of artifacts potentially encountered with CR are minimized with the latest technology improvements, but may still occur with older systems.

Lead backing added to the aluminum-framed, carbon-fiber cassettes has eliminated the so-called light-bulb effect—darkened outer portions of a film caused by backscattered radiation (Solomon 1991). High sensitivity of the CR plates renders them extremely susceptible to scattered radiation or inadvertent exposure; therefore routine erasure of all CR plates on the day of use is recommended, as is the storing of imaging plates on end, rather than stacking cassettes one on top of the other (Volpe 1996). The occurrence of persistent latent images after high exposures or after prolonged intervals between plate erasure and reuse (Oestman 1991, Solomon 1991) has been lessened by the improved efficiency of the two-stage erasure procedure used in the latest CR systems (Volpe 1996). Improved recognition of the collimation pattern employed for a given image allows varied collimation fields (including off-angle) and in turn, improves histogram analysis and subsequent processing of the imaged region (Volpe 1996), although these algorithms can fail in some instances. Plate cracking from wear-and-tear can also create troublesome artifacts (Volpe 1996).

Inadvertent double exposures can occur with the present CR systems, potentially masking low-density findings such as parenchymal consolidation, or leading to errors in interpreting line positions. Such artifacts are more difficult to detect than with screen-film systems because CR's linear frequency processing response optimizes image intensity over a wide range of exposures (i.e., due to its wide dynamic range). Figure 6.7 shows an example of a double exposure artifact; additional examples are included in Volpe

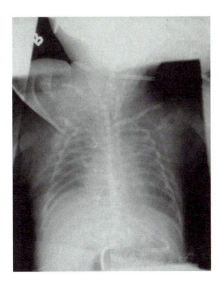

FIGURE 6.7

Example of inadvertent double exposure.

(1996). Laser scanning artifacts can still occur with current CR readers; a linear artifact across the image is caused by dust on the light source (Volpe 1996). Proper and frequent cleaning of the laser and light guide apparatus as well as the imaging plates themselves can prevent such artifacts.

The ability of CR to produce clinically diagnostic images over a wide range of exposures depends on the effectiveness of the image analysis algorithms applied to each data set. The specific processing parameters are based on standards tuned to the anatomic region under examination. Incorrect selection of a diagnostic specifier or anatomic region can result in an image of unacceptable quality. Understanding the causes of some of these CR imaging artifacts as well as maintaining formal, routine quality assurance procedures helps one to recognize, correct, and avoid future difficulties.

SUMMARY OF CR

CR can be used for the digital image acquisition of projection radiography examinations into a PACS. As a result of its wide exposure latitude and relative forgiveness of exposure technique, CR can improve the quality of images acquired in difficult imaging situations, such as portable or bedside examinations of critically ill or hospitalized patients. As such, CR systems have been successfully used in the intensive care unit (ICU), in the emergency room (ER) or trauma center, as well as in the operating room (OR). CR can also be cost-effective for a high-volume clinic setting or in a low-volume setting for input to a teleradiology service, and it has successfully reduced retake rates for portable and other examinations.

Technologic advances in computed radiography hardware and software have contributed to the increased acceptance of CR as the current counterpart to conventional screen-film projection radiography, making its use for clinical purposes more widespread. CR is compatible with existing X-ray equipment, yet separates out the functions of image acquisition or capture, image display, and image archival vs. traditional screen-film radiography, in which film serves as the image detector, display, and storage medium. This separation of functions by CR enables optimization of each of these steps individually. Potential benefits are improved diagnostic capability (via the wide dynamic range of CR and the ability to manipulate the exam through image processing) and enhanced radiology department productivity (via networking capabilities for transmission of images to remote digital softcopy displays and for storage and retrieval of the digital data).

DIGITAL RADIOGRAPHY (DR)

In addition to the current clinical devices for digital image acquisition of projection X-rays, such as computed radiography (CR) or imaging with photostimulable or storage phosphors, are the direct digital detectors, which fall under the general heading of digital radiography (DR). (Film scanners for digitization of existing analog film are discussed elsewhere in this chapter.)

Unlike conventional screen-film radiography in which the film functions as the imaging sensor, or recording medium as well as the display and storage media, DR—like CR—eliminates film from the image recording step, thereby separating image capture from image display and image storage. This separation of functions potentiates optimization of each of these steps individually. In addition, both CR and DR can capitalize on features common to digital or filmless imaging, namely, the ability to acquire, transmit, display, manipulate, and archive data electronically, overcoming some of the limitations of conventional screen-film radiography. Digital imaging benefits include remote access to images and clinical information by multiple users simultaneously, permanent storage and subsequent retrieval of image data, expedient information delivery to those who need it, and efficient, cost-effective workflow with the elimination of film from the equation.

In this chapter, DR refers to devices in which the digitization of the X-ray signal occurs within the detector itself, providing an immediate full-fidelity image on a softcopy display monitor. Compare this with CR, which uses a photostimulable phosphor imaging plate detector in a cassette design that must be processed in a CR reader following X-ray exposure for conversion to a digital image. DR devices may be classified as direct or indirect based on their detector design and conversion of absorbed X-rays into an image. Note that the acronym "DR" may be used by some to refer to direct radiography, also called direct digital radiography (DDR), as a subset of digital radiography in which X-ray absorption within the detector is converted into a proportional electric charge without an intermediate light conversion step.

Recent technologic advances in CR and DR have made digital projection radiography more prevalent in the clinical arena, with CR currently having a greater clinical install base. Hardware and software improvements in detector devices, in image reading-scanning devices, in image processing algorithms, and in the cost and utility of image display devices have contributed to the increased acceptance of these digital counterparts to conventional screen-film radiography.

The purpose of this section is to provide an overview of state-of-the-art digital radiography systems. A basic description of the data acquisition process is given, followed by a review of system specifications, image quality, and performance, including signal-to-noise, contrast, and spatial resolution characteristics. Advantages and disadvantages inherent in CR and DR, and a comparison with screen-film radiography is given with respect to system performance, image quality, workflow, and cost.

REVIEW OF THE FUNDAMENTALS

PROCESS DESCRIPTION: INDIRECT VS. DIRECT CONVERSION

DR refers to devices for direct digital acquisition of projection radiographs in which the digitization of the X-ray signal takes place within the detector. DR devices, also called flat-panel detectors, include two types: (1) indirect conversion devices, in which light is first generated using a scintillator or phosphor and then detected by a charge-coupled device (CCD) or a thin-film-transistor (TFT) array in conjunction with photodiodes; and (2) direct digital radiography (DDR) devices, which consist of a top electrode, dielectric layer, selenium X-ray photoconductor, and thin-film pixel array (Lee 1995). Figure 6.8 shows a comparison of the direct and indirect en-

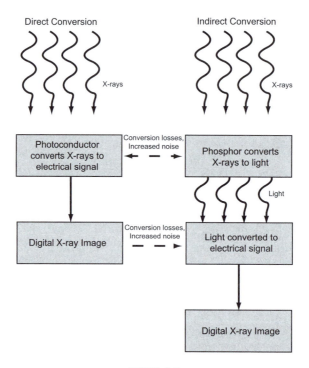

FIGURE 6.8

The image production steps involved in direct and indirect digital radiography detectors.

ergy conversion steps in the production of a digital X-ray image. DDR devices offer direct energy conversion of X-ray for immediate readout without the intermediate light conversion step.

The basis of DR devices is the large area thin-film-transistor (TFT) active matrix array, or flat panel, in which each pixel consists of a signal collection area or charge collection electrode, a storage capacitor, and an amorphous silicon field-effect transistor (FET) switch that allows the active readout of the charge stored in the capacitor (Lee 1995). Arrays of individual detector areas are addressed by orthogonally arranged gate switches and data lines to read the signal generated by the absorption of X-rays in the detector. The TFT arrays are used in conjunction with a direct X-ray photoconductor layer or an indirect X-ray sensitive phosphor-coated light-sensitive detector/photodiode array.

The DDR device diagramed in cross-section in Figure 6.9 (Lee 1995) uses a multilayer detector in a cassette design; the X-ray energy is converted

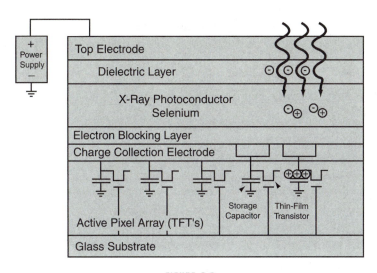

FIGURE 6.9

Cross-sectional view of an example direct digital radiography (DDR) detector panel.

directly to electron-hole pairs in an amorphous selenium (Se) photoconductive conversion layer. Charge pairs are separated in a bias field so that the holes are collected in the storage capacitors and the electrons drift toward the Se-dielectric interface. At the end of exposure, the image resides in the pixel matrix in the form of charges, with the charge proportional to the absorbed radiation. At the end of readout, the charges are erased to prepare for another detection cycle.

An example of an indirect DR device uses an X-ray sensitive phosphor coating on top of a light-sensitive flat-panel amorphous silicon (Am-Si) detector TFT array. The X-rays are first converted to light and then to a proportional charge in the photodiode (typically a cesium iodide (CsI) scintillator), which is then stored in the TFT array where the image signal is recorded.

DR detectors have high efficiency, low noise, good spatial resolution, wide latitude, and all the benefits of digital or filmless imaging. These sensors are not yet widely used clinically because of their high cost of production and the one-room-at-a-time technology, as well as portability issues and other impracticalities.

SYSTEM CHARACTERISTICS DR devices have the same wide exposure latitude and effective linear detector characteristic curve as CR devices, enabling use under a broad range of exposure techniques. Similarly, DR has a wide dynamic range of quantization to thousands of gray levels. Detectors have thus far been designed only for the X-ray room table or wall bucky, and their fragility and poor portability makes them difficult to use in the bedside X-ray environment. The short DR imaging cycle time, however, lends itself to combined static radiographic and dynamic fluoroscopic uses. This is especially true for the indirect devices—the direct Se detector, for example, has a ghosting problem due to charge trapping, which introduces a lag time at the end of each cycle, lengthening the time between readiness for the next exposure.

IMAGE QUALITY   The image quality of DR devices is competitive with CR and screen-film. DR devices have very high DQEs, capturing roughly 80% absorption of the X-ray energy at optimum exposures. Thus, DR is a very high efficiency, low noise detector, converting much of the incoming X-ray signal into useful output. However, a major factor limiting DR efficiency involves the packing fraction, or active detector area to dead space taken up by the data readout devices (transistors, data lines, capacitors, etc.). The smaller the pixel size, the smaller the packing fraction, with a larger proportion of dead area overwhelming the active area, in some cases reducing the active area to 30% or less (Lee 1995). The overall effect is a reduction in geometric and quantum efficiency.

The spatial resolution of DR is comparable to CR, which is still less than that for analog X-ray. Typical matrix sizes are on the order of 2000 to 2500 pixels × 2000 to 2500 pixels. The pixel size of the TFT array detector is the limiting factor for spatial resolution, with the direct Se detector yielding a better inherent spatial resolution than indirect detectors. This can lead to better signal modulation and superior contrast.

DR design presents a delicate trade-off between detector efficiency, which is inversely proportional to pixel size, and spatial resolution, which is affected directly by pixel size. Typically, DR devices are specified for higher detection efficiency at a cost of much less spatial resolution than screen-film, compensated by a wide dynamic range or high contrast resolution. Design complexities requiring further development include wiring configurations to minimize dead space and maximize the detector packing fraction, fast and robust signal readout methods, and better error correction matrices for more accurate signal readout.

COMPARISON OF CR AND DR

Table 6.2 lists the advantages of CR and DR, including all the benefits of digital images that can be electronically processed, manipulated, distributed, displayed, and archived. The superior contrast resolution of the digital

TABLE 6.2
Summary of Advantages of CR and DR Systems

▶ Digital images capable of being electronically processed, manipulated, distributed, displayed, and archived

▶ Large latitude system allowing excellent visualization of both soft tissue and bone in the same exposure image

▶ Superior contrast resolution can compensate for lack of spatial resolution

▶ Decreased retake rate

▶ Potential cost savings if film is eliminated

▶ Improved radiology department workflow with elimination of film handling routines

modalities can compensate in many cases for the lesser spatial resolution as compared with screen-film. Both CR and DR can be used for digital image acquisition of projection radiography examinations into a PACS.

As for any digital image acquisition device, CR and/or DR would be the first point of entry into a PACS. Errors may propagate from here, with the quality of the PACS output being directly dependent on the quality of the signal input. In addition to image quality, the following features are essential for successful clinical implementation of CR or DR systems for a PACS. DICOM conformance is essential and includes compliance with the image data and header format, as well as the DICOM communication protocol. Equally critical is interfacing with the radiology information system (RIS)/hospital information system (HIS). Integrating the CR/DR system with the RIS-HIS can reduce human errors in patient demographic information input and improve efficiency. Ease of integration of the device into the daily workflow routine and simplicity and robustness of the user interface are very important. Reliability, fault tolerance, and capabilities for error tracking are also major issues to consider, as are device speed and performance.

DR devices have more efficient detectors, offering direct energy conversion of X-ray for immediate readout. These detectors have low noise and good spatial resolution, wide latitude and all the benefits of digital or filmless imaging. But cost is still high because detector production is difficult and expensive, and DR is a one-room-at-a-time detector. DR may be cost-effective in high-volume sites and for imaging examinations requiring high quality, such as upright chest exams and bone work.

The ease of use, straightforward integration, and proven reliability of CR systems vs. DR systems, adds to the attractiveness of CR as a replacement for screen-film systems in general radiography in a picture archiving and communications system (PACS) digital imaging network. DR, however, has potential for excellent image quality available immediately at the time of exposure. It is likely that CR and DR devices will coexist for some time.

Several technical limitations still remain such as CR's and DR's decreased spatial resolution compared to conventional screen-film methods, preventing its use in certain clinical applications such as mammography. Meeting the cost competitiveness of screen-film systems is difficult unless film printing is eliminated from the cost equation. Future improvements in image processing algorithms, with a better understanding of optimum display settings for softcopy viewing, have the potential to greatly facilitate and standardize softcopy reading of digital projection radiographs and further the acceptance of CR and DR in the clinical arena.

QUALITY ASSURANCE/QUALITY CONTROL (QA-QC) FOR ACQUISITION

The current trend for radiology departments and medical imaging within healthcare enterprises is increasingly moving toward the all-digital or filmless medical image management system or PACS. Operational concerns with PACS implementations can arise at all stages of the process, from design specifications, to installation, to training, and acceptance (Honeyman 1997b). Quality control procedures necessarily become modified in the filmless radiology department, and new processes must be developed (Honeyman 1997a) to better prepare for the total digital clinical department.

Forming and maintaining a continuing quality improvement (CQI) committee may facilitate PACS installation and training periods, workflow modifications, quality assurance, and clinical acceptance. This committee should include radiologists at all levels (resident, fellow, attending), radiology technologists, film library personnel, emergency department and intensive care unit clinician end-users, and PACS team members. The CQI committee may assist in the creation of new management procedures, provide a means for user feedback and education, and contribute to the overall acceptance of and user satisfaction with the system (Andriole 1998).

PROBLEMS OCCURRING AT ACQUISITION

The imaging modality is the first entry point into the PACS and any errors in data input here can propagate throughout the system. Thus, interfacing a PACS to the RIS-HIS and better yet, having DICOM Modality Worklist capability at the imaging device, are essential. When a PACS is properly interfaced to the RIS-HIS, input data can be verified by comparison of pertinent demographic data (name, date, time, medical record number (MRN), accession number, exam type) at the PACS acquisition gateway with the data recorded in the RIS. Thus, any imaging exam entering the PACS will be RIS-verified prior to archival and distribution.

Several imaging modalities are tightly coupled with the RIS (i.e., some CR manufacturers) and provide automatic downloading of demographic information from the RIS via bar code readers, to the modality and hence the DICOM header. This eliminates the highly error-prone manual entry of data at acquisition. Unfortunately for manual data entry devices, any errors in data may result in the image data being held in a queue pending human inspection and resolution. Continuous feedback should be given to technologists making repeated errors in data entry.

The well-designed PACS holds newly acquired studies in a restricted area (fix-queue or "penalty box") until the demographic data in the header is matched to a pending exam request from the RIS-HIS. If any failure occurs, such as an incorrect MRN or DOB (date of birth), the new exam does not pass automatically into the system to be archived (although it may be displayable) until the discrepancy has been resolved by human intervention. However, the inverse test has not been implemented. Pending exam orders held in the RIS-HIS that do not relate to any incoming PACS image data within a certain time frame should be flagged. Full PACS acquisition quality assurance (QA) requires this bidirectional process monitor to ensure that data in the PACS is valid and verified with data in the RIS-HIS, and that all data in the RIS-HIS is acquired into the PACS. This may also assist QA procedures in determining which studies that have been ordered and completed have no associated report and therefore may not have been read.

Some DICOM transfer of imaging exams (i.e., from CT and MR scanners) to the PACS require autosend-networking pathways to be enabled at the scanner. Unfortunately, these features can be turned off easily (frequently by the service manufacturer) resulting in missed real-time transfer of images to the PACS. Stressing the importance of having the autosend enabled at the time of imaging to the imaging technologists, as well as the manufacturer's service personnel can reduce this problem.

Although many digital angiographic/fluorographic systems are DICOM-compliant, few have been integrated into a PACS. The large volume of data typically generated by angiographic procedures is one reason for this. One way to reduce the data volume, and perhaps facilitate connection to a PACS might be to store only key images of an angiographic run much the way they are filmed. Some manufacturers allow operators to create summary series of the examinations, which could then be transmitted to the PACS for viewing on display workstations. A second problem for incorporation of angiographic images into a PACS arises from the inability of most PACS to do the subtraction, pixel shifting, and rapid mask selection features used in most angiographic examinations.

QC PROCEDURES/TROUBLESHOOTING

Involving anticipated users of the system during the PACS planning, specification, and lab testing phases can be beneficial. User awareness of the goals of a PACS implementation and its system features prior to clinical installment can affect the overall success of the system. Installation of system components are most successful when scheduled during low-volume periods and when all affected users are notified well in advance of the install date. Backup contingency plans must be in place prior to going live in the clinical environment.

Among the many roles of the medical physicist and/or PACS engineer in incorporating an imaging modality into the diagnostic imaging department are acceptance testing of the device and quality assurance/quality control (QA-QC). The medical physicist should be involved in the citing and planning of the imaging system, as well as the installation, testing, tuning, and training. Formal QA-QC procedures are still evolving, particularly for the newer modalities such as CR. In fact, substantial efforts have been underway to standardize CR QA-QC, such as the American Association of Physicists in Medicine (AAPM) Task Group #10 draft document "Computed Radiography Acceptance Testing and Quality Control." (See also Seibert [1994] and Willis [1995].)

In spite of the fact that CR is more forgiving of a broad range of exposures, the use of this modality is not an excuse to employ poor radiographic technique. CR exposures should be routinely monitored as well as the image quality on a per-exam basis. Understanding the causes of possible CR imaging artifacts as well as maintaining formal, routine QA procedures can help personnel to recognize, correct for, and avoid future difficulties with this relatively new modality, just as with the proven modalities. Formal QA-QC procedures should be put in place and diligently adhered to.

Maintenance, QA-QC, and workflow procedural modifications continue to be developed as incidents occur, and system troubleshooting is carried out as more radiology departments implement PACS technologies. Documentation of events and CQI committee review and analysis of system functioning in conjunction with review of user suggestions is extremely important to the successful clinical operation of the PACS.

FUTURE TRENDS IN IMAGE ACQUISITION

Although the types of imaging modalities probably will not change all the much in the next several years, anticipated trends in image acquisition for digital radiology and PACS include changes in the image data sets, changes in the imaging devices themselves, and improvement in image processing for softcopy display of digital images.

IMAGE DATA SETS

No new types of imaging modalities are foreseen for the near future. However, it is anticipated (and has to a certain extent already begun) that image data sets acquired from the existing modalities will increase in overall study file size, in some cases dramatically. For example, many radiology departments have begun installing multiple detector array CT scanners, which generate a greater number of individual images than do single detector array scanners. This occurs because of the smaller slice thickness in helical acquisition ($\sim$5 mm) vs. the thickness acquired with single detector arrays ($\sim$7 to 10 mm) and the clinical imaging protocols used.

Image matrix sizes for the digital projection radiography devices (CR and DR) have gone up from roughly from 1000 and 2000 square matrices to 4000×5000 pixels squared. This was done in an attempt to improve the spatial resolution by increased sampling and to improve the look of X-rays printed on 14 in $\times$ 17 in film. Most laser film digitizers can now vary their spot sizes from 200 μm down to 50 μm, greatly improving the inherent spatial resolution of the scanned images, with a concomitant increase in file size.

The bit depth representation of grayscale pixel values has also increased from 8 bits to 10, 12, and 16 bits, and color images are stored as 32-bit or 4 byte/pixel data files. Furthermore, the addition of postprocessing results or slice reconstructions and cinegraphic sequences to the image data set, while improving the overall quality of the image, may greatly increase the amount of data acquired into a PACS.

DEVICES

While image data sets and file sizes are getting larger, the physical footprint of the imaging devices themselves will continue to get smaller. This has occurred most dramatically with CR devices, going from requiring roughly 36 m^2 of floor space and special electrical power and cooling, to desktop devices that can be placed in almost any location. CT and MRI devices are also becoming smaller, more portable, and more robust. It is also hoped that all of these devices will continue to become less costly.

IMAGE PROCESSING

An important area receiving increased attention is image processing capability for softcopy image display. Future processing techniques will most likely go above and beyond the simple window and level (or contrast and brightness) manipulation techniques. These postprocessing algorithms are currently available and tunable at the imaging modality, or accompanying modality acquisition workstation, but in time may be manipulable in real-time at the display station.

Image compression is currently being debated, but may in time be available at the modality to reduce image transmission time and archival space. Some techniques, such as the wavelet transform, may become more widely used not only as a compression technique but also for image enhancement at the imaging devices.

It is anticipated that the percentage of all imaging devices used by healthcare enterprises that are digital will increase greatly. The percentage of digital image acquisition from all devices should also increase, thereby decreasing the amount of film used as an acquisition, display, and archival medium.

CONCLUSION

Image acquisition is the first point of data entry into a picture archiving and communications system (PACS); errors generated here can propagate throughout the system, adversely affecting clinical operations. General predictors for successful incorporation of image acquisition devices into a digital imaging department include:

▶ ease of device integration into the established daily workflow routine of the clinical environment,

▶ high reliability and fault tolerance of the device,

▶ simplicity and intuitiveness of the user interface, and

▶ device speed.

Conformance with the digital imaging and communications in medicine (DICOM) standard is critical. DICOM consists of a standard image format as well as a network communications protocol. Compliance with this standard enables an open architecture for imaging systems, bridging hardware and software entities, allowing interoperability for the transfer of medical images and associated information between disparate systems.

▶ Compliance with the DICOM standard has greatly facilitated image acquisition for PACS and digital radiology departments.

▶ DICOM compliance should be required from the modality and PACS vendors.

▶ Most modalities today do comply with the DICOM standard.

▶ Interface boxes are available to convert legacy devices to DICOM.

Equally essential, particularly at acquisition, is interfacing the RIS-HIS with the PACS. This greatly facilitates input of patient demographics (e.g., name, date, time, medical record number, accession number, and exam type), and imaging parameters and enables automatic PACS data verification, correlation, and error correction with the data recorded in the RIS-HIS. Several imaging modalities are tightly coupled with the RIS (i.e., some CR manufacturers) and provide automatic downloading of demographic information from the RIS by bar code readers to the modality and the DICOM header. This eliminates the highly error-prone manual entry of data at acquisition. Some vendors also provide the capability to download RIS-HIS schedules and worklists directly to the imaging modality:

▶ RIS-HIS-PACS database integration is essential for a clinically functioning digital department and is intelligence added,

▶ HL-7 compliance is desirable,

▶ RIS-HIS databases are typically patient centric, enabling query and retrieval of information by the patient, study, series, or image data hierarchy, and

▶ Modality Worklist capability at the imaging device can greatly improve departmental workflow and efficiency.

Digital image acquisition from the inherently digital modalities, such as computed tomography (CT) and magnetic resonance imaging (MRI), just makes sense. There are two methods for accomplishing this: direct capture and frame grabbing. Direct digital interfaces allow capture and transmission of image data from the modality at the full spatial resolution and bit depth or grayscale inherent in the modality, while analog (video) frame grabbers digitize the video signal voltage output going to an image display, such as a scanner console monitor, and image quality is limited by the process to only 8 bits (or 256 gray values).

Direct capture of digital data from the inherently digital modalities is the preferred method of acquisition.

Digital acquisition of images already on film can be accomplished using a variety of image digitization devices. These include the infrequently used analog video cameras with analog-to-digital converters (ADC), digital cameras, charge-coupled devices (CCD), and laser scanners. Laser scanners use a fine laser beam of generally variable or adjustable spot sizes down to 50 μm. They have maximum resolution of $4096 \times 5120 \times 12$ bits, can accommodate the full optical density range of film, and are semi- or fully-automatic in operation.

Laser scanners are the film digitizer of choice for most PACS needs, with an adjustable spot size to meet the application.

CR and DR are modalities that digitally acquire projection radiographs without the use of film. CR utilizes a photostimulable phosphor (PSP) imaging plate in a cassette design similar to that of screen-film cassettes. The PSP imaging plates have the property that, when exposed to X-ray, a latent image is formed in the plate until it is subsequently stimulated to luminesce by a laser. The emitted light is then captured and converted to a digital image. DR converts X-ray energy to charge collected by a thin-film transistor pixel array, offering electronic readout initiated immediately at the time of exposure.

Both CR and DR have:

▶ all the benefits of digital (filmless) images, including the ability to acquire, transmit, display, manipulate, and store data digitally;

▶ wide latitude response detectors, potentially reducing retakes resulting from poor exposure as in the screen-film based environment;

● equivalent spatial resolution capabilities;

● CR has superior procedural flexibility, can accommodate portable bedside examinations, and is a proven clinical modality; and

● DR has a higher efficiency detector and immediate image readout.

Some current DR problem areas include ease-of-use and portability issues, the requirement for a single device per radiographic room ("one-room-at-a-time technology"), and its high production cost. It is likely that CR and DR will coexist as digital radiographic devices for a long time.

Quality assurance/quality control (QA-QC) procedures become necessarily modified in the filmless radiology department, and new processes must be put in place. Forming and maintaining a continuing quality improvement (CQI) committee may facilitate PACS installation and training, workflow management, quality assurance, and clinical acceptance.

The major problem occurring at acquisition is inaccurate data input at the modality. This source of (human) input error can be greatly reduced by integrating the RIS-HIS with the PACS. This allows RIS-verification of PACS data prior to archival, and an image audit monitoring of what is in the PACS with what is in the RIS, and vice versa.

QC for the imaging modalities is as essential in the digital world as it is in the film-based arena. Proper planning and communication with end-users early and often as to system status can reduce dissatisfaction with the system.

TABLE 6.3
Summary of Future Trends in Image Acquisition

Image matrix size	↑
Image quality	↑ ↑
Spatial resolution	↑
# Image slices	↑ ↑
Size of imaging examinations	↑ ↑
Size of devices	↓ ↓
Portability of devices	↑
Cost of devices	↓
% of Image devices that are digital	↑ ↑
% of Image acquisition that is digital (elimination of film)	↑

Future trends anticipated in image acquisition for digital radiology and PACS are summarized in Table 6.3 and include changes in image data sets such as:

▶ increased matrix sizes,

▶ increased inherent spatial resolution,

▶ increased slice numbers and study sizes, and

▶ improved image quality.

Imaging devices themselves will continue to get smaller in physical footprints, become more portable and robust, and possibly less costly.

An important area receiving increased attention in the future will be the image processing capabilities for softcopy display. Many of these techniques will be driven by the image acquisition modality vendors and by research teams to develop the optimal softcopy display of digital images for diagnosis and review.

In time, the percentage of images acquired digitally will increase, and less film will be printed for medical imaging.

▶ REFERENCES

Agfa. *The Highest Productivity in Computed Radiography.* Agfa-Gevaert N.V. Report. Belgium 1994.

Andriole KP et al. *Analysis of a high-resolution computed radiography imaging plate versus conventional screen-film radiography for neonatal intensive care unit applications.* SPIE Physics of Medical Imaging 2163:80–97, 1994.

Andriole KP et al. *Continuing quality improvement procedures for a clinical PACS.* Journal of Digital Imaging, 11:111–114, 1998.

Andriole KP. *Anatomy of picture archiving and communication systems: Nuts and bolts—image acquisition: Getting digital images for imaging modalities.* Journal of Digital Imaging, 12:216–217, 1999a.

Andriole KP et al. *PACS databases and enrichment of the folder manager concept.* Journal of Digital Imaging, 12(suppl 1):216–217, 1999b.

Andriole KP. *Computed Radiography Overview.* In *Practical Digital Imaging and PACS.* Seibert JA, Filipow LJ, and Andriole KP (Eds.) Medical Physics Publishing, 1999c. Pp. 135–155.

Barnes GT. *Digital X-Ray Image Capture with Image Intensifier and Storage Phosphor Plates:*

Imaging Principles, Performance and Limitations. Proceedings of the AAPM 1993 Summer School: Digital Imaging. Monograph 22:23–48, University of Virginia. Charlottesville, VA 1993.

Berg GE, Kaiser HF. *The X-ray storage properties of the infra-red storage phosphor and application to radiography.* Journal of Applied Physics 18:343–347, 1947.

Bogucki TM, Trauernicht DP, Kocher TE. *Characteristics of a Storage Phosphor System for Medical Imaging.* Kodak Health Sciences Technical and Scientific Monograph, No. 6. Eastman Kodak Co. New York 1995.

Gringold EL, Tucker DM, Barnes GT. *Computed radiography: User-programmable features and capabilities.* Journal of Digital Imaging 7:113–122, 1994.

Honeyman JC et al. *PACS quality control and automatic problem notifier.* SPIE Physics of Medical Imaging 3035:396–404, 1997a.

Honeyman JC, Staab EV. *Operational concerns with PACS implementations.* Applied Radiology, August: 13–16, 1997b.

Ishida M. *Fuji Computed Radiography Technical Review, No. 1.* Fuji Photo Film Co., Ltd., Tokyo 1993.

Kodak. *Digital Radiography Using Storage Phosphors.* Kodak Health Sciences Technical and Scientific Monograph. Eastman Kodak Co., New York 1992.

Kodak. *Optimizing CR Images with Image Processing: Segmentation, Tone Scaling, Edge Enhancement.* Kodak Health Sciences Technical and Scientific Monograph. Eastman Kodak. New York 1994.

Kotera N et al. *Method and Apparatus for Recording and Reproducing a Radiation Image.* U.S. Patent 4,236,078. 1980.

Lee DL, Cheung LK, Jeromin LS. *A new digital detector for projection radiography.* SPIE Physics of Medical Imaging. 2432:237–249.

Luckey G. *Apparatus and Methods for Producing Images Corresponding to Patterns of High Energy Radiation.* U.S. Patent 3,859,527. June 7, 1975. Revised No. 31847. March 12, 1985.

Matsuda T et al. *Fuji Computed Radiography Technical Review, No. 2.* Fuji Photo Film Co., Ltd., Tokyo 1993.

Oestman JW et al. *Hardware and software artifacts in storage phosphor radiography.* Radio-Graphics. 11:795–805, 1991.

Ogawa E et al. *Quantitative analysis of imaging performance for computed radiography systems.* SPIE Physics of Medical Imaging. 2432:421–431, 1995.

Seibert JA. *Photostimulable phosphor system acceptance testing.* In Specification, Acceptance Testing and Quality Control of Diagnostic X-ray Imaging Equipment. Medical Physics Monograph No. 20. Seibert JA, Barnes GT, Gould RG (Eds.) AAPM. Woodbury, NY 1994. Pp. 771–800.

Solomon SL et al. *Artifacts in computed radiography.* AJR 157:181–185, 1991.

Sonoda M et al. *Computed radiography utilizing scanning laser stimulated luminescence.* Radiology 148:833–838, 1983.

Storto, ML et al. *Portable Chest Imaging: Clinical Evaluation of a New Processing Algorithm in Digital Radiography.* 81st Scientific Assembly and Annual Meeting of the Radiological Society of North America. Chicago, November 26–December 1, 1995.

Volpe JP et al. Artifacts in chest radiography with a third-generation computed radiography system. AJR 166:653–657, 1996.

Vuylsteke P, Dewaele P, Schoeters E. *Optimizing Radiography Imaging Performance.* Proceedings of the 1997 AAPM Summer School. pp 107–151, 1997.

Willis, CE et al. *Objective measures of quality assurance in a computed radiography-based radiology department.* SPIE Physics of Medical Imaging, 2432:588–599; 1995.

Wilson AJ, West OC. *Single-exposure conventional and computed radiography: The hybrid cassette revisited.* Investigative Radiology 28:409–412, 1993.

CHAPTER 7

IMAGE WORKFLOW

ELIOT L. SIEGEL • BRUCE REINER

"Mr. Abrahams, Mr. Abrahams! I can find you another two yards."
Sam Mussabini (Olympic trainer), *Chariots of Fire*

Diagnostic radiology departments have a dual mission. One is to provide the highest quality of care possible for their patients. The second is to maximize income (or at least, minimize loss). To a large extent, this is not too dissimilar from the role and goals of an industrial assembly line environment in which the goals are to maintain a high level of quality and consistency while maximizing efficiency and productivity. During the past few years, the increased penetration of managed care, increased competition among diagnostic imaging providers, and other factors have resulted in decreased reimbursement rates. This has resulted in the need to decrease personnel and other operating expenses while maintaining or in most cases, increasing the volume of studies. Imaging departments have been asked to absorb these reductions in resources without any compromise in the quality of services.

Although this has been achieved to some extent by asking radiologists and other personnel to work "harder and faster and longer" and by cutting "excess fat," these exhortations will only work to a limited extent, if at all. The optimal way to realize further reductions in costs and to maximize efficiency without compromising patient care is to study, modify, and if necessary completely redesign the workflow process in the imaging department.

In many ways, this workflow analysis and reengineering is analogous to the process in which an Olympic sprinter or swimmer can be evaluated. His or her movements can be broken down into small components and analyzed in detail to determine how to make the athlete's performance even better. In some cases this might involve relatively small changes such as having a swimmer shave his arms and legs before the race to minimize friction. In other cases this analysis might reveal major ways to improve performance that might involve a completely new swimming stroke or starting or finishing strategy and so on.

Unlike most modern day "industrial assembly lines," radiology departments are notoriously inefficient. An inordinate number of steps are typically required in the workflow process from the time a patient is registered until an imaging report is made available to the referring clinicians. These functions are performed by a variety of clerical, technical, and professional personnel in a process that often evolves over a period of years into a confusing, illogical, and disorganized process.

Although there is a relatively large amount that has been written about the process of workflow optimization (process analysis) in the industrial engineering literature, there has been relatively little that has been published in the radiology literature. This is particularly true with regard to the transition of radiology from a film to a filmless environment. Relatively few attempts at the equivalent of process analysis have been made in radiology prior to the introduction of PACS.

Several investigators have attempted to estimate the average time required to perform various radiological examinations. However these procedure times have been found to vary widely by as much as 300% due to a number of difficult-to-control variables, such as uneven, unpredictable patient flow, personal and fatigue time, and additional time requirements for administrative, supervisory, and educational activities.

A radiology department can perform formal or informal time-motion studies and can create a work flow diagram. For example, prior to the introduction of PACS at the Baltimore VA Medical Center, a workflow analysis was performed by Booz-Allen & Hamilton, which enumerated 57 steps in the process from when a clinician initiated an order for a radiology study until the transcribed radiology report was available in the patient's chart for review.

There are a number of consultants who currently provide this service. It is often amazing to radiologists and administrators in the department to see how inefficient most practices have become over time. However, even with a careful redesign of the workflow process, there are a number of limitations of a manual system of keeping track of patients and a number of major constraints that are associated with the use of film. If used properly, a Radiology Information System (RIS) and a Picture Archival and Communication System (PACS) can provide major improvements in image workflow.

The RIS typically refers to a computer system that supports patient registration (or transfer of registration information from another system), exam ordering and tracking, and film management, and in most cases scheduling, reporting, billing, and statistics as well.

In common usage, the term PACS refers to a computer system that is used to capture, store, distribute, and then display medical images. However, a medical PACS can be redefined as the use of computer technology to re-engineer and improve the efficiency and quality of services in the delivery of healthcare services, particularly when integrated with a radiology information system. The term "workflow" refers to the movement of patients, images, and information throughout the imaging department and healthcare enterprise. In order to optimize patient care and efficiency, it is critical to understand the potential for PACS to improve workflow.

A PACS should not be used merely as a computerized substitute for current processes that are performed in a conventional film-based department; it provides the opportunity to creatively re-invent the workflow process. This requires an understanding of how the radiology department operates and a thorough understanding of the capabilities of the PACS, the operations of the radiology and hospital information systems, and a complete understanding of the current workflow process and of the jobs of the staff members in the department.

Workflow in an imaging department consists of a number of different processes and can be characterized in multiple ways. These processes include subprocesses, each of which consist of a number of steps including patient registration, exam ordering, image acquisition or procedure performance, transportation and storage of images, interpretation and reporting of examinations, and review of results.

Workflow analysis can be used to study the movement of the patient and images throughout the healthcare enterprise. An alternative approach would be to focus on the staff members themselves, including the radiology clerk, technologist, administrator, or radiologist.

PACS AND WORKFLOW: EFFECT ON PERSONNEL

CLERICAL PERSONNEL

The time-motion study that was developed for the Baltimore VA Medical Center's imaging department prior to the introduction of PACS demonstrated that a large percentage of the steps in the workflow process were clerical in nature. These included a number of steps in the completion and submission and handling of an order or "requisition" for the examination as well as the process of handling that request in the radiology department, in addition to the steps involved in the interface of the clerical staff with the technologists. The clerical functions also included the many steps required in the handling of film by the film library staff and people who were involved in the movement of film throughout the medical center. One particularly labor intensive task was the daily requirement to retrieve over 500 film jackets for patients that were to be seen in the various outpatient departments and then attempt to retrieve these studies later so that they could be returned and then organized in the film library. The film library staff were also responsible for finding old patient film jackets and matching these to new studies with the old and new examinations then being transported to the reading rooms for interpretation by the radiologists. Once the radiologists interpreted the study, then the clerical staff was again involved in transporting the films back to the film room or various other areas of the medical center. They were also responsible for delivery of the audiotapes that were used by the radiologists for dictation to the report transcription area.

CLERICAL REDESIGN

The transition to the use of a hospital information system and radiology information system (HIS-RIS) and a PACS at the Baltimore VA Medical Center had a profound impact on workflow in the clerical areas of the department. The use of the computer systems resulted in a dramatic reduction in the number of steps required and the amount of time required to perform these.

The use of an integrated HIS-RIS reduced the process of submission of a radiology request to a much faster and simplified process in which the healthcare provider identifies the patient to be studied and the exam to be performed, and enters the reason for the examination on a computer workstation using a graphical user interface. Additionally, other "demographic" patient information, such as patient age, sex, patient location, the requesting clinician, and patient's primary care provider, are automatically sent by the HIS to the radiology department and to the PACS. This information is also available to the technologists in the radiology department, who interact with the system to schedule the patient examination and edit the request when it is appropriate.

The ordering information is sent to the PACS, which then creates an electronic image "folder" entry in its database and initiates a request to the long-term image storage device to retrieve previous examinations for comparison. This "prefetch" of old studies from the archive is thus initiated prior to the new study being performed, well in advance of interpretation by the radiologist or review by the clinicians. Additionally, the "prefetch" of comparison studies can be initiated by other events in addition to a request for a new study, such as a patient admission, patient transfer, or a scheduled appointment for an outpatient visit. Thus all patient images can be routed from long-term to short-term storage or can be sent to a particular workstation or group of workstations according to predefined rules. The elimination of film and integration of the PACS with the HIS-RIS have thus obviated the need for a paper request for the ordering clinician or for the clerical staff, radiologists, or transcriptionists. With the exception of mammograms, which are still performed using film, and films that come from other institutions or are sent to facilities that are still using film, the dramatic reduction in the number of films has reduced the need for film file room personnel. At the Baltimore VA Medical Center, all but one of the film room librarians have been eliminated (and subsequently found other jobs within the medical center).

The workflow process has also been redesigned for the transcriptionists using a digital dictation system in combination with the hospital information system. Radiologists' dictations are recorded digitally and made available immediately to the transcriptionists as well as to clinicians. The transcriptionists now work at home and connect to the digital dictation system and hospital information system using separate phone lines. Reports are typed at home directly into the HIS-RIS radiology reporting module and are then made available to clinicians to review the preliminary report immediately and for radiologists to verify and finalize their reports. This process has resulted in substantial reductions in report turnaround times from approximately 24 to 48 hours to approximately 2 hours.

The substitution of a digital storage system for film has resulted in eradication of one of the most vexing problems in an imaging department. This is the phenomenon of "lost" or "missing" films. Our rate of "missing" (or more specifically rate of undictated studies) dropped from an unacceptable 8% to less than 1% within a year after the implementation of the PACS

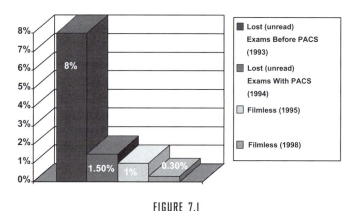

FIGURE 7.1

Lost films diagram.

and has subsequently dropped to approximately 0.3% (Figure 7.1). This 0.3% rate represents a drop of more than 25-fold but indicates the continued presence of unreported cases that "slip through the cracks." At our institution, we run a management report using the radiology information system that identifies these unreported studies. There are a number of explanations for these 0.3% of cases that are unreported, including the occasional inadvertent misidentification of an unread case as dictated by our radiologists, network transmission failures, and other miscellaneous causes.

The elimination of the majority of steps previously required for clerical operations has not only resulted in much faster patient and report throughput in the department, which has resulted in improved patient care, but has also resulted in the reduction in our clerical staff by 56%. This has resulted in substantial savings, which alone are greater than those achieved by the elimination of film in the department. Time-motion analysis with activity sampling and interviews to estimate savings in film handling times associated with PACS show the estimated time savings for film library (clerical) staff to be 55%; for technologists, 10%; and for radiologists, 10%.

TECHNOLOGISTS

TECHNOLOGIST WORKFLOW BEFORE PACS

Prior to the transition to the use of PACS and the HIS-RIS at the Baltimore VA Medical Center, the technologists had a number of responsibilities that overlapped with those of the clerical and film library staff. This resulted in the requirement that the technologists perform a large number of manual processes that added to the number of workflow steps in this section of the department. These included responsibility in some areas, such as in the Computed Tomography (CT) department, for making sure that old studies were pulled for comparison with new examinations and that films were brought to the radiologists for preliminary checking and subsequent interpretation. Patient information was re-entered into the computers on the various imaging modalities, such as CT, using the information from the physician order forms. This resulted in a relatively (~15%) high rate of error in the entry of patient identification numbers or the spelling of patient names.

TECHNOLOGIST WORKFLOW AFTER PACS

The elimination of film and the transition to the PACS and HIS-RIS resulted in enormous improvements in the workflow of the technologists. This resulted in a 40% increase in technologist productivity for general radiography (Figure 7.2). These comprise 65% of the total number of studies performed in the imaging department

We performed a prospective study in which we reverted to conventional, film-based operation for a period of one week to perform detailed time-motion studies of the CT technologists and compared the data with similar time-motion studies performed subsequently of the technologists using the PACS in a filmless environment. The study documented that filmless operation resulted in the elimination of a large number of steps that were necessary in a conventional CT department (Figure 7.3).

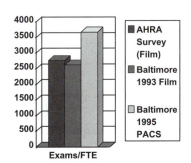

➥ **AHRA Survey (Film)**
 ➥ **2,760 exams/FTE**
➥ **Baltimore 1993 (Film)**
 ➥ **2,622 exams/FTE**
➥ **Baltimore 1995 (PACS)**
 ➥ **3,670 exams/FTE**

FIGURE 7.2

Technologist productivity increased by 40% after the transition to the use of computed radiography and PACS.

These eliminated steps include those related to the creation of multiple versions of the images in different window or level settings, which can be performed by the radiologist at the computer workstation, as well as those related to the handling and distribution of films. This resulted in a 60% reduction in the amount of time required for a CT technologist to perform an examination (Figure 7.4 and Figure 7.5).

Additionally, there has been a dramatic reduction in the examination retake rates for the general radiographic studies performed in the department. This reduction has been due to a combination of the very wide dynamic range of computed radiography, which has replaced film, and to the ability to modify the window and level (contrast and brightness) settings at the computer workstation. This drop from a 5% to a 0.8% repeat rate has resulted in the elimination of 84% of the retakes, which has also improved the technologists' workflow.

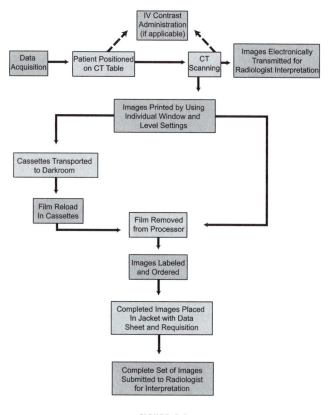

FIGURE 7.3

CT technologist workflow diagram comparing film and filmless operation.

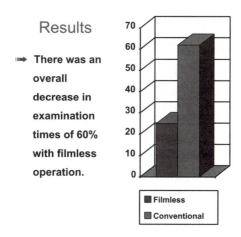

Results

⇒ **There was an overall decrease in examination times of 60% with filmless operation.**

FIGURE 7.4

Comparison of time required to scan and transfer images and total time for film-based and filmless operation.

One of the benefits of integration of an imaging modality, such as a CT scanner, an HIS-RIS, and a PACS is the ability to reduce workflow steps and improve accuracy using the feature known as "Modality Work-list." This refers to a program with which a modality can communicate with a PACS or HIS-RIS to obtain the list of examinations to be performed. This

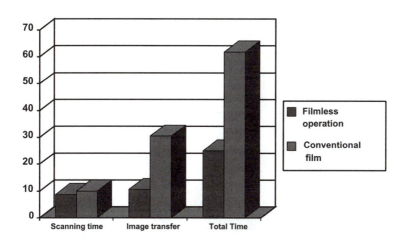

FIGURE 7.5

Reduction in CT technologist scanner time with filmless operation.

"worklist" can be displayed on the technologist operator console and allows the technologist to select a particular examination or combination of studies. This both speeds entry of patient information and increases the accuracy of the data. This has reduced the modality transmission error rates to below 1.5%, in comparison to the approximately 15% rate of patient entry errors by technologists that has been described in the literature (Figure 7.6).

This sort of integration requires a level of communication and integration between the HIS-RIS and the imaging modality that is currently not available in most institutions. The two most common standards used in this communication are DICOM (Digital Imaging and Communications in Medicine) and HL7 (Health Level 7). Unfortunately, the vast majority of HIS-RISs do not support DICOM and the implementation of HL7 varies widely, making it very difficult for any particular imaging modality to provide a Modality Worklist solution that would support all of the HIS-RIS systems. Fortunately, the RSNA and the Health Information Management Systems Society (HIMSS) have become partners in sponsoring a "phased series of public demonstrations of increasing connectivity and systems integration" that has brought together imaging vendors with HIS-RIS vendors. This effort, known as the IHE (Integrating the Health Care Enterprise) Initiative, has resulted in the creation of a consensus on the use of both DICOM and HL7 to communicate information between an imaging modality, hospital or radiology information system, and a PACS. This initiative may also facilitate the ability to communicate information between two PACS systems or two HIS-RIS systems, which would have a major positive impact on the ability to share patient medical records and images from one facility to another.

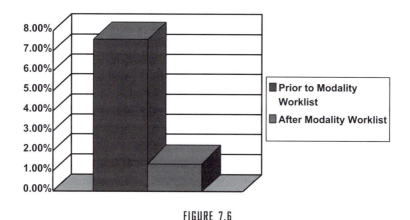

FIGURE 7.6

Reduction in CT transmission rates with use of modality worklist.

RADIOLOGIST WORKFLOW

For a number of reasons, including the fact that they are the most expensive members of the imaging department's staff, radiologists' workflow has been studied extensively to determine which factors influence productivity and accuracy. Studies performed at the Baltimore VA Medical Center have documented an increase in radiologist productivity by more than 50%. The marked improvement occurred despite the fact that radiologist reading times only decreased by approximately 8 to 15%. This increase is believed to be due to a combination of complex factors, including more effective sharing of the workload by the radiologists, fewer interruptions, immediate availability of old examinations and reports for comparison, and the elimination of the film library and the inefficiencies and time delays associated with it.

WORKLOAD SHARING

Filmless operation utilizing an enterprise wide-PACS has resulted in the ability of radiologists to read from a shared, enterprise-wide worklist (list of unread examinations). This worklist acts as a database filter that allows a radiologist to view images defined by anatomic regions (e.g., chest, neuroradiology, or musculoskeletal), or modality (e.g., ultrasound, nuclear medicine, angiography, and special procedures), or any combination of these. Unlike the situation in a conventional, film-based department in which a group of films is brought to a single radiologist or location, unread examinations can be interpreted anywhere in the enterprise served by the PACS. Thus a stack of films brought to a radiologist does not remain unavailable for interpretation when the radiologist is performing a procedure, or talking on the telephone for example. Radiologists are also more easily able to decrease their unproductive time when walking from one location to another in order to retrieve films, or when waiting for films to be brought to their reading area.

FEWER INTERRUPTIONS

The transition to filmless operation at the Baltimore VA Medical Center was associated with an 82% reduction in the "in-person" consultation rate for general radiography and a 44% reduction for the cross-sectional imaging section, despite an increase in the volume of studies. This decrease in the general radiography consultation rate from 13% (pre-PACS) to 2.4% (1996) was even greater than we had anticipated (Figure 7.7).

This decreased rate of consultation has resulted in a higher percentage of the radiologists' time available for image interpretation rather than clinical consultation and has similarly resulted in time savings for the clinicians as well. The change in the mode of communication between radiologists and clinicians has had a major impact on this aspect of radiologist workflow. The expectation by clinicians for decreased report turnaround times that occurred after radiologists began reading studies within a few minutes after they were completed resulted in the purchase of a digital dictation system for the radiologists. With this system, clinicians are able to access radiology reports via the telephone. Additionally, radiologists are much more likely to use the telephone to discuss urgent findings such as a pneumothorax in the intensive care unit than before the transition to filmless operation. This is because the decreased time from when the study is done until it is reviewed makes it much more likely that the radiologist is the first one to review the images. This has resulted in the ability to perform "real time" radiology in which radiologists can review studies at the time that they are most clinically important. This is much better than the previous situation with a film-based department, in which the studies were reviewed at a later time or even at a later date after clinicians have already reviewed them and formed their own impressions based upon the images. This use of the telephone, voice mail, E-mail, and the digital dictation system has changed the workflow paradigm to an electronic one, in which there is more rapid and often better documented communication of findings to clinicians. The

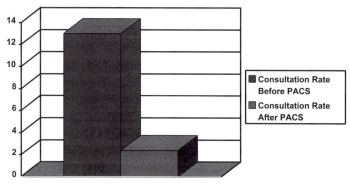

FIGURE 7.7

There was an 82% reduction in clinician consultations for general radiology cases.

negative effect of this decrease in the number of "in-person" communications between radiologists and clinicians is the potential for radiologists to be perceived as having a less important role in patient care. One of the ways that this concern has been addressed has been by the addition of more conferences and teaching sessions with the clinical staff.

NO WAIT FOR FILM ROOM PERSONNEL

One of the major limiting steps in the radiologist's workflow prior to the introduction of the PACS was the dependence on the radiology film room personnel. Radiologists would have to wait for films to be brought to the film library, matched with previous studies and reports for comparison, and then brought out to the radiologists for interpretation. In some instances, such as portable ICU radiographs, the radiologists were required to wait for the films to be "hung" on a film alternator and then retrieved when they were no longer needed. This dependence on the film room meant that prior to PACS, radiologists were unable to begin reading early in the morning before the first film librarian started his or her shift. Additionally, they were not able to come in during "off hours" in the evening, at night, or on the weekends except when a film librarian was also scheduled to work.

AVAILABILITY OF OLD EXAMS AND REPORTS

As radiologists are taught during residency, old films and old reports are a radiologist's "best friend" when interpreting a new examination. In a film-based department, these old reports and studies are often not available and if they are, they are typically not well organized in a patient's film jacket. The ability of a PACS workstation to provide immediate access to old reports and old imaging studies has resulted in much more efficient workflow and has also been a major factor in the improved productivity of radiologists.

RADIOLOGIST READING TIMES

Although radiologist image interpretation speed has been only one of a number of factors that have resulted in increased productivity, the workflow improvement that has been associated with PACS in this area has been significant. At the Baltimore VA Medical Center, we found that radiologist reading times decreased by 19% in the interpretation of portable chest radiographs from the intensive care unit. Another study performed at our facility demonstrated that radiologists were 8% faster in the interpretation of musculoskeletal radiographs using computer workstations and computed radiography in comparison to interpretation using conventional film. Similarly, radiologists were found to require 15% less time to interpret CT examinations using a computer workstation than with film. This was, for the most part, associated with the decreased amount of time required to display the images, particularly in multiple window and level combinations. The advantage of softcopy interpretation over film for CT studies was even greater for examinations in which there were prior CT examinations for comparison. This increased speed of CT interpretation was not associated with any decrease in the accuracy of interpretation, and in fact accuracy was seen to increase to a statistically significant degree.

"HANGING" PROTOCOLS

One of the more complex components of the process of reading conventional film is the arrangement of images from a current and previous study on a view box or film alternator. In a film-based department, radiologists typically function in one of two ways. The first mode is one in which radiologists are responsible for taking a new study and finding the comparison studies from a film jacket. Often, the film librarian places these outside the film jacket. The radiologist then takes these examinations and arranges them on a series of "view boxes." The radiologist must then find any relevant old reports, interpret the study, and take the films back down and place them back into the film jacket. In the second mode, the study to be read is placed on a film "alternator" with any relevant films and reports. The film librarian must learn how most radiologists like to have the films arranged, or in many cases may place the films in a way specific to the preferences of the particular radiologist who will be interpreting the studies. The rules for how the films are placed on a film alternator are often referred to as "hanging protocols." Having the file room personnel arrange the films results in improved workflow for the radiologists but, of course, requires additional time from the file room staff. The hanging and removal of the studies also creates delays in the radiologists' workflow because the radiologists often must wait for the studies to be hung, taken down, and for new studies to be put up.

A PACS softcopy workstation can automate many of these manual workflow steps, eliminating delays in the display of imaging studies and performing this task much more rapidly and reliably than would be possible in a conventional film-based department. These PACS hanging protocols can range from relatively simple ones, such as "new studies on the right, older ones on the left," to much more complex ones. The system can define, for all users or for specific radiologists or clinicians, specific rules that determine which previous studies, if any, are retrieved for comparison and precisely how current and old studies are displayed. Images can be displayed, for example, in frame mode, which closely emulates film (e.g., nine images on one monitor) or can be displayed in what is known as "stack" mode, in which images are "stacked" on top of each other and displayed sequentially as one would might view a cartoon on a series of stacked cards. The stack mode has been found to result in increased reading times and a number of authors have suggested advantages associated with this mode of image interpretation that might result in increased accuracy as well.

The PACS at the Baltimore VA Medical Center uses a series of algorithms for display on a multimonitor workstation that are known as Default Display Protocols (DDPs). The use of the DDP, which can be toggled off or on, was found to result in an increase in radiologist productivity of between 10% and 20%, depending upon the imaging modality (Figure 7.8).

Additionally, radiologists reported less fatigue subjectively with the use of the DDP in comparison with electronic but manual selection of the prior studies to be retrieved and manual (electronic) or nonintelligent placement of the images on the workstation. Reading times are also decreased somewhat by the reduced amount of time required to review previous reports. Using the PACS, these are organized in chronological or another organized format to make review of these previous reports rapid and easy.

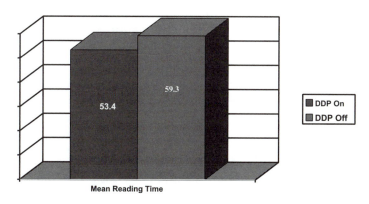

Mean Reading Time

DDP On
DDP Off

FIGURE 7.8

Radiologist reading times for general radiography decreased by 10% with display default protocol.

PAPERLESS RADIOLOGY AND MODALITY WORKLISTS

In order to maximize the efficiency of the workflow of diagnostic radiologists, early PACS adopters have discovered that it is important to achieve paperless as well as filmless operation. Many PAC systems in operation continue to be significantly hampered with regard to efficiency because they have not been able to eliminate paper in the radiologists' workflow process.

In a paper-based department, even in a filmless environment, the radiologists are given a stack of forms that contain information about the patient, the examination, and the reason for the study, in addition to limited additional information such as the name of the ordering physician or service, patient location, and so on. The radiologist must then take these paper forms and enter the patient or study identification manually or must use a bar code reader or other mechanism to identify the patient and study to the workstation. This requires additional steps that can be eliminated with a paperless softcopy reading environment.

In a paperless radiology reading room, the radiologist uses what are referred to as "worklists," which define the type of unread studies that are to be presented for interpretation and their order of presentation. For example, a radiologist can read studies from a worklist limited to a particular modality, such as CT or nuclear medicine studies, or from an anatomic area, such as all chest studies regardless of modality (e.g., CR of the chest, CT of the thorax, MR of the thorax, V/Q scan of the lungs). The worklist thus represents a "filter" into the PACS database of studies yet to be interpreted.

The advantages of a worklist for radiologists include the ability to sign in at any location and have full access to all unread examinations in the radiologists' area or areas of expertise at any time, the ability for multiple radiologists to share responsibility for reading similar types of studies, and the performance improvement that is associated with the elimination of the need to manually key in or bar code patient or study information. A prerequisite for a paperless environment is either an automatic (or much less preferably, a manual) interface between the hospital or radiology information systems and the PACS.

WORKSTATION PERFORMANCE

One of the most important determinants of radiologist and clinician performance is the time required for a PACS workstation to retrieve one or more imaging studies, to display them for interpretation, and to use workstation tools to reveal as much clinically significant information as possible about the images. The studies that we have performed at the Baltimore VA Medical Center have suggested that the first image from an 8 MB computed radiography study should take less than 3 sec to display. Additionally, cross-sectional images, such as a 512×512 pixel CT image, should display at a rate of at least 5/sec or faster. Our data suggest that image display performance significantly slower than that may result in a significant decrease in radiologist reading speed, with increased levels of fatigue.

Manufacturers of PACS have taken two general approaches to the delivery of images to a radiologist's workstation. The first is one in which images are stored on a single, large, short-term storage unit, typically a redundant array of inexpensive disks (RAID). With this approach, workstations communicate directly with this centrally located storage device over a very fast network for image retrieval. The major advantage of this approach is the flexibility to rapidly retrieve any images at any location for both radiologists and clinicians. This approach optimizes the ability of the PACS to support shared reading worklists at multiple locations. The major disadvantage of this approach is that it requires a very fast network and that there tends to be a "single point of failure." Consequently the system becomes vulnerable to a major loss of function in the event of failure of the short-term storage device.

The alternative PACS architecture for delivery of images uses a model that more closely emulates (and has many of the disadvantages of) a film-based environment, in which films are sent to or placed on a film alternator. With a PACS, this is accomplished electronically by "routing" the appropriate images to one or more workstations that are likely to be used to review those images studies. With this architecture, images to be read and comparison studies are stored locally on the hard drives (local storage) of the workstations themselves. Images can be intelligently routed to a workstation or any number of workstations that are likely to retrieve these studies. For example, all CT examinations can be routed to one or more workstations dedicated to interpretation of CT examinations, or they can be routed to the workstations or radiologists who are likely to read those studies on any particular day. Relevant comparison CT or general radiographs or other studies deemed to be likely to be needed for comparison can also be routed to those workstations automatically, using pre-defined rules determined by the radiologists. The major advantage of this system is the independence from failure of any one component of the PACS or even the network itself. With this architecture, images are available locally for interpretation even in the event of a major network malfunction. The disadvantage of this approach, which is based upon local routing of images to workstations, is the difficulty in selecting rules that will anticipate the often unpredictable and spontaneous requirements of radiologists for comparison studies and for review of older imaging studies that may be requested by clinicians for review. The relatively limited amount of space in local storage on a given workstation may result in the need for a radiologist to perform a number of additional steps, often requiring additional time in order to retrieve additional studies. Consequently the selection of optimal algorithms to anticipate which images should be routed to a particular workstation are critical to the success of this type of PACS with regard to optimizing the radiologists' workflow. The other disadvantage of this architecture is the tendency for the workstations to require a greater amount of local storage and the requirement that images be stored in multiple locations, which can be relatively inefficient.

Fortunately, the current trend in PACS is to create a hybrid system that can minimize the disadvantages and optimize the benefits of each approach. For example, PACS that use a central hard drive (or RAID) are beginning to employ mirrored or back-up systems to further decrease the likelihood of a general system failure. Additionally, those systems that use local workstation storage are tending to create more central "nodes" or short-term image servers that are used to store images for a cluster of workstations. This can result in more efficient storage and retrieval and can decrease the need for very specific algorithms for routing images to a particular workstation. It is likely that this trend will continue in the future and will significantly blur the differences between the two approaches to short-term image storage and distribution.

The combination of the use of Modality Worklists, the use of the Display Default Protocols, and a fast image retrieval and display system (less than 2 sec for a computed radiography image and less than 0.25 sec/cross-sectional image) is optimal. Given these workflow and performance features, radiologists should be substantially more productive and exhibit a lesser degree of fatigue than would be achievable with a conventional film-based environment.

IMAGE PREFETCH

One of the workflow rate limiting steps in the process of image retrieval and display is related to the fact that retrieval of images from long-term storage from an optical, magneto-optical, or tape archive is very slow. In fact, retrieval times can be 10 to 100 times slower from long-term compared to short-term storage, depending upon the PACS architecture and equipment.

Although retrieval times using currently available long-term archive technology are becoming much shorter, the discrepancy between long- and short-term retrieval times has mandated the use of strategies to minimize the likelihood of a delay in image retrieval. This requires a set of algorithms that attempt to maximize the likelihood that the required images are available in short-term storage. This process is an excellent example of the advantage of a PACS that is integrated with the hospital and radiology information systems and of an "intelligent" system.

One of the most straightforward examples of image prefetch is with workstations that store new and historic examinations locally at the workstation. With this PACS architecture, images and predefined prior studies (e.g., last two studies that match both modality and anatomic location) are routed to a particular workstation or workstations. This prefetch strategy can also be used in a system in which the workstations share a single RAID server. In this type of system, the predefined prior studies are retrieved from long-term storage automatically when a new imaging study is performed.

Other prefetch strategies can substantially increase the likelihood that images that are likely to be needed by the radiologist or clinician are available on a local workstation or server. For example, image prefetches can be triggered by a scheduled or new admission to the hospital, by a scheduled outpatient appointment, and by transfer of a patient from one location to another (e.g., to the intensive care unit). Our analysis of the radiology information system database at the Baltimore VA Medical Center indicates that a relatively small number of studies can be pulled to achieve a high likelihood that the required studies will be available in short-term storage. For example, we found that if a PACS retrieved the most recent 30% of a patient's previous examinations into a short-term storage area prior to an outpatient appointment, there was a 91% probability that the required images would be available on the server rather than waiting for the long-term archive. This prefetch can be used as the digital equivalent of the practice of pulling film jackets in advance for outpatient visits and can be very effective in optimizing radiologist and clinician workflow in the review of imaging studies.

WORKSTATION TOOLS

The retrieval of the images to the workstation is only the first of several workflow steps in the interpretation of an imaging study. In order to extract as much clinically useful information as possible from the images, a number of steps are required for image manipulation and image enhancement.

1. Images must be optimized with regard to window and level (brightness and contrast) settings.

2. They can be displayed in frame mode in formats such as 1, 4, 9, 12, 15, or more images per monitor.

3. They can be displayed in stack mode, sequentially in a single window in a movie or cine-like format.

4. The images can be zoomed or magnified.

5. Images can be arranged in a logical format to make it as easy as possible to compare various sequences (e.g., enhanced vs. unenhanced, or T1 vs. T2 vs. contrast-enhanced MR images) or a current study with comparable images from a previous study.

6. Images can also be enhanced with tools such as edge enhancement, smoothing, or interpolation algorithms that "smooth" the image to give it a less boxy or "pixely" appearance, or those that enhance the ability to display a wide range of contrast on an 8-bit monitor or film, such as Fuji's Dynamic Range Control (Fuji Medical Systems, Stamford, CT) or Agfa's MUSICA processing (Agfa-Gevaert, Mortsel, Belgium).

Current PACS workstations vary tremendously in the success of their graphical user interface and the number of steps required to use these and other tools. Most workstations in current use do a relatively poor job of optimizing radiologist workflow. The best of these workstations have a relatively simple (elegant) graphical user interface and require a minimum number of keystrokes and steps to retrieve, optimize, compare, remove, and then proceed to the next imaging study. The most challenging requirement in the optimization of radiologist workflow seems to be in the area of comparison of one or more historical examinations with a new exam. This requires an intelligent display or hanging protocol for these studies as well as tools that make it as easy as possible for the system to facilitate comparison of new and old images. As the PACS industry continues to develop and mature, vendors are spending an increasing amount of time obtaining feedback and performing studies of radiologist work flow in the interpretation of imaging studies, which has and will continue to result in improvements in the radiologist-machine interface. We have found that the use of workstation tools by radiologists changes with increasing experience with the system. Initially, radiologists have a tendency to use tools such as image zoom and magnify less frequently as they gain additional experience with the workstation. However, we have found that even experienced radiologists utilize the window and level adjustments in the majority of cases. We are currently performing studies to determine the impact of dynamic range control, which is an algorithm that attempts to translate 10-bit computed radiography data into an 8-bit grayscale for display on the frequency the window/level tool is adjusted by radiologists.

One of the more hotly debated issues with regard to optimization of radiologist reading performance and workflow has been the question of the optimal number of monitors that are required when using a PACS workstation for various modalities, such as CR, CT, MR, and sonography. This is particularly important given the substantial expense of these monitors and the high percentage of the total workstation cost associated with the number of monitors. At the Baltimore VA Medical Center, we performed a prospective study of the impact on radiologist performance and levels of fatigue as a function of the number of monitors. We found that radiologist reading speed increased approximately 25% with a four-monitor workstation compared to a one-monitor workstation in the interpretation of portable chest CR images when we took into account the number of prior studies reviewed. Interestingly, the number of historical studies reviewed tended to decrease as the number of monitors decreased. There was very little difference (differences were not statistically significant) in the amount of time required to read the studies when comparing two- and four-monitor workstations and the largest increase in performance was seen between one- and two-monitor workstations. Although we have not yet performed this study, our expectation would be that the use of stack mode for CT and MR studies would substantially decrease the added value of four- or even two-monitor workstations for the interpretation of these studies. Anecdotally, this seems to be particularly true when the workstation permits images from multiple examinations to be "linked" according to anatomic section, which facilitates easy comparison of current and previous cross-sectional images.

The degree of radiologist fatigue was also subjectively rated for one-, two- and four-monitor configurations. We found that using a one-monitor configuration, for example, 39% of the studies were rated as "low fatigue" and 24% as "high fatigue," while with a four-monitor workstation, 57% were rated as "low fatigue" and only 1% as "high fatigue" examinations.

Given the extensive attention that has been paid to PACS monitors and workstations, surprisingly little attention has been paid to the radiologist (and clinician) reading room environment. Our research at the Baltimore VA Medical Center has indicated that a number of factors, including monitor and ambient room lighting levels and a number of other factors, play a critical role in radiologist productivity and fatigue. We found that radiologist performance decreases significantly and fatigue increases as monitor brightness drops or as ambient room lighting increases.

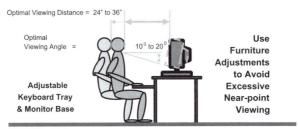

Position Monitor & Body Within Optimum Parameters

FIGURE 7.9

Workstation ergonomics. (Source: Bill Rostenberg, AIA Principal, SMP/SHG Inc.)

Research laboratories such as those at the Carnegie Mellon Intelligent Workplace in Pittsburgh, Pennsylvania have documented the tremendous importance that factors such as the workstation chair design, the availability of individual lighting and temperature controls, and the room acoustics have on performance and fatigue. Architects, who have responsibility for designing workplace environments have also recognized the vital role of workstation ergonomics (Figure 7.9).

CLINICIANS

Although most of the PACS literature has focused on the imaging department, at our institution (and probably in most academic facilities), the majority of requests to access imaging studies from the PACS are from clinicians. Although dictation and report turnaround times are very fast (20 minutes and 2 hours during the working day at the Baltimore VA Medical Center), clinicians continue to access imaging studies and access them more in a filmless than a film-based environment. Several other studies have also demonstrated that the increased access to images made possible by a PACS has a significant impact on patient care.

DeSimone, Kundel, and Arenson et al. evaluated the impact of PACS on clinical practice in the ICU setting and showed statistically significant reductions in time to perform clinical actions following the diagnostic examination. Using PACS, significant alterations were demonstrated in the processes of obtaining radiological information, viewing exams, and consulting between ICU physicians and radiologists. The results of the study suggest that a PACS has a major effect on both patient management and radiology department workflow in the ICU setting.

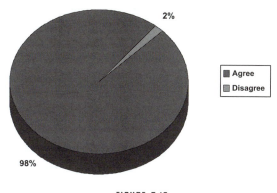

FIGURE 7.10

Survey of clinician perception of time savings with PACS.

Of clinicians surveyed at the Baltimore VA Medical Center, 98% indicated that the use of the PACS contributed to more effective use of their time (Figure 7.10).

This was largely due to the improved access to current and previous imaging studies and the convenience of accessing these images in patient care areas. The typical clinician indicated that he or she accessed the PACS 3 to 5 times/day, with 22% accessing the system more often. The average estimate of the amount of time saved because of the PACS, according to clinician surveys, was approximately 50 minutes, suggesting that the system substantially enhanced their workflow.

This increase in access to images and time savings related with the PACS has been associated with an increase in the clinical utilization of radiology services by more than 30% (Figures 7.11 and 7.12).

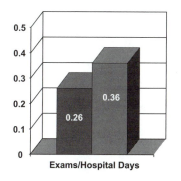

There was a 39% increase in inpatient utilization when evaluating exams/hospital days in 1993 vs. 1996

FIGURE 7.11

Increase in inpatient utilization with PACS.

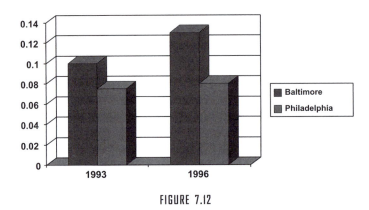

FIGURE 7.12

Increase in outpatient utilization with PACS in comparison to Philadelphia VAMC.

The increase in utilization at our facility after the introduction of PACS has been out of proportion to the increase at a matched VA facility and in the VA system-wide.

Focused studies of PACS use by surgeons, emergency room physicians, and other clinicians have consistently demonstrated a preference for film-less in comparison to film-based delivery of imaging services (Figure 7.13).

This preference has largely been due to the improvements in work-flow associated with the use of PACS in these areas. One example of this improved workflow has been in the communication of abnormal findings by emergency room physicians. One of the challenges in a paperless and filmless environment has been the communication of preliminary impressions of ER physicians to radiologists. This has been addressed at our institution by giving the ER clinicians the ability to view an indicator on their workstation that allows them to determine whether a study has been interpreted by a radiologist. For those studies that have not yet been dictated by a radiologist by the time the ER physician reviews the imaging study, the ER physician can type a preliminary impression directly into the PACS workstation. The radiologist is then able to alert the ER physicians when there is a discrepancy between their preliminary impressions and the radiologist's interpretation of the images. This is an example of the use of the PACS for bidirectional communication not only from radiologists to clinicians but also from clinicians to the imaging department.

The tendency of clinicians to "line up" to use the PACS and to not sign off when they have reviewed their own images has increased their efficiency but has resulted in a potential security and patient confidentiality compromise. Clinicians and radiologists often object to PACS security mea-

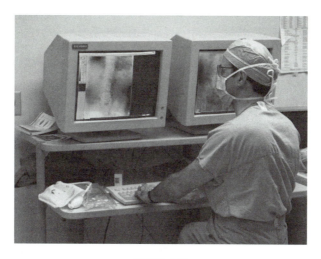

FIGURE 7.13

Surgeon using PACS in the operating room.

sures as interfering with their workflow, and it is often a challenge to overcome this tendency of clinicians to bypass security recommendations. This challenge can be addressed in a number of ways, including the use of biometric recognition devices that utilize fingerprint, voice, or retinal patterns to determine the identity of a person using the workstation. Portable radiofrequency devices could also provide automatic sign-in and sign-out functionality at PACS workstations. Unfortunately, none of these automatic security systems has been satisfactorily implemented in current generation PAC systems.

Although it is intuitive that adequate training of radiologists and clinicians is important in optimizing their efficiency and potentially even their accuracy in the use of the computer workstation, this hypothesis has not been tested extensively. We performed a prospective study in which a subset of new interns received training and the remainder did not receive any formal training in PACS. Subsequent testing was performed one and then four weeks after they had worked at our medical center. Although all members of both groups were able to pass a basic "survival" skills test after four weeks, there were significant differences in their ability to perform more "sophisticated" tasks. Additionally, the amount of time required to retrieve, review, adjust window and level, and close a study was significantly less (78 sec in comparison to 113 sec) for the group of interns that had received formal training in comparison to the untrained group (Figure 7.14).

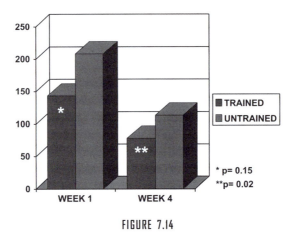

FIGURE 7.14

The trained group of interns was still significantly faster than the untrained group in the use of the PACS workstation, even four weeks after the training session.

MULTI-INSTITUTIONAL PACS

The market forces that have created the strong impetus to increase efficiency and productivity have also resulted in the formation of imaging networks in which large radiology groups provide imaging services for multiple facilities. Although this can result in substantial savings by taking advantage of centralized administration, scheduling, purchasing, and other functions, there are also inherent challenges to a multi-facility practice. These challenges include issues related to distance, different equipment and information systems, communications, and personnel with different "cultures" and a variety of approaches to the operation of the department. Optimizing the workflow with a radiology information system and PACS can be very difficult but can be extraordinarily beneficial in a multi-facility environment. Radiology coverage and subspecialty expertise can be shared across multiple hospitals. This has been particularly helpful in the situation in which one or more radiologists provide night-time coverage for multiple facilities—the so called "Nighthawk" radiologist. The workflow efficiency that is possible by having a single radiologist provide network coverage across multiple facilities has been a major impetus for many radiology groups to install a teleradiology or PACS.

These groups have experienced a number of challenges in the creation of these multi-facility systems. One of the biggest problems has been the fact that it is rare that a group of these facilities all share a single radiology information system. Consequently, the group is faced with the requirement to have a RIS and/or PACS keep track of multiple patient identification systems and multiple methods of communicating information from one system to another. Other difficulties encountered with multi-facility teleradiology or PACS environments include problems with interfacing equipment from multiple vendors, communications difficulties using conventional phone lines or special high-speed communication systems, difficulties with hospital credentialing, privileging, and licensure, and suboptimal communication with clinicians at other facilities.

Despite these challenges, however, the potential workflow advantages of a multi-facility shared or complete virtual radiology department are tremendous, both to the radiology department and to the clinician. The potential to share the radiology caseload in a more effective manner made possible by PACS in a single institution is even greater in a wide area networked virtual department, particularly with regard to subspecialty expertise. The ability to access images obtained at other institutions within the network can eliminate many of the delays associated with film transportation as well as decrease the number of unnecessarily repeated examinations. Technologist functions such as quality control can be performed network-wide rather than having this function performed at each facility.

In the VA Maryland Health Care System, the transition to a wide area network virtual radiology department has resulted in savings of approximately $800,000 to $1,000,000 per year, largely in personnel costs. The network is set up in a "hub-and-spoke" configuration in which images are sent to Baltimore for storage on the VA Baltimore commercial PACS and are then made available throughout the healthcare network. This hub-and-spoke configuration is also used for the hospital and radiology information systems, resulting in the need for a central computer system in Baltimore and reliable, high-speed networks connecting the facilities. This "central" architecture for the PACS has been successful in our environment.

However, other more sophisticated, distributed PACS architectures will be required as the number of facilities or the volume of studies performed increases, to ensure system reliability and to minimize the likelihood of network and image server bottlenecks.

The Department of Defense has taken this concept of a virtual radiology network one step farther in its Virtual Radiology Environment project. This project will use the virtual radiology environment to "optimize the use of radiology resources in the Army" by taking advantage of a high-speed ATM-based network to connect the various Army PACS installations. The Virtual Radiology Environment utilizes a sophisticated "agent-based system" that monitors the activity and resources (including radiologists) at each facility and makes images available in such a way as to maximize the workflow of the networked facilities as well as the level of subspecialty expertise available for image interpretation. This represents an excellent example of the potential for workflow improvement in a multi-facility network that will likely become commonplace in the next 10 years.

Perhaps the biggest challenge of all with regard to integration of multiple healthcare facilities is the need to have a common, agreed upon method for exchange of patient images and other patient information. Currently, a large number of steps are required when images from one facility are required at another. Even (or perhaps particularly) when two facilities operate in a film-less environment, it is very cumbersome to share images between them. There are no agreed upon standards or solutions that currently address an automated solution to this requirement. We're even farther away from a solution that would make processes such as patient identification, Modality Worklists, and management of image interpretation automated in a multivendor, multi-HIS-RIS hospital system or between two or more healthcare systems. Fortunately, the RSNA's Integrating the Healthcare Enterprise (IHE) effort has made some promising strides in bringing the modality imaging vendors to the table with both RIS and HIS vendors to discuss and formulate solutions to these challenges. Over the next few years this effort is likely to make true integration across one or multiple healthcare enterprises much more practical.

"DOWN TIME" AND WORKFLOW

The concept of "down time" is almost always addressed in a PACS request for proposal and in the vendor response. This is, of course, absolutely necessary because of the inevitability of failure of one or more of the major components of a PACS at some point and the relative vulnerability of currently available systems. One definition of down time is a state in which there is a significant workflow disruption that is associated with failure of one or more components of the system. The severity of the down time with regard to both clinical and financial implications is related to this disruption in the departmental workflow. It is absolutely imperative that an imaging department and hospital that uses a PACS have a detailed contingency plan for an alternative workflow process in the event of failure of the PACS. Additionally, PACS vendors should design their systems to minimize the workflow disruption in the event of a failure and should provide detailed recommendations about how the department should handle a failure of certain types of components.

There has been very little written concerning PACS down time in the imaging literature. At the Baltimore VA Medical Center, we have reported a study of our system maintenance requirements over the past five years. During this interval, we experienced a 1% down time that was unscheduled and have also experienced an approximately 1% scheduled down time for system maintenance and upgrades. Fortunately, the overall down time (both scheduled and unscheduled) has decreased over the past few years, although our current expectations continue to be that we will experience a significant system failure at a rate between 0.25% and 0.5% per year. As PACS vendor software and hardware offerings become more mature, and as more and more redundancy is built into the system architectures, our expectation is that down time will continue to decrease. Our recommendation would be that when issuing a request for proposal for a PACS, a reasonable down-time period to require would be 0.5% or less.

WORKFLOW: THE FUTURE

During the past few years, the importance of understanding workflow for RIS and PACS vendors has resulted in substantial improvements in the development of intelligent software and its integration with other information systems. This trend will undoubtedly continue. Universal adoption of communication protocols such as the IHE and standards such as DICOM and HL7 will continue the trend toward the elimination of paper and will result in further reductions in the number of steps in the flow of information to and from the imaging department. Future versions of PACS software will record and analyze workflow patterns by clerical, technical, radiologist, and clinical staff members and will anticipate their requirements in such as way as to continue to decrease the number of steps, time, and frustration associated with routine tasks. For radiologists, this will be augmented by the incorporation of technologies such as voice recognition integrated into the PACS, the ability to have real-time televideoconferencing with clinicians and other radiologists, and the use of improved radiology reporting systems, which will be an outgrowth of current research on structured reporting systems. Computer-assisted diagnosis, which is now just being implemented commercially for detection of pathology on mammograms, will provide both a prescreen and a double-read for radiologists in the interpretation of a much wider array of imaging studies in a number of different modalities. The use of computer workstations will enable radiologists to more readily compare current and previous examinations which, as is the case with multi-slice CT studies, will require review of a greater number of images. Computer workstations will also permit a greater degree of interactivity with the images themselves, which will be important in the interpretation of general radiographic images obtained in new ways such as the "tomosynthesis," which will be able to create tomographic images by obtaining multiple rather than one or two projections for a general radiographic study. Both disease-specific and indication-specific processing will be applied by PACS, which will both maximize the quality of the clinical information displayed on a workstation as well as decrease the amount of time required to review the images.

CONCLUSION

The benefits of digital over conventional radiology have been extensively documented and include the elimination of lost and misplaced imaging studies and easier and more reliable access to those studies by radiology and hospital staff. However, based on our seven-year experience with PACS, by far the greatest benefit of digital radiology has been the improvements in workflow that are made possible by the new paradigm. It has not only been great fun to respond to the challenges with PACS as a toolkit and to use the technology to reinvent and re-engineer our entire radiology and nuclear medicine departments, but it has resulted in major gains both economically and in our ability to deliver timely, high quality care. Now that PACS has gotten past the "early adopters" phase, both vendors and customers have learned that success will be predicated on the ability of the vendor and imaging department to work together to take advantage of the tremendous potential that PACS provides to re-engineer the workflow process. This new understanding will serve to accelerate the development and acceptance of PACS during the next several years.

▶ WEB REFERENCES

http://www.ece.arizona.edu/~cerl/VREProject.htm
http://www.hl7.org
http://www.rsna.org/IHE/ihemiss.html
http://www.rsna.org/REG/practiceres/dicom/index.html

WORKSTATIONS

STEVEN C. HORII

The practice of medicine involves viewing a vast amount of visual information. Whether it be seeing a patient's overall appearance at the start of a physical examination or interpreting a computed tomographic study of the abdomen, physicians and their co-workers rely on their visual sense to gather the data they need to make a diagnosis or establish an appropriate treatment. Increasingly, the images used to support these tasks are in digital form. With rare exception, the digital image data itself (which is, after all, just an array of numbers) is not reviewed because the analog nature of human visual perception requires modulations of light intensity and wavelength. That is, we need variations in brightness and color to see things.

A workstation for medical imaging is a device at which the images necessary for diagnosis, treatment planning, and treatment management are viewed. For many years, this role was fulfilled by transparency film illuminated by a light box or by an opaque piece of paper viewed by light reflected from its surface. Films were made by direct exposure to light or X-radiation, and subsequent development made the image visible through deposits of opaque salts or pigments in the film. For paper prints, a piece of film was used as a negative with light shined through it onto photosensitive paper. With the advent of laser film printers, the basic process remained the same, but exposure occurred by modulating a laser beam rather than exposing the film directly to the image source. Laser paper printers for reflection images use a xerographic process. An electrostatically charged photosensitive drum is discharged by a laser beam scanned over its surface, and the remaining static charge picks up pigment particles (toner), which are then heat-fused onto paper.

As more of medical imaging uses digital processes, conversion to film for viewing involves the extra steps of exposing and processing the film. In addition, film has to be managed or it is rapidly lost, or is not sent where it is needed when needed. Medical imaging workstations are a component of picture archiving and communications systems (PACS) that handle the management of the images as well as their distribution and archival storage. Because workstations act as the human interface to PACS, they have a difficult task to perform: a workstation represents a major change for those who have used film for their image viewing for many years.

This chapter describes workstations for medical imaging, specifically for diagnostic radiology, in detail. It gives information about how these devices work, what their important functions are, and how one can go about specifying workstations in system requests for proposals (RFPs).

A BRIEF HISTORY OF WORKSTATIONS

Workstations, as they relate to devices used to interact with computers, have a history that extends back at least to the 1950s (Bell 1988). Some workstation development also closely paralleled technology advances of the Cold War. Today, these early workstations would be considered a terminal rather than a computer in its own right. The computers of the day, after all, were room-sized devices. However, a workstation used as part of an air defense system known as Cape Cod (developed in the 1950s) was the first example of a hand-held device (a "light gun") that could interact with information displayed on the screen (a CRT) (Ross 1988). The importance of this early work is perhaps not so much the hardware that resulted from it, but the experience gained by engineers who worked on these projects whose careers had a major influence on workstation philosophy and design.

To some extent, workstations were the antithesis of the computer paradigm of the day—a large, centralized mainframe computer system operated in a "batch" mode. Users brought their programs and data (usually in the form of punched cards or magnetic tape) to operators who ran these and returned any output some time later. The workstation paradigm, on the other hand, allowed users to interact with the computer directly. In effect, the power of the computer could be distributed to users rather than concentrated in the "computer center."

In the history of workstations, two facilities in the United States stand out: Xerox Palo Alto Research Center (Xerox PARC) and the Massachusetts Institute of Technology's Digital Computer Laboratory. Many of the developments that make up what we think of as modern personal computers and workstations evolved at these pioneering institutions. From MIT came the Cape Cod system mentioned previously, plus early concepts for software to support distributed users (Ross 1988; Licklider 1988). Xerox PARC first pioneered networked computing with the development of Ethernet (Thacker 1988), and graphical user interfaces, with the Alto workstations (Lampson 1988). While Apple Computer (Apple Computer Corporation, Cupertino, CA) is to be credited with first popularizing the graphical user interface with its "Finder," many of the concepts used by the Apple system were first developed at Xerox PARC. Microsoft followed with the Windows operating system (Microsoft Corporation, Redmond, WA). Key to the operation of the Alto workstation was the user's interaction with icons displayed on the CRT screen—by pointing at them and clicking the pointing tool button, what happened next depended on what the icon represented, either a program to be started or a file to be opened. The concept of "windows" that could be moved, resized, and overlapped was also first developed in various software suites written for the Alto.

Any discussion of graphical user interfaces would be incomplete without a mention of the essential "pointing tool," most commonly a "mouse." This invention comes from another early pioneer, Douglas Engelbart, who actually holds the patent on the computer mouse. In early work at Stanford Research Institute in the 1960s, he developed many of the ideas behind human-computer interaction devices (Engelbart 1988).

This description of early contributors is necessarily superficial. If you want to explore this topic further, you will find the book from which many of the references have been drawn an excellent resource (Goldberg 1988).

MEDICAL IMAGING WORKSTATION HISTORY

Less has been written about medical imaging workstations than about devices used in more general computing applications. For this chapter, we use the definition of a medical imaging workstation as a computer graphics-intensive device intended to support interactive display and manipulation of images by physicians or other health care professionals. Given this definition, the first workstations were the "independent console" devices used in conjunction with computed tomography (CT) machines. Nuclear medicine departments were also early adopters of workstations, as they could support the computing-intensive image processing typically used when they interpreted many of the examinations. Involving an independent workstation for this task meant that the computer associated with the imaging equipment could be used instead for acquiring studies, allowing for improved patient throughput.

The earliest references seem to date to the mid- to late 1970s. In 1976, Larsen described a workstation that could be used for the image processing of CT brain scans (Larsen 1976). An important aspect of Larsen's work is that it described an interactive display. This allowed the user to see immediately the result of the image processing done on that image. Lemke et al. (1979) described what may be the earliest description of a PACS (1979). The system description includes workstations for image processing of head CT images, a filing system for storing the images, and a computer network for communicating the results. It also includes concepts of management of the resulting image files and incorporation of other information, such as text reports and voice annotations.

By the early 1980s, workshops and conferences devoted to PACS were held. The first of these occured in 1982 (Duerinckx 1982), at which a system for networked image processing was described (Maguire Jr. et al. 1982). A prototype of the workstation for the author's system was constructed and tested. The system had similarities to the one described by Lemke earlier. Its limitations were the result of the high cost of graphics display subsystems at the time and the lack of standards for digital medical image formats. The fundamental requirements for a PACS were described by Dwyer et al. (1982). Included in Dwyer's paper was a discussion of retrieval rates over time of radiological examinations, a set of data that has formed the basis for many subsequent PACS archive designs.

In these early PACS papers, significant recurrent themes are: user interfaces, integration with other information systems, and understanding the fundamental tasks performed by radiologists and radiology operations and support personnel. These topics are still widely discussed, and the realization of integrated information systems and workflow-aware PACS are just emerging.

ENABLING DEVELOPMENTS FOR WORKSTATIONS: HARDWARE

If computer technology had not advanced rapidly, workstations of the sort used in medical imaging today would not be possible. As an example, the memory needed to store a single computed radiographic image is about 10 MB. In the mainframe computers of the 1970s, the entire system memory was typically less than 100 KB. That memory, usually magnetic core, filled a cabinet 2 m high $\times$ 1 m wide $\times$ 1 m deep. The memory had to be temperature-controlled, and the air conditioning system for the computer was often nearly as massive as the computer itself. A single integrated circuit memory chip easily holds well over 100 KB; in fact, capacities are over 1 MB/chip. This progress, rapidly increasing memory capacity, follows Moore's law, named for the engineer who proposed it. What Moore's law says is that the memory capacity of integrated circuits doubles every 18 months. The law has held true since the first integrated circuit memory chips were made. A corollary, less well known, is "Bell's Model," named after C. Gordon Bell. It notes that the price per bit for semiconductor memories has declined at a rate of 36%/year (Bell 1988).

Integrated circuit fabrication techniques not only yielded low-cost memory devices, but also made possible the microprocessor. Microprocessors are ubiquitous, found in consumer devices ranging from automobiles to sewing machines. The microprocessor is also the basis for the personal computer. Prior to the microprocessor-based personal computers of today was the minicomputer. Historians (Augarten 1984; Bell 1988) argue that the minicomputer is the forerunner of the personal computer, mostly because it fostered the idea of decentralized computing. Users who needed computing power could usually meet their needs with a department-level minicomputer rather than by using the mainframe computer that the facility typically owned and controlled.

A major factor in expanding of the use of computer workstations in general was the development of network technology. Local area networks allowed the workstations to communicate with each other and with servers that stored large amounts of information or had specialized processing hardware. Workstations could also access shared service devices, such as printers, over networks. The development of Ethernet was a major advance for workstation interaction. More recently, internet technology has further affected workstation design because of the effort to decentralize computing power even further through the use of distributed software.

How vast amounts of information are stored is yet another facet of computer technology that advanced the cause of workstations. Medical imaging is one of the largest generators of digital information, and it requires fast access as well as very large capacities. The growth in the capacity of mass storage devices has also risen exponentially. In the early days of minicomputers, removable cartridge disks typically had capacities of .25 MB to 5 MB. These disks were about 25 to 30 cm in diameter and cost hundreds of dollars each. Contrast that with the newest generation of removable media for personal computers. Capacities range from 1.4 MB for a conventional floppy disk to 4 GB or more for a Digital Versatile Disc (DVD). Fortunately, while capacity of media has risen exponentially, the cost has not. The result is that the cost per bit of storage has fallen dramatically.

Most minicomputers and personal computers today still use cathode ray tube (CRT) displays for the main display device. An important aspect of these CRTs, however, is their increasing display matrix size; that is, the number of pixels that can be shown on a screen. The earliest personal computers typically displayed 24 lines of 80 characters each on a CRT that was essentially a television monitor. The 640 × 480 pixel display of the first PCs grew out of video monitors. As the memory needed to store the pixel array got less expensive, the pixel array sizes increased rapidly. Color monitors made it far easier to differentiate functions and controls on graphical user interfaces. At the time of this writing, most PCs have display sizes of 1024 × 768 pixels up to 1600 × 1200 pixels. Specialized CRTs and display electronics for medical imaging now achieve matrix sizes of 2000 × 3000 pixels. A branch of the display "family tree" developed as a result of the push toward portable computing. Early machines, such as the Osborne and Kaypro systems, continued to use CRTs. However, flat panel displays, at first low-resolution black and white units, were much better suited to a computer no thicker than a notebook. The most recent laptop computer displays use active matrix (each pixel has a transistor driving its gray or color level) liquid crystal flat panels that are up to 15-inch (38cm) diagonal size with 1024 × 1280 pixel matrices. These displays are larger than many of the early PC CRTs.

Flat panel displays are currently more costly than CRTs, and units with the display resolution needed for plain radiographic images are just becoming available. Nonetheless, it is likely that the flat panel, with its higher luminance and thin form (allowing it to be used in small spaces), will make a significant contribution to medical imaging workstations.

The technology enabled by scientific and engineering advances has made a variety of workstation designs possible. A "generic" workstation is shown in a block diagram in Figure 8.1.

ENABLING DEVELOPMENTS FOR WORKSTATIONS: SOFTWARE

Most users of a medical imaging workstation would probably refuse to use it if it required extensive typing of arcane commands. Behind the graphical user interfaces that many radiologists and other physicians now rely on is a

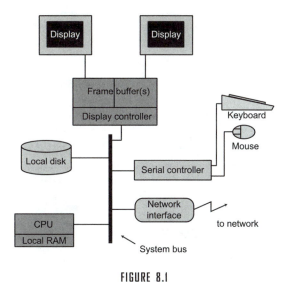

FIGURE 8.1

Generic workstation.

huge number of person-hours of programming time. The whole idea of distributed computing required new types of operating systems that would allow multiple, simultaneous users to share information over networks. These advances speak to the importance of software development as a technology enabler.

THE ROLES OF A MEDICAL IMAGING WORKSTATION

Within a picture archiving and communications system (PACS), the workstation has the unique function of serving as the human interface for the display. As such, it has to support a user interface that is readily learned and easily used, yet flexible enough to meet the varied needs of different healthcare professionals. The film-based environment familiar to radiologists has evolved to the point where the "user interface" is well known and the roles played by support personnel are transparent unless there is a problem (see Figure 8.2). Workstations also must be able to faithfully display the information they are sent, or if they cannot, provide an indication to the user that some change from original data may have occurred. The speed of workstation operations has to be high enough so as not to cause user frustration,

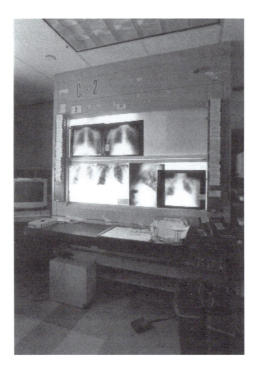

FIGURE 8.2

Film alternator.

but not so high as to drive costs for the hardware to impractical levels. We believe that workstations have to provide a clear advantage over film for users, whether in speed, functions performed, or ability to perform tasks not possible with film. If this is not the case, much of the motivation to switch from hardcopy to softcopy will be absent.

Two fundamental roles are apparent, each with variations to suit particular applications. One is the primary interpretation (diagnostic) role of workstations designed for use by the radiologist or other medical imaging specialist, who interprets the imaging study at the request of the referring physician. The second is the review (or secondary diagnostic) role of workstations that support the features used for viewing images that have already been interpreted. We conducted a study comparing medical intensive care unit (MICU) physicians with radiologists (Horii et al. 1996) using a workstation for portable chest radiographs done on CR plates. Some functions were used more frequently by the radiologists than by their MICU colleagues. In particular, the radiologists used the grayscale adjustment ("window" and "level") more frequently than did the MICU physicians. However, the MICU physicians used the other workstation image manipulation functions (zoom, invert, and full-resolution display) more often than did the radiologists. In the task evaluated, which was reading portable chest radiographs, the radiologists were performing primary interpretation of the images. Such studies tend to be limited to specific image categories or reading conditions and should not be used to generalize a list of workstation functions. They are useful in determining which functions are most readily selected for the different workstation roles.

The secondary diagnostic role is also performed by radiologists. Examples include comparing previously interpreted examinations with current ones or correlating one examination type with another. These uses require that workstations for radiologists support both a primary and secondary diagnostic role. They also imply that workstations should be able to display diverse image types.

Although this chapter emphasizes the radiological role of workstations, other medical specialists who use imaging, such as ophthalmologists, dentists, and pathologists, often have workstation requirements very different from those of diagnostic radiology. The role, however, is similar in that a primary diagnosis is rendered based on the images viewed.

Aside from the primary and secondary diagnostic roles, there are also roles for consultation, teaching, and special imaging. The consultation and teaching role also involves viewing images that have previously been interpreted. For consultation, the goal is to answer specific clinical questions that a referring physician may have about the imaging studies performed on his or her patients. Consultation may be conducted by the radiologist for groups of physicians, so such workstations need to be able to support viewing by groups larger than the ones usually involved in primary diagnosis. The teaching role is for training resident physicians in interpreting imaging examinations. Because it is desirable for such residents to have access to libraries of "teaching files," workstations oriented to the teaching task may have a user interface that makes such access simple and fast.

The application of powerful computer graphics hardware and software to diagnostic imaging has resulted in new capabilities (Robb 1998). Systems to support such applications often act in another role for workstations, that of special imaging. Since these workstations have additional processing electronics for manipulation of volumetric or surface-rendered images, their user interfaces are quite different from those for conventional two-dimensional imaging. Computer-aided diagnosis (CAD) is an application that applies image processing and classification to radiographs for automated detection of candidate abnormalities. Applications include the detection of lung nodules

and breast lesions (Xu et al. 1997; Huo et al. 1998). While the user interface for particular CAD applications is different from that used for primary
interpretation, the inclusion of CAD software in existing workstations has
been a goal. The reason for integrating such software into diagnostic workstations is to avoid making the radiologist move from one workstation to
another to use CAD applications.

WORKSTATION ADVANTAGES AND PROBLEMS

ADVANTAGES OF WORKSTATIONS
OVER CONVENTIONAL FILM

It is reasonable to ask why one should switch from interpreting film on light
boxes (or multiviewers) to images on workstations. Film has the advantage
of being viewable almost anywhere there is a light source—whether a light
box designed for the purpose or a ceiling light that is not. Use of a workstation ties the viewer to the location of the hardware, unless a portable
computer is being used. This debate has endured since workstations for radiology first appeared.

DYNAMIC DISPLAYS

Perhaps the most advantageous aspect of workstations compared to film is
the dynamic nature of workstation displays. This pertains both to dynamic
alteration of grayscale display properties ("window width" and "level" adjustments) and spatial or temporal dynamic displays. Adjustments of window width and level change the display relationship between the information contained in the pixels of the image and the gray level assigned to the
pixels. This is necessary because most imaging done in radiology results in
images with more information in the pixels than can be displayed simultaneously on a display device (or on film, for that matter). For film, this is the
reason why a CT examination of the chest must have the lung-optimized
window width and level images photographed along with the same images
adjusted to best show the mediastinal anatomy. For workstation displays,
which typically also cannot simultaneously display all of the grayscale information of radiographic images, the adjustment of window width and level
simply determines which portions of the pixel data will be displayed and
with how much contrast. The advantage for workstations is that these parameters can be adjusted continuously in real time.

In dynamic spatial displays, the typical mode is to "stack view" cross-sectional images (e.g., CT, MR); that is, to allow rapid movement from image to image. In this mode, a single image is usually displayed, and operating the controls moves to the next or previous image on the stack. Rapid movement has a movie-like effect. With dynamic temporal displays, cross-sectional images obtained at a fixed location but at different times are displayed sequentially. Again, the movement is controlled by the user. Such displays are useful for showing temporally evolving events, such as the enhancement of solid organs when intravenous contrast is used.

A variation on the dynamic display is the cine loop. This is quite commonly used in ultrasound and nuclear medicine for both spatial and temporal displays. A form of cine loop is a stack view of images that are all displayed automatically (i.e., the user does not need to manipulate a device to move through the stack).

IMAGE PROCESSING

Workstations also allow image processing. Simple forms of image processing apply an operation to all individual pixels. Window width and level adjustments are a simple example. In addition to the tables used for translating pixel values (such as Hounsfield Units in CT or counts in nuclear medicine) into gray values displayed, another simple form of image processing is to alter those tables (called lookup tables). For example, the display characteristics of the CRT might be compensated for in the lookup table so that equal steps in pixel value result in equal changes in displayed brightness. More complex forms of image processing involve operations that use multiple pixel values to compute each new pixel value. For example, the values of the eight neighboring pixels around a central pixel might be used to adjust the value of the central pixel. Such operations can increase or decrease "sharpness" or enhance edges. Image processing is possible with film, though cumbersome: the use of a "hot light" to look at dark areas of a film is an example of analog image processing.

INFORMATION ORGANIZATION

Throughout this chapter, the term "comparison examination" is used to refer to a prior study of the same type as that being interpreted or reviewed. The term "correlation examination" refers to a study of a different type from the one being interpreted or reviewed, but covering the same or related anatomy. These concepts are well-established in radiology and workstations need to support them.

A potentially powerful feature of workstations over film and light boxes is the improved organization of the information related to the images as well as the images themselves. With film and light boxes, the multiple films of an examination are sorted into the correct order and oriented by someone, then "hung" on the light boxes or multiviewers. Many workstations now have the capability of doing this arranging automatically, at least for an examination with multiple images and for comparison examinations. File room clerks and residents, however, excel at organizing images when rules for putting up the films become complex or when a correlation examination is desired, for example, hanging a prior abdominal ultrasound when a CT of the abdomen is to be read.

Having reports of previous examinations available is also extremely important. With conventional film, prior reports are typically printed out and supplied with the paperwork accompanying the examination. Some workstations can retrieve relevant reports from a radiology information system (RIS) and display them along with the images. The advantage over the conventional method is that the process is automatic and does not require using paper.

A novel application on workstations is to provide "similar images" with information about them. This is cumbersome to do with film, though it is the basis of the film-based teaching files that most radiologists still maintain. Taira and colleagues (1995) showed a letter prototype workstation application that could find and display images or image features similar to the ones being interpreted. This requires establishing a database of images with cataloged features, but once done, it provides both a teaching tool and diagnostic aid. A radiologist seeing an unusual finding on a film could ask to be shown other cases with similar findings. Along with them would be displayed information about each patient and diagnosis.

Better information organization can also mean that nonradiological information sources are made available to the workstation user. Laboratory values, pathology reports and images, endoscopic images, and even patient schedules are all potentially useful to the radiologist. Having to find these on paper or from other file rooms is time consuming and, more often than desired, unsuccessful.

NOVEL IMAGE DISPLAY TECHNIQUES

Aside from dynamic displays, some image display techniques are either impossible with film-based images or extremely difficult. The creation and display of shaded-surface and volumetric images is one example. A related one is "virtual endoscopy." By creating shaded-surface or volumetric displays of organs such as the colon or bronchial tree, it is possible for a workstation to compute the view would look from inside (Vining 1996). Whereas it is possible to produce still photographic hardcopy from such images, the value of the workstation display is the ability to move through the structures in real-time, much as an endoscopist would see the actual anatomy.

We have done some experiments with a type of display used for photoreconnaissance. It is known as a "window shade" display, but the author calls it the "overlapped image" display (Horii et al. 1994). This technique involves displaying two images on a single monitor, but with one overlying the other. The user moves a line with a computer mouse to reveal more of the image "underneath" as more of the image "on top" is "covered." This avoids the user's having to remember the location of a finding to be compared when viewing two films side by side. Particularly for small abnormalities or structures, it avoids the radiologist's having to keep a finger or pointer on the finding on one film when looking at the other so it can be easily found again. With the overlapped image display, even without registration of the two images, the locations of findings on the images are closer than they would be on separate monitors or light boxes. Figure 8.3 shows an example of this sort of display. Another helpful technique is to superimpose a movable rectangle as a "window" to the image "underneath."

MacMahon and colleagues at the University of Chicago have experimented with a temporal subtraction technique to highlight changes in comparison examinations (Kano et al. 1994). Their method involves registering a prior image with the current one and then subtracting them. The result-

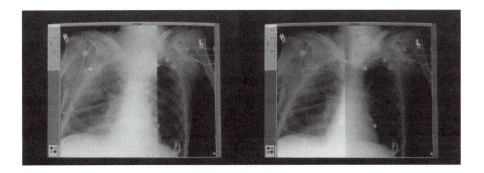

FIGURE 8.3

Overlapped image display.

ing image shows areas that have changed (since areas that have not changed will subtract or drop out). The remaining image can be used to guide the radiologist to examine those areas in the original image more closely. The image registration aspects of this technique, in particular, are not possible with film, because the methods involve nonlinear "warping" of the comparison image, if needed.

With workstations increasing in power and decreasing in cost, it is likely that other new image display methods will become part of the radiologist's "tool kit."

DISADVANTAGES AND PROBLEMS WITH WORKSTATIONS

To understand the description of some workstation problems, a distinction should be made between two terms often used interchangeably. The terms "brightness" and "luminance" are often used to describe how much light comes out of a CRT or light box. Strictly speaking, luminance describes how much light is emitted from a display and brightness describes what is perceived by the human visual system. Because human vision is so adaptable, it is better to use luminance when comparing the light output of two displays.

The successful replacement of film and light boxes with workstations and softcopy depends on whether diagnostic accuracy is compromised. A number of comparison studies have addressed this topic.

Kundel (1993) did a meta-analysis of a number of comparison studies of film and digital hardcopy. In this method of analysis, studies done by different groups can be combined if certain assumptions are made and if the studies meet certain statistical criteria. Although this analysis did not compare film against softcopy because of the spatial resolution issues of digital plain radiography, it does provide a useful comparison. The study could not show a statistically significant difference between conventional and digitally produced film except for skeletal abnormalities imaged with a 512×512 pixel matrix (which rated significantly poorer in observer performance than their conventional film equivalents). In the studies used by Kundel in his meta-analysis, the digital hardcopy was produced from digitization of an analog hardcopy original. An interesting finding is that all of the studies favored analog film to a slight degree, and although this was not statistically significant, the fact that the differences in observer performance were not equally distributed around zero does suggest a slight overall disadvantage of digital imaging.

In a study by Slasky et al. (1990), observer performance with conventional film, digitally produced film, and workstation viewing was evaluated by receiver operating characteristic (ROC) analysis. For individual observers, no significant differences between the digitally produced film and workstation viewing could be identified. However, when observer data were combined, the workstation viewing had poorer diagnostic accuracy (judged by the area under the ROC curve, called Az) for pulmonary interstitial disease and pneumothoraces. Performance was not significantly different for pulmonary nodules.

Scott et al. (1995) did a study on film and workstation viewing that compared observer performance of radiologists and emergency room physicians at different levels of training. This study also showed that observer performance on the workstation was inferior to that with film. However, in this study, the workstation display resolution was 1200×1600 pixels—less than the 1536×2048 pixels used by Slasky et al. The major reason for this difference is that the Scott study was directed at an evaluation of a teleradiology workstation, and the conclusion was that the workstation was unacceptable for primary diagnosis of the class of radiographs used for the study (primarily emergency department musculoskeletal, abdominal, and thoracic images). For teleradiology applications in which primary interpretation of the images is done from a workstation, the American College of Radiology (1994) has recommended in its standard that pixel array size and display monitor size should be such that the displayed resolution of the image is not of lower spatial resolution than the original image. The author notes that with very fast zoom and roam techniques (which allow viewing of a section of the image at full resolution), this recommendation may be met with lower spatial resolution displays.

Not all workstation comparisons show a disadvantage to film. A study by el-Saden et al. (1997), examined observer performance in detecting intra- and extra-axial brain lesions on CT scans. They found no statistically significant differences overall, and slightly better observer performance with workstations for assessment of low attenuation lesions. The monitors used in this research study displayed 1024×1250 pixels.

Reasons for the poorer diagnostic performance of workstations compared to conventional film are not all known. A reduction in spatial resolution is one possibility, although in studies in which the monitors matched film resolution [e.g., some of those cited in Kundel (1993)], observer performance was still inferior with workstations. One likely factor is the difference in luminance. High luminance grayscale CRT monitors may have an output of 100 to 200 foot-Lamberts (ft-L) (343–685 candelas m^2), still less than the 400 to 600 ft-L (1370–2056 candelas m^2) of conventional fluorescent-tube illuminated light boxes (Sezan, Yip, and Daly 1987). Human visual perception is known to have a contrast-detail response in which the contrast required to see some level of detail decreases as luminance increases (Taylor 1973), until very high luminance levels are reached. Less luminous flux for an image also means that the signal-to-noise ratio is inferior to that for the same image displayed with higher luminous flux. Rossman (1969) has noted that the signal-to-noise ratio of an image is likely to be a major determinant of both perceived image quality and observer performance. The lower luminance of workstation monitors also makes the effects of glare more dominant. Extraneous illumination is well known to degrade observer performance in detecting abnormalities on radiographic images (Baxter, Ravindra, and Norman 1982; Alter et al. 1982; Ravindra, Norman, and Baxter 1983; Rogers and Johnston 1984), making consideration of the environment of workstations more important than for film-based reading.

DISPLAY RESOLUTION LIMITS

There are currently few electronic display devices in production that can display the full image matrix (about 4000×5000 pixels) of a mammogram (Asher and Martin 1968). Conventional CRTs are currently limited to about 2000×3000 pixels by the physics and electronics of CRT displays. What this means is that for some examination types, the full resolution image cannot be viewed all at once. Most proposals for solutions to this problem are to use "roaming" or "panning" around the image matrix so that the maximum display spatial resolution available is used.

The luminance of CRTs compared to film on light boxes was noted in the prior section. Newer CRTs have luminance levels that overlap the lower end of light box outputs. Active matrix liquid crystal displays (AMLCDs) are beginning to approach CRTs in both display spatial resolution and with potentially even higher luminance. Lower resolution AMLCDs, up to 1024×1280 color pixels, are currently in use with personal computers as alternatives to CRTs. At high luminance levels, existing AMLCD flat-panel displays do not yet achieve a contrast ratio (full luminance to black) as high as that of CRTs. This is primarily because the "black" is not optically dense enough. As AMLCD flat panels mature, however, the contrast ratio is likely to improve. High contrast is also desirable for nonmedical applications that are chiefly responsible for increasing flat-panel display popularity.

In addition to spatial resolution, display devices must also be able to show variations in gray level. This is known as contrast resolution. Few electronic display devices intended for direct viewing can exceed 8 to 9 bits of contrast range (translating into 256 to 512 discrete gray levels). Because of the density/exposure properties of film (the Hurter-Driffield, or H-D curve), film resolution is also limited to the equivalent of an 8-bit contrast range. Digital images have pixel values that, when translated to gray values for display, range up to 12 bits or 4096 values (e.g., computed tomographic images). For both film and electronic displays, then, an operation to map the pixel values into gray values is needed. The "window" width and level operations do this for CRTs; for film, the same image can be photographed at different levels (e.g., mediastinal and lung settings for CT).

With CRTs and other displays, the image has to be redisplayed at some interval unless the display has a "memory." There is a type of CRT that does store an image, but it is not used in medical imaging. When the image is being redisplayed, or refreshed, it may appear to vary in brightness or "flicker." If this flicker is noticeable, it is at best irritating and at worst, results in headaches. The threshold at which flicker is perceived varies with brightness. The brighter the display, the higher the frequency at which it must be refreshed to prevent the perception of flicker. Perceptible flicker should be an important deciding factor when evaluating workstation displays. The displays should also be run at a high luminance level when trying to determine whether or not flicker is perceptible.

DISPLAY SPEEDS

The rapid display of images, particularly for cross-sectional imaging with its generation of multiple "slices" (e.g., MRI and CT), is of great importance during the reading process. For comparison purposes, a film multiviewer that can change four or eight films in 2 sec is operating at an equivalent of 20 to 40 MB/sec (assuming 10-MB images). This is a very high data rate and requires specialized hardware (parallel transfer disk drives or large image memory display buffers) to achieve on workstations.

Workstations can readily exceed film-based operational speed when a prior study that is not already "preloaded" is requested. With film, this necessitates a trip to the file room. On a workstation, provided it is part of a PACS, this request goes to the electronic archive. Retrieving images from electronic archives is generally faster than finding, pulling, and putting up the same images on film.

New techniques for compressing images (reducing their size while being stored or sent to a display buffer) may help increase display speed without requiring special hardware. An example of such techniques has been described by Chang and colleagues at the University of Pittsburgh (Chang and Hoffman 1993). They showed that, using wavelet-based compression, a very fast display of images is possible on conventional personal computers. Their methods also take maximum advantage of available display resolution, but if this is less than the spatial resolution of the original image, the full-resolution image is available by panning the display window around the full image. An advantage of the method is that it can also be used over the Internet, allowing for wide-area, fast-image distribution. Commercial software that performs some of these functions is also available.

THE USER INTERFACE AND WORKLOAD ISSUES

There is little doubt that the most heavily discussed aspect of workstations for medical imaging is the user interface design, partly because opinions vary about how such an interface should work. The "classic" idea has been to emulate the operation of a film multiviewer. The idea that workstations can perform functions not possible with film is a counterargument to the use of the "classic" paradigm in user interface design. Manufacturers have tended to use the user interface "look" to differentiate one product from another, as the hardware is often the same or similar across multiple manufacturers.

One problem with user interface design is that objective study of the resulting interface is difficult and time consuming. Users find the obvious problems with a design almost immediately; it is the more subtle difficulties that may not have readily evident impact, and only thorough examination will reveal them. At best, they may cause problems such as longer reading time or complaints of fatigue. At worst, they may degrade diagnostic accuracy.

Another problem with interface design is that, to some extent, a user interface works at competing goals. A good user interface should be simple to learn (often, because it follows a simple mental model). On the other hand, it should also allow a user to operate quickly. The features that make a user interface simple to learn (graphical elements, pull down menus, etc.) often slow down the experienced user. This is the reason for the popularity of the "F-keys" in the Windows operating system and shortcuts with the "command" key in the Apple Macintosh operating system. This sort of solution, providing shortcuts for the experienced user, is one method of building an adaptable user interface.

Readers are urged to become familiar with the work on workstation user interfaces done by groups at the University of North Carolina (Beard et al. 1993; Beard et al. 1994) and the University of Arizona (Krupinski and

Lund 1996). These groups have applied well-validated methods of industrial psychology to the evaluation of user interfaces for medical imaging workstations. The results are sometimes counter-intuitive. Beard and colleagues at UNC Chapel Hill, for example (Beard et al. 1987), found that a very fast single-screen workstation could be as effective for reading CT studies as multiple films on light boxes, despite the widely held opinion that multiple monitor workstations are needed for CT reading.

Krupinski and Lund at the University of Arizona conducted an important study of visual gaze fixation during the image reading task (Krupinski and Lund 1996). They found that it took longer to fixate on an abnormality on workstation displays, and that overall viewing time was longer on the workstation. Of considerable importance, they also found that, for film all eye fixations were confined to the image area, while for the workstation display about 20% of the fixations were in the area of the menu that displayed the image processing functions. In other words, the radiologists set their gaze on a nonimage area for about a fifth of all fixations. If they were to spend the same amount of overall time looking at the image, those additional gaze fixations would add to the viewing time per image. A more serious potential problem occurs if the gaze fixations on the control menus decrease the number of fixations on the image, possibly decreasing detection of abnormalities. This should give some pause to workstation designers who have continued to raise the complexity of controls and functions of on-screen menus and buttons in efforts to increase the number of user functions available.

The study of how humans interact with computers is not new. The scientific study of human-computer interaction (HCI) grew out of earlier industrial psychology methods for examining human-machine interactions of other types. Applications of such studies resulted in improved safety and efficiency of industrial machinery. The keys to such studies are in quantitative examination of time and motion and in detailed task analysis. For studies of viewing images, eye-tracking experiments are added to time-motion studies. Such examinations can tell experimenters what it is that radiologists and others do in viewing images. As different user interface elements are added or changed, repeat measurements can show whether the change is likely to have a positive or negative impact.

From such research, several key points have emerged. A basic principle of HCI is that the user interface should follow a logical and simple mental model. Because the task of reading from a workstation is likely to differ from the film reading task, the mental model of the workstation interface should also be simple to learn. If radiologists are confronted with an unfamiliar film multiviewer, they are likely to make a few mistakes until they learn how to advance or back up the films and how to turn the separate illuminators on and off. The number of errors they make until they become facile with the system is a measure of how simple the interface is to learn.

A common user interface control is the familiar computer mouse. On a flat desk, moving the mouse away from the user generally moves the cursor on the screen upward while mouse movement toward the user moves the cursor down, and right and left movements correspond as well. Switching these directions is very difficult for almost all users to adjust to; the controls run counter to the mental model. This sort of control inversion can have disastrous consequences. Aircraft that use a "stick" for flight control respond to pulling back on the stick by climbing and to pushing forward by diving. If the airplane becomes inverted and the pilot disoriented, the reversal of the control responses may not be realized; pulling back on the stick would then put the airplane into a dive.

This author has often proposed a good test of a user interface: if a person can figure out how to use it without having to refer to a manual, it is probably based on a good mental model. The popular personal computer operating systems, Apple's Mac OS and Microsoft's versions of Windows, try to have software developers adhere to a set of standards. Although the mental model may not be entirely intuitive, once learned, new software that conforms to the design guidelines will conform to that model and be much simpler to use.

CONTROLS

From the mental model question, "How do I make this thing do what I want?" comes the development of logical controls to perform those tasks. It is this process of turning operations done in a conventional, noncomputer system into controls and outcomes in the computer-based system that constitutes development of a user interface. The trend in medical imaging workstations has been to adopt the GUI-based user interface. As noted from the work by Krupinski and Lund, however, that may not be the best possible choice. There have been significant departures from the GUI paradigm mostly in historical workstations. Examples include the General Electric Medical Systems Independent Console (G.E. Medical Systems, Milwaukee, WI), for which multiple keys were traded off against a GUI. The plasma panel of that console did allow flexible "soft" buttons to be used as well, vastly increasing the number of things that could be done without making the number of function keys impossibly large. The idea used for this console—that commonly used functions would be represented on dedicated keys and those that were needed for specific operations would be on the plasma display—has also been translated into more modern workstation designs. Many current systems have "soft" keys displayed in a fixed portion of the menu on the monitor(s) to perform the common functions. Operation-specific functions are selectable from menu portions that change with the task. The most common functions, such as window width and level adjustment, are usually available under mouse (or other cursor) control. The work by Krupinski and Lund for display of radiographic images on workstations and that of Beard (1994) for CT images would argue for minimal controls that can be operated without the user's having to look at them. Such a set of controls is not, as of this writing, available from medical imaging workstation manufacturers, though one manufacturer (Aurora Technology, Lake Forest, IL) has incorporated a foot pedal allowing the user to change to the next or prior examination on the worklist.

NAVIGATION

Finding the examination to be reviewed and a specific examination when there is more than one for a patient is known as the navigation task. The navigation method most commonly used is based on the model of the film jacket. In a hierarchical display, the electronic patient "jacket" is shown with the studies it contains. The user then selects the study (and sometimes the series) to be displayed (see Figure 8.4). An additional organizational layer on top of this is the worklist. This model parallels the lists or index cards kept at film multiviewers to show which examination is on which panel. On most workstations, the worklist shows a list of patients, and selecting a patient then displays the "jacket."

The worklist is potentially a very powerful tool; with appropriate workstation software and an interface of the PACS to a radiology information system, worklists could be used to help manage workflow. That is, examinations to be read could be directed to particular workstations or shown on the worklist of a particular radiologist when he or she logs on. A worklist could also be used to show referring physicians which examinations have been read and have reports available. Information such as the length of time the patient has been waiting, the "stat" status, and the patient's appointment time with the referring physician could be used to help the radiologist prioritize reading order. A "lockout" could prevent two radiologists from trying simultaneously to read the same examination while still allowing "viewing" access.

Some of these features are currently implemented in commercial workstations, but others are still on our "wish list." Beard (1990) developed a

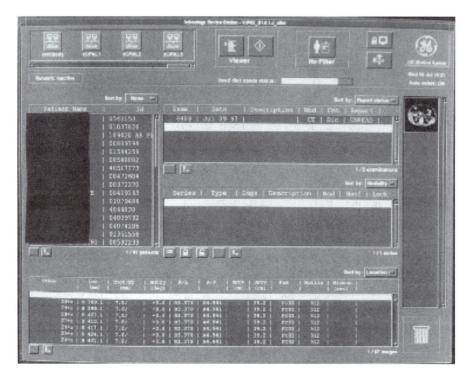

FIGURE 8.4

Workstation screen shot.

rapid prototyping and evaluation method in part for examining the human-computer interactions involved in the navigation process. A significant part of image navigation is some form of automated arrangement of the images in an examination when there are multiple images. This has come to be called the "hanging protocol," after the manner in which films are arranged on light boxes or multiviewer panels for reading. For sectional imaging, such as CT, MR, and nuclear medicine PET and SPECT, the ability to sort images by series, by time of acquisition, by anatomic location, and by imaging protocol (such as pulse sequence for MR) is of great importance. In the conventional film-based operation, this sorting is often done by the technologist as the examination is filmed. Automation of such sorting will facilitate interpreting these examination types at workstations. For plain radiographic images, the "hanging protocols" are also of some importance. In the scenario of a trauma patient who has multiple radiographs, sorting them by examination time may be wholly inadequate. Other criteria, such as anatomic area being radiographed, also have to be considered. In addition, the sorting of sectional images and the arrangement of radiographic ones is also governed to some extent by the individual desires of the radiologist. All these requirements dictate that such sorting and arrangement be both automated and customizable.

Controls and displays in general could benefit the user if they were customizable. The number of images displayed simultaneously for sectional imaging, the window width and level preset values, the initial image display parameters (very useful for MR imaging), and even the location and arrangement of on-screen controls could all be based on who logs in, so that personalized "setups" are automatically set. If this sounds extravagant, readers should recall that many such functions are done currently in film-based operations in a fashion "transparent" to the radiologist by technologists, file room clerks, and radiology residents who quickly learn the preferences of the radiologist with whom they are working.

ERROR RECOVERY

An important aspect of user interfaces is error recovery. In the best of circumstances, users will still make mistakes. How a user interface allows the correction of such errors is important; if the error correction process is deemed too taxing by the user, it may be ignored and errors may propagate. Aside from preventing erroneous conditions that are detectable, there is the matter of reversing a function or operation that was inadvertently selected. There are two levels of such reversal; the "undo what I just did" version that can be thought of as allowing a user to back up a step, and the "take me back to where I started" choice that resets starting conditions.

In the case of the undo function, some things, such as selecting a preset image arrangement, can be reversed fairly simply. Others, particularly operations that manipulate pixel data, may be irreversible. Some forms of edge sharpening, for example, cannot readily be reversed, nor can erasing images. In some instances, warnings to the user prior to executing such an operation may be warranted, and a well-designed user interface will provide a safety option for even the erasing of an image.

The "reset" function, analogous to a "panic button," is useful when a user has gotten so far off the desired functional direction that only resetting to the starting conditions will be helpful. Such a reset, however, should ordinarily not be the equivalent of shutting down and restarting the workstation; a well-designed reset should just re-establish starting conditions quickly.

A manner of quantifying the user effort required to invoke undo and reset functions is based on a model proposed in the MDIS Specification (1991). This model relies on the number of keystrokes or their equivalent (a mouse button click) used to implement workstation functions, and it has also been used by Beard (1989) in developing workstation designs. For users contemplating the purchase of PACS workstations, determining the number of "keystroke-equivalents" needed to perform common functions is a good method of comparing the effort involved in using different workstations. For example, a workstation that requires six keystroke equivalents to perform the window width and level functions is far too cumbersome by almost anyone's measure. Typically, such a commonly used function should be always available, or require at most a single keystroke.

User interfaces are a complex subject, and—as many believe—a matter of personal choice. Nonetheless, principles including simplicity of the mental model behind the interface and minimum actions to perform common functions are applicable across many users and levels of experience.

WORKSTATION FUNCTIONS AND FEATURES

FUNCTIONS

No matter the workstation role, workstations have some basic functions that need to be supported if users are to gain desired information from the images displayed.

A basic requirement for workstations is speed. Some types of film multiviewers can move films so fast that they go by in a blur (the transparent band types). Even the slower film alternators can move a four-over-four set of films (amounting to some 96 to 120 images for many of the cross-sectional imaging methods) in about 3 to 5 sec. This is a very high performance to match in a workstation. In general, a desirable target speed is an image display time of less than 2 sec from the time the image is selected for display. Most users do not tolerate display times longer than this for routine displays. If they understand that an ad hoc request is taking longer because of the time needed to fetch the study from the archive, they are more willing to tolerate a longer delay. It is desirable to provide either a progress indicator, or a notice that lets the user know how long such a retrieval will take. This avoids the problem of the user's not being sure whether the system is working. With a multitasking workstation, a retrieval can be done in the background while other processes (for example, reading another study) can take place in the foreground.

A feature that was implemented on the workstation developed at the University of Pennsylvania (van der Voorde et al. 1986) took advantage of common user actions to support viewing comparison studies. Kept on local disk were the current examination plus up to four prior studies. However, icons for up to seven studies older than the first were also displayed. The software automatically displayed the current examination plus the most recent previous study, and users could select older examinations by clicking on the icons. Once a user selected the third prior study, the software assumed that even earlier studies might be desired and would initiate a request from the archive for the older studies. In this way, if the user got to the fifth older examination, that image would either have already been loaded from the archive or the retrieve would be in process. Since most users did not request studies beyond the second or third, this avoided filling local storage with examinations that were unlikely to be reviewed.

Workstations also have to provide a navigation method for finding examinations to be read, compared, and correlated. This navigation process is related closely to the user interface and the mental model assumed. Table 8.1 lists commonly encountered navigation functions (Feingold, Seshadri, and Arenson 1991; Greenes 1984; Jost et al. 1984; Arenson et al. 1990; Leung et al. 1995).

A method for adjusting grayscale is evident from most workstation designs and studies of those designs (Horii et al. 1996). Adjustment of "window width and level" has consistently been shown to be the most frequently used image manipulation tool. Other image manipulation tools typically provided include some form of magnification (an overall magnification or the analog of a magnifying lens), roaming (either moving around in the magnified image or moving the magnifying window), video inversion ("black bone"), and rotation and flipping of the image. Some workstations also perform fast image processing to support edge enhancement, grayscale histogram equalization, and image arithmetic (adding or subtracting images). Specialty workstations may have additional image manipulation functions. Table 8.2 summarizes these image manipulation functions (Sezan, Yip, and Daly 1987; Feingold, Seshadri, and Arenson 1991; Greenes 1984; Jost et al. 1984; Arenson et al. 1990; Hohman et al. 1994).

Measuring features on images and calculating pixel statistics are two commonly available functions. These are deemed a necessity for computed tomographic workstations because of the heavy use of these operations on dedicated CT display consoles. Such measurements are diagnostically important, and in film-based operations they are often filmed as overlays on the image. Workstation controls for this include a method to place a region of interest (ROI) of selectable shape on the image, to move it around on the

TABLE 8.1
Navigation Functions

Worklist	Display a list of examinations to be interpreted (should be reachable by a single keystroke equivalent). The user should be able to sort the worklist chronologically, by patient name, or by examination type with sub-sorting by date or patient name.
List all	Display a list of all the current day's examinations—the daily list (also reachable by a single keystroke equivalent). It should be possible to sort this list as for the worklist.
Folder display	For each patient, show the analog of the master jacket.
Image icons	In exam folders (within the patient folder), show icons of images in studies.
Next patient (exam)	Moves to the next patient or examination on the worklist.
Previous patient (exam)	Moves to the prior patient or examination on the worklist.
Consult	Interrupts current display, brings up "List all" or "Worklist," and allows selection and display of another patient or examination for consultation purposes.
Consult remote	For consultation between workstations. Invokes the display of the same study on two workstations and two cursors, one controlled by each workstation so that the two users may point to different areas on the image.
Resume last	Returns to exam interrupted by the Consult or Consult remote function (should return to images, format, and grayscale settings as prior to invoking either Consult mode).
Mark as read	Marks the examination as "read." This should alter the appropriate flag in the image database so that others looking at the worklist or patient list will see the marked examinations displayed as "read." This function should also: a) be restricted to use by those permitted to read examinations, and b) prevent more than one person marking the examination as "read."
Compare	Brings up the patient folder so that a prior exam of the same type or other examination can be displayed for comparison and correlation purposes. Note that some examination types should have a site-configurable automatic display of prior examinations (e.g., chest radiographs will almost always be displayed with the prior examination). Display formats should be both site- and user-configurable.

image, and to resize it. Once the radiologist believes the position and size to be correct, the function to compute pixel statistics is invoked. The need is to support multiple ROIs on any image, so the functions should not be limited to a single ROI. Some orthopedic applications, for plain film and cross-sectional imaging, require the measurement of angles as well as distances.

TABLE 8.2
Image Manipulation Functions

Window width	Adjusts range of pixel bits sent to the display system. Should always be accessible.
Window level (center)	Sets center of window width in the bits of the pixel. Should always be accessible.
Grayscale reset	Resets window width and level settings to initially displayed values.
Zoom/magnify	Invokes an operation that maps the displayed image into a larger area (zoom is typically by pixel replication; magnify uses pixel interpolation).
Place ROI	Places a pre-shaped (circle, square), or hand drawn region of interest on the image. The controls should allow for the user to move the ROI around the image and change its size.
ROI magnify	Magnifies within a movable region of interest. This should allow for variable degrees of magnification (may be in discrete steps) and should be movable in real time using the manual input control.
Gray scale invert	Reverses the meaning of the highest and lowest pixel values in terms of gray scale; for example, white bones would be displayed as black.
Window width and level presets	Single keystroke equivalent selectable preset WW/WL combinations. For example, lung, mediastinum, and bone for CT.
Image processing	Image processing functions are not commonly used while reading cases; however, access to such functions as edge enhancement, histogram equalization, and application of user-defined filters could be provided through a button that brings up a menu of such functions available.
Undo	At least one level of being able to undo the function just completed. This should be accessible with a single keystroke equivalent. Note: An undo of some image processing functions may be difficult to implement unless a copy of the "original" image is maintained.
Pixel statistics	Reports the number, mean, and standard deviation of pixels in an ROI.
Measure	Provides linear, area, and angle measurements on an image.
Annotate	Allows a user to add text annotation to an image. This function can be used with the display of an ROI or graphics arrows. Users should be able to toggle the annotation on and off. Such annotation should be saved with the image.

A method for displaying the radiology reports of the examinations being viewed is also important. Although this is often thought of as a feature primarily for review workstations, the utility of reports for radiologists should not be underestimated. In subspecialty radiology practices, it is very useful to know how a correlative study was read when interpreting an examination of a different type. In more generalist practices, it is still important to know how a colleague read a prior examination. Displaying reports usually requires that some form of interface to the radiology information system (RIS) or hospital information system (HIS) be operational.

To a large extent, a successful conversion from film-based reading to the use of workstations for the same work also involves replacing of many of the functions now done manually with automated equivalents. Selection of prior studies to display, arrangement of images when displayed, and clearing of films from the alternator when the readings are done are all examples of image management functions that need to be supported in the workstation environment. If not, the transition to workstations means the migration of support tasks to the radiologist. While this might seem attractive at first because of potential personnel reductions, the radiologist's time is very expensive and his or her productivity depends on these support functions being accomplished. Simply moving these operations from clerks and other personnel to the radiologist will have a negative impact on productivity. Table 8.3 lists a set of these basic image management functions.

OTHER USERS, OTHER FUNCTIONS

It is important that the workstation designer take into account the needs of users in addition to radiologists. Orthopedic surgeons, for example, need to measure angles much more frequently than do radiologists. Also, having digital versions of templates for orthopedic appliances (joint replacements, various pins and fasteners) available for placement on the digital image and scaled so that they are in the proper relationship to the digital image would be very useful for surgical planning. At least one workstation manufacturer has shown a prototype workstation that allows these functions (Sectra Imtec AB, Linkoping, Sweden).

Reconstructive plastic surgeons use powerful computer graphics workstations. For a number of years, they have been employing such workstations for reconstructing a patient's anatomy in three-dimensional form so that surgery can be planned and the results approximated (Fujino 1994). Many plastic surgery departments have their own workstations, but they rely on a PACS connection or removable media to get the image data from radiology. Chiefly, they use CT and some MRI imaging.

Radiation oncologists do treatment planning on specialized workstations, but they also rely on diagnostic imaging. Their workstations have to support both image review functions as well as the treatment planning soft-

TABLE 8.3

Image Management Functions

Delete exam (local)	Provides for deletion of an examination from the local storage (with appropriate warnings).
Autodelete	Provides for automated deletion of examinations from local storage based on user-set criteria.
Mark for teaching file	Flags the examination being read as one useful for teaching purposes.
Mark for nondeletion	Flags the examination being read as one not to be autodeleted. Note that a site-configurable expiration time for this "protection" is useful.
Redirect	Allows sending of an examination to a particular workstation.
Scrapbook	Saves selected images (or pointers to images) in a file. Retrieving this file later would (optionally) first display the scrap images while providing access to the full study, if requested.
Print	Provides hardcopy printing of selected images (e.g., the Scrapbook) or a whole study. Print options (film, paper, 35mm slide) depend on devices in the system. Print function permission should be configured by type of user.
Local storage statistics	If the system uses local storage for images, this function should display the percentage of capacity currently used.
In progress notice	For time-consuming operations (such as retrieving an archived case) this function should display a progress indicator to give the user some idea when the operation will be completed.
Hanging protocol	Allows for site- and user-customizable arrangements of images, series, etc. as defaults for initial displays. For example, some radiologists prefer to read chest cases with the current films in the center two of four light boxes and the prior study on the outer two light boxes; others prefer the pair of frontal images on two adjacent light boxes and the pair of lateral images on the other two. It should be possible using electronic hanging protocols to support both of these possibilities and others. The arrangement used should be based on user login.
Associate report	If a radiology report is available for an examination on the daily list or for prior studies that will be displayed, a method for displaying that report should be implemented. An entry on the daily list should show report status (none, preliminary, reviewed, finalized or signed, referring physician reviewed). The latter status is one that is being added to the others at many institutions.

ware. The DICOM Standards Committee has approved a new part of the standard that allows treatment plans to be handled on electronic communications networks, much as diagnostic images are.

Surgeons need workstations that can function in an operating room environment. Such equipment needs to meet certain electrical safety standards, as some anesthetics can create a potentially explosive atmosphere. To operate the workstation, either a nonscrubbed person is needed or the controls must be usable while maintaining aseptic conditions. Membrane keyboards, disposable keyboard covers, and voice-recognition systems are all potentially useful in meeting this need.

Within diagnostic radiology, certain applications need specialized workstations. For training residents, a workstation should support an Internet connection plus a CD-ROM or DVD drive for educational material on removable media. Conference rooms need a workstation that can drive a video projection system so large groups can see the images. Guided-biopsy systems in mammography have application-specific workstations with controls and a user interface designed for the task.

In general, the important idea is not necessarily to design a workstation for each special application, but to understand that such applications exist and that they may need hardware or user interface elements outside of the general design.

WORKSTATION ERGONOMICS

A major principle of ergonomic design is to take into account the physical and mental abilities of the user so as to minimize effort and errors when using a device. For computer workstations, having a good user interface is a key element of ergonomic design as it helps reduce fatigue during long periods of use and minimizes the error rate of the user. Beyond this, the physical layout of the workstation itself, such as the placement of dedicated controls and location of components that need to be reached (e.g., removable media drives), can contribute to or detract from the goal of an ergonomic design.

FURNITURE

Good ergonomic design also dictates that the environment in which work is done needs to be a major factor in planning. Unfortunately, reading rooms for workstations tend to be designed using principles based either on multiviewers or on an ad hoc basis. A frequent error made by those planning a PACS installation is to place a low priority on furniture for workstations and reading rooms. The utility of a well-designed, ergonomically correct workstation will be counteracted by tables that set the monitors too low or high and by chairs that are too uncomfortable to sit in for more than a few minutes. Adjustability of workstation furniture and seating is important because the users vary in their physical dimensions. It follows that such adjustments should be simply and quickly made. There are a few literature references to designing reading rooms for workstations. The earliest reference we know of is by ter Haar Romeny (1995), who wrote one paper on the subject of reading room design for workstations (Horii et al. 1989) and one on user interfaces and ergonomics (Horii 1992). Since then, Rostenberg (1995) has written a comprehensive book on architectural design for medical imaging.

LIGHTING

In part because of the lower luminance of workstation CRT monitors compared to light boxes, glare control and ambient lighting are more important considerations in the design of workstations. We caution readers that architects may be tempted to work from designs developed for offices in which large numbers of video display terminals are used. However, the tasks at such video display terminals (now mostly replaced by personal computers) are generally for text-based operations. Text on a monitor represents a very high-contrast display and does not present the problem for users that the low contrast of medical images tends to present.

A number of studies (Baxter, Ravindra, and Norman 1982; Alter et al. 1982; Ravindra, Norman, and Baxter 1983; Rogers and Johnston 1987) have shown the detrimental effects of ambient light on visual discrimination tasks. The study by Rogers and Johnston (1987) was done with electronic displays; the others are film-based and involve light box-bases. The lower luminance of workstation CRTs suggests that ambient light effects are even more pronounced. The effects of glare are also more evident. Turning off all lights reduces both ambient and glare light sources, but it is impractical as some task lighting is needed during most reading sessions. The best solution lies in careful lighting design. Use of indirect lighting (light reflected and diffused by bouncing it off a wall or ceiling) can greatly reduce glare as there are no point sources to reflect.

Figure 8.5 is an example of a reading area designed for workstations

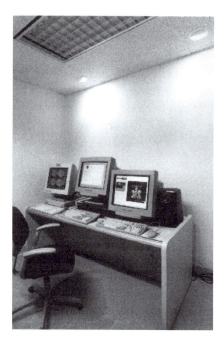

FIGURE 8.5

Example reading room.

that incorporates indirect lighting to good advantage. Most reading rooms need two sets of lights, one set for use during reading sessions and the other for use by the housekeeping staff or others doing nonradiologic work in the room. The set used during reading sessions provides too low an ambient level for most housekeeping or maintenance tasks. The second set of lights provides sufficient illumination for such work and can be switched off during reading sessions. If possible, even indirect lighting should be controlled by dimmers. Local fire and building codes may limit how low room illumination may be, and exits and doorways may have to remain more brightly lit than desired. The help of an architect is of great value when it comes to such issues.

HEAT

An often-overlooked consideration of reading environments is the large amount of heat that can be generated by workstations and associated equipment. It is important to let the architects and engineers know the approximate additional heat load that can be expected from the equipment. People are also a heat source to be considered, so the number of individuals projected to occupy the room is also important. A tendency of hospital administrators is to design for average, rather than peak, heat loads, as doing so helps keep construction and operating costs down. This makes proper estimation of heat load all the more important.

NOISE

As for noise, most workstation computers contain fans that generate noise. Most reading rooms are also be used by several groups of people simultaneously. These are two of the factors that enter into the consideration of noise in the reading space. The building's heating, ventilation, and air conditioning (HVAC) also generates noise. Placement of an imaging room can affect the amount of noise transmitted from the outside. Acoustic design is of considerable importance in reading rooms, as background noise can make it difficult for transcriptionists to understand the speaker, or can contribute to problems with voice recognition systems. Methods that help reduce the levels of noise (Lawrence 1989) include the use of sound-deadening materials (carpeting, acoustical ceiling tiles), surfaces that diffuse sound (textile-covered or texture painted walls), and partitions between workstations.

Architects and interior designers can also help with the siting of reading rooms. New construction makes this simpler than renovating existing space. Location of the reading room is otherwise influenced by two major factors: who will be working in it and who needs access to the personnel or equipment within it. Architects can help by siting the reading room and its entrances and exits to make the flow of people through the room as unobtrusive as possible.

SELECTING A WORKSTATION

Selecting a workstation begins with the fundamentals of selecting any system: it should meet the needs of the intended user as efficiently as possible. However, determining this requires a very careful and thorough needs analysis. Most often, a needs analysis is part of preliminary work of specifying a PACS. In this effort, generating the functional specification is most important. The functional specification is usually developed from a functional model. The functional model is based on the tasks performed to carry out the work of the facility. This is one of the most difficult aspects of developing a functional specification, because it is surprisingly hard to find out exactly what happens in a facility. Be aware of the difference between what job descriptions and supervisors say happens and what is actually done. We recommend being sure that the end-users of systems are fully consulted about their role in operations and encouraged to describe actual activities and difficulties, even if these are at odds with "official" work descriptions. It is especially important to discover any "workarounds" or "shortcuts" that users develop, as these tend to show where there are problems or bottlenecks.

STARTING WITH AN (ALMOST) BLANK SHEET

It is very difficult to develop a workstation functional specification independent of that for the PACS as a whole. The workstation interacts with the archive and sometimes with printers and external information systems. Ideally, the functional specification for a PACS is developed as a whole, or at least as a series of components with a master plan, rather than as separate parts that are assembled after the fact.

A suggestion for developing workstation specifications is first to establish the requirements. This should be done for each anticipated workstation role and should involve the end users (radiologists, other physicians, technologists, physicists, and others) in drafting the requirements. This can be done as part of the work of a "PACS committee" or other local body organized to plan for a PACS acquisition. A set of fundamental questions should be answered for each workstation role. Table 8.4 provides a basic set of such questions. Please note that this list is not meant to be exhaustive; the way your facility operates will likely add questions to this list. It is very important to keep a standard set of three questions in mind throughout the process of developing a functional model.

What operation(s) is (are) done at this step?

Who does this (these) operation(s)?

How long does it take to do this (these) operation(s)?

For workstations, the answer to the second question is almost always "the radiologist" or other user. However, for each step done with film that will need a workstation analog, the answers to the first and third questions are important in establishing criteria for the functional specification. For example, the process of bringing up the next examination to be read on a multiviewer might take 5 sec. A functional specification for a workstation to perform the analog of this function might be that "the time from requesting the next examination to the start of its display shall be no longer than 5 sec." Note that this statement is too generic; in the functional specification the type of examination would have to be specified as well.

The process of creating a functional model and translating it into a functional specification is time-consuming and difficult. It may well be worth the expense for a facility to hire someone experienced in this process to help. The next step, creating the request for proposal, or RFP, is also critically important. The language used in RFPs is very specific (and very stilted) to avoid the risk of getting systems that do not meet needs. A guideline for preparing an RFP has been written by Perry and Prior (1999), and it acquaints the reader with the typical sections of, and language used in, RFPs for PACS.

FUTURE DEVELOPMENTS IN WORKSTATIONS

"It's tough to make predictions. Especially about the future."—Yogi Berra

IMAGE DISTRIBUTION

As PACS move from academic medical centers and research implementations into diverse medical treatment facilities, workstations must address the problem of image availability in widespread locations. Dr. Haskin (1985) noted some years ago that most hospitals possess a large number of light boxes, which implies a large number of locations in which images are viewed. Contemporary healthcare systems involve large networks of facilities of varying sizes, from physician offices to large medical centers (Greenes and Bauman 1996). Since the patient population is served by combinations of these facilities, some manner of distributing images and other information is needed to support the level of service that such networks are advocating.

One choice that is receiving increasing interest is the use of the Internet or a private version of it (often called an intranet) to share images. A good history of the Internet is provided by Hafner and Lyon (1996) and serves to provide some scale for this world-wide "network of networks." The advantages of an open and readily accessible network, especially the multimedia World Wide Web that operates on the Internet, are diminished for

TABLE 8.4

Basic Workstation Questions

Question	Comments
Who is going to use this workstation? Please answer with a list of all users and about what percent of the time they will use the workstation.	Establishes the user population to consider.
What types of examinations will be interpreted or reviewed at this workstation?	A list of examinations normally read/reviewed. This helps establish display system requirements and number of monitors needed.
What comparison and correlation examinations are needed?	This list should be exhaustive—failing to include, for example, color flow ultrasound may mean that the workstation will have no color display capability.
With what frequency will: a) comparison, and (b) correlation examinations be used?	May need data from existing work patterns.
How many examinations per day will be read or reviewed at this workstation?	To determine workload.
What is the projected growth rate in this number per day?	To allow for growth—failure to consider this may result in obsolete workstations very quickly.
About how many hours per day do you spend reading the examinations you are answering these questions about?	This helps establish a reading rate—how many examinations per unit time need to be read.
Do you have a relatively "set" way of arranging the films of an examination?	This helps determine if automated hanging protocols can be used.
If so, who does this arranging now?	This will determine if this task is done by the viewer or by someone else.
At present, does the way films are arranged vary from user to user in your setting?	To determine if hanging protocols need to be customized on a per-user basis.
Do you work from a list of examinations to be read/reviewed?	Establishes need for a worklist.
If so, who or what system creates this list?	Manual or automatic worklist at present—determines if an interface to an external system may be needed for this. For example, the worklist is generated from the RIS.
Once an examination is read or reviewed, do you need to notify someone or some system of that?	Determines how the user notes an examination as "read." This may be automatic—see the follow-up question next.

What system, or whom, do you notify, or is this triggered from your dictation?

Most RIS software includes a function that changes the status of an examination when a report on it is dictated, when that report is transcribed, and when it is finalized. This question is to determine if a workstation would need to communicate with the RIS about this so that the examination will be marked as "read" or removed from the worklist. If the user reports this to a person, that person's tasks need to be elaborated.

How do you get comparison and correlation examinations?

To determine who does this—this function likely needs to be automated. This question is to help make sure that this function is not left out.

What image manipulation (window width and level, bright light, gray scale alteration, etc.) do you, or someone else, do presently? Please make the answer to this question a list of things done.

Establishes image manipulation functions used with film. Tell the user that window width and level changes or presets used by technologists when filming an examination is an example of image manipulation done by someone else for the user.

What measurements do you make, or are made for you, on the examinations you read/review? Please make the answer to this question a list of measurements done.

Example, pixel statistics (ROI) for CT.

If an error is made in the process of performing the examination (for example, the wrong patient name is "flashed" on the film or the right/left marker is incorrectly placed) who corrects such errors and about how long does that process take?

To establish how quality control/assurance is done in some PACS, the QC/QA steps may take longer than for conventional film.

Are most errors with examinations caught before you see the films to read?

Helps determine control points for image movement—that is, the QA/QC workstation the technologist uses may be used to correct errors so that they are rarely sent to the reading work-station.

Do you now, and will you be, reading/reviewing examinations with others? If so, how many?

Determines the need for group viewing and teaching functions.

Have you used electronic workstations for reading or reviewing examinations before.

Helps establish the experience of the user.

medical information by a lack of security and privacy. Although technological solutions are available for some of the problems posed by the general issue of security "gaps," moving the technology of the Internet to a private intranet helps solve the problem. Any connection between the private network and public communications carriers (necessary for wide-area service) can be carefully controlled. The development of virtual private network (VPN) technology also provides a high level of security for connections between facilities over public networks.

The advantages of Internet technology for workstations are that "browsers," or the software used to retrieve information from remote World Wide Web (WWW) servers, are available for multiple types of machines, are capable of handling images, and have a user interface well-understood by a large segment of the population. The use of personal computers with a browser to access medical information has been described by several authors (Li et al. 1995; Mascarini et al. 1995; Feingold et al. 1997) (see Figure 8.6). The low cost of personal computers and the wide variety of communications choices to access the Internet or an intranet mean that images

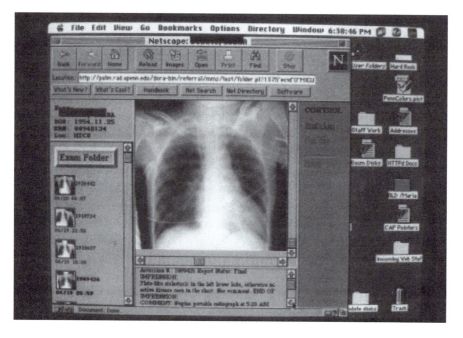

FIGURE 8.6

Web browser workstation.

and other medical information can be made widely available. The majority of future workstations used outside of radiology, or other specialties that do not perform primary diagnosis from workstations, are likely to be personal computer-based and access information using an Internet browser. Movement of the Internet WWW search service software to intranets (DeJesus 1997) means that anyone using an intranet can search even very large databases.

Workstations also permit on a desktop what used to require a mainframe computer: reconstruction of two-dimensional slice data into three-dimensional images that may be manipulated in real-time. This is, in itself, a large topic deserving of much greater explanation than can be given here. The reference by Vannier (Vannier and Marsh 1996) provides a thorough overview of the subject.

HARDWARE ADVANCES

Workstation-class graphics performance is already available on personal computers. This trend is driven by the computer game market, which in recent years has seen major advances in performance. If workstation software is written to take advantage of the graphics processors available, personal computer performance is more than adequate for most medical image displays. The future of hardware for workstations is likely to follow the mass-market trends: faster microprocessors, less expensive memory and long-term storage, and more powerful special-purpose (graphics and communications) "chips."

Display devices are likely to show continued improvement. Prototype flat-panel liquid crystal displays at resolutions needed for medical imaging are already available. Cathode ray tubes have also made progress, chiefly with increased luminance without decrease in tube life. Plasma panel displays with enough resolution for high-definition television are currently on the market. These are color displays, although the early implementations were monochromatic (Say et al. 1986). Experimental displays have some potential to serve as diagnostic displays and include field emission (Derbyshire 1994), light emitting diode (LED) (Sherr 1993), and digital micromirror devices (Sampsell 1993). Plasma panels operate by a gas fluorescing when excited by a potential applied across transparent electrodes on glass.

Field emission displays (Spindt et al. 1976; Gray, Sune, and Jones 1993) use a series of electron-emitting points fabricated with integrated circuit technology. These points are surrounded by an aperture grille that accelerates the emitted electrons. Because the electric field intensity around a point increases as the radius of curvature of the point decreases, very high field intensities can be achieved around the points with fairly low potentials applied to them. A phosphorescent screen placed in front of the emitter array serves as the display surface, and like a CRT, it fluoresces in response to the electron bombardment. Because the points are microscopic and spaced at close intervals (on the order of 10 μm), the resulting spatial resolution can be very good. Recently, experiments using diamonds deposited as an array of microscopic thin-film patches have shown promise as electron emitters (Shyankay 1995). This is a result of diamond's property of repelling electrons. The result is that a very low potential applied to the array releases more electrons than does the same potential used with silicon points.

Arrays of light-emitting diodes (LEDs) have also been built as laboratory demonstrations for flat-panel displays and large panels for poster-sized displays. The availability of blue LEDs means that full color displays are possible. Making small LEDs with enough luminance is one problem; for color displays, each pixel would have to have three LEDs. Cost is high for these displays, and though LEDs use far less power than incandescent lamps for the same luminance output, they still use much more power than electroluminescent (EL) displays or a backlit LCD panel.

Another potential alternative also uses integrated circuit manufacturing techniques. The digital micromirror display (DMD) (Motamedi, Wu, and Pister 1997) uses such techniques to produce a panel of small mirrors, each with a pivot and drive electrodes. The drive electrodes produce oscillations of the mirrors that modulate light reflected from them. These mirrors are also quite small; on the order of 17 μm^2. This form of display operates by reflecting light rather than emitting it. Because the DMD uses reflected light, the resulting display is not a flat-panel, but more the size and shape of a projection television system. Some current computer projectors use this technology.

Perhaps the ultimate in workstations is the "wearable" one. Serious work has been done on computers worn on the body with head-mounted miniature displays. One of the originators of this concept, Steve Mann (1999), has been experimenting with the idea since it became possible to build a computer one could wear. While not likely to be an attractive option for most radiologists, such a device has potential advantages for interventional radiologists and surgeons. Using sensors of head and eye position, it is possible to superimpose a medical imaging view of anatomy over the actual patient. Image-guided surgery could take on new possibilities using such technology.

It is likely that other advances, such as improved voice recognition, biometric identification, and ultraportable electronics, will alter the workstation "landscape." Voice recognition could provide "Star Trek"-like computer control. Biometric identification would enable very high levels of security for computer systems (a system simply would not work for a user it didn't recognize). Ultraportable electronics are, to quite an extent, already here, but further advances might yield display devices in an eyeglass frame for a truly "wearable" computer.

CONCLUSION

Workstations for medical imaging are a key component of a PACS because they form the system-to-user interface. A fortunate situation for PACS is the steady decline in the cost of workstation hardware with an equally steady rise in performance. Nonetheless, major advancements in the software for workstations are still necessary in user interfaces that adapt to the user and in integration with other information systems that enable automation of processes.

Although questions about diagnostic accuracy using workstations have been raised, workstations are in use now for primary diagnostic interpretation. The situation is similar to that during the introduction of intensifying screens for radiography. The spatial resolution of the resulting radiographic films decreased, but the tradeoff against reduced dose was thought to be well worth this loss. Again, radiologists are being asked to change the way they do things, and work on evaluating and improving PACS workstations will help minimize negative effects.

▶ REFERENCES

Alter, AJ et al. *The influence of ambient and view box light upon visual detection of low contrast targets in a radiograph.* Invest Radiol 17:402, 1982.

American College of Radiology: *ACR Standard for Teleradiology.* Reston, American College of Radiology, 1994.

Arenson, RL et al. *The digital imaging workstation.* Radiology 176: 303–315, 1990.

Asher, RW, Martin, H. *Cathode ray devices.* In: Luxenberg, HR, Kuehn, RL (eds), Display Systems Engineering. New York: McGraw-Hill, 1968: 237–276.

Augarten, S. *Bit by bit: An illustrated history of computers.* New York, 1984; Ticknor and Fields: 263–281.

Baxter, B, Ravindra, H, Norman, RA. *Changes in lesion detectability caused by light adaptation in retinal photoreceptors.* Invest Radiol 17:394, 1982.

Beard, D et al. *A prototype single-screen PACs console development using human-computer interaction techniques.* Proc SPIE 767:646–653, 1987.

Beard, DV et al. *Evolved design of a radiology workstation using time-motion analysis and the keystroke model.* SPIE Physics of Medical Imaging 1091:121–131, 1989.

Beard, DV. *Designing a radiology workstation: A focus on navigation during the interpretation task.* J Digit Imaging 3(3):152–163, 1990.

Beard, DV et al. *Interpretation of CT studies: Single-screen workstation versus film alternator.* Radiology 187(2):565–9, 1993.

Beard, DV et al. *Eye movement during computed tomography interpretation: Eyetracker results and image display-time implications.* J Digit Imaging 7(4):189–192, 1994.

Bell, CG. *Toward a history of (personal) workstations.* In: Goldberg, A (ed), A History of Personal Workstations, 4–36, ACM Press, New York, 1988.

Chang, PJ, Hoffman, E. *Multimodality workstation featuring multiband cine mode and real-time distributed interactive consultation.* RSNA 1993; InfoRAD Exhibit 9507WS.

DeJesus, EX. *The searchable kingdom.* Byte 22(6):92NA1–92NA12, 1996.

Derbyshire, K. *Beyond AMLCDs: Field emission displays?* Electronics Design, October, 1994: 56–66.

Duerinckx, AJ (ed). *Proc. SPIE v 318: Picture archiving and communications systems for medical applications, Parts I and II.* SPIE, Bellingham, WA, 1982.

Dwyer III, SJ et al. *Salient characteristics of a distributed diagnostic imaging management system for a radiology department.* SPIE Physics of Medical Imaging 318:194–204, 1982.

el-Saden, SM, Hademenos, GJ, Zhu, W. *Assessment of intraaxial and extraaxial brain lesions with digitized computed tomographic images versus film: ROC analysis.* Academic Radiology 4(2):90–95, 1997.

Engelbart, D. *The Augmented Knowledge Workshop.* In: Goldberg, A (ed), A History of Personal Workstations, 187–232, ACM Press, New York, 1988.

Feingold, E, Seshadri, SB, Arenson, RL. *Folder management on a multimodality PACS display station.* SPIE Physics of Medical Imaging 1446:211–216, 1991.

Feingold, ER et al. *Web-based radiology applications for clinicians and radiologists.* SPIE Physics of Medical Imaging 3035;60–71, 1997.

Fujino, T. *Simulation and computer aided surgery.* Chichester; John Wiley and Sons, 1994.

Greenes, RA. *Toward more effective radiologic workstation consultation: Design of a desktop workstation to aid in the selection and interpretation of diagnostic procedures.* Proceedings of the Eighth Conference of Computer Applications in Radiology; American College of Radiology 1984: 554–561.

Greenes, RA, Bauman, RA. *The era of health care reform and the information superhighway.* Radiol Clin of North Amer 34(3):463–468, 1996.

Goldberg, A (ed). *A History of Personal Workstations,* ACM Press, New York, 1988.

Gray, HT, Sune CT, Jones, GW. *Silicon field emitter arrays for cathodoluminescent flat-panel displays.* J Soc for Info Display 1(2):143–146, 1993.

Hafner, K, Lyon, M. *Where wizards stay up late: The origins of the Internet.* New York, Simon and Schuster: 1996.

Haskin, ME et al. *Data versus information: Which should we exchange?* SPIE Physics of Medical Imaging 536: 37–42, 1985.

Hohman, SA et al. *Radiologists' requirements for primary diagnosis workstations: Preliminary results of task-based design surveys.* SPIE Physics of Medical Imaging 2165:2–7, 1994.

Honeyman, JC et al. *Functional requirements for diagnostic workstations.* SPIE Physics of Medical Imaging 1899:103–109, 1993.

Horii, SC et al. *Environmental designs for reading from imaging workstations: Ergonomic and architectural features.* J Dig Imaging 2(3):156–162, 1989.

Horii, SC. *Electronic imaging workstations: Ergonomic issues and the user interface.* RadioGraphics 12:773–787, 1992.

Horii, SC et al. *Overlapped image display method: A technique for comparing medical images on a workstation.* SPIE Physics of Medical Imaging 2164:456–466, 1994.

Horii, SC et al. *PACS workstation usage differences between radiologists and MICU physicians.* SPIE Physics of Medical Imaging 2711: 266–271, 1996.

Huo, Z et al. *Automated computerized classification of malignant and benign masses on digitized mammograms.* Academic Radiology 5(3):155–168, 1998.

Jost, RG et al. *An electronic multiviewer.* Proceedings of the Eighth Conference of Computer Applications in Radiology; American College of Radiology 1984: 304–311.

Kano, A et al. *Digital image subtraction of temporally sequential chest images for detection of interval change.* Med Phys 21(3):453–461, 1994.

Krupinski, EA, Lund, PJ. *Comparison of film vs. monitor viewing of CR films using eye-position recording.* Proc SCAR '96; 1996:269–274.

Kundel, HL. *How much spatial resolution is enough?* A meta-analysis of observer performance studies comparing plain films and digital hard copy. SPIE Physics of Medical Imaging 1899: 86–89, 1993.

Lampson, BW. *Personal distributed computing: The Alto and Ethernet software.* In: Goldberg, A (ed), A History of Personal Workstations, 293–335, ACM Press, New York, 1988.

Larsen, GN. *Interactive image processing for computerized tomography (Ph.D. Thesis).* Department of Electronics and Electrical Engineering, University of Missouri at Columbia. August, 1976.

Lawrence, A. *Acoustic design.* In: Ruck, NC (ed), Building Design and Human Performance. New York: Van Nostrand Reinhold, 1989: 117.

Lemke, HU et al. *Applications of picture processing, image analysis, and computer graphics techniques to cranial CT scans.* Proceedings of the Sixth Conference on Computer Applications in Radiology and Computer/Aided Analysis of Radiological Images; 341–354. IEEE Computer Society Press, 1979.

Leung, KT et al. *Image navigation for PACS workstations.* SPIE Physics of Medical Imaging 2435:43–49, 1995.

Li, X et al. *World Wide Web telemedicine system.* SPIE Physics of Medical Imaging 2711:427–439, 1995.

Licklider, JCR. *Some reflections on early history.* In: Goldberg, A (ed), A History of Personal Workstations, 117–130, ACM Press, New York, 1988.

Maguire Jr, GQ et al. *Image processing requirements in hospitals and an integrated systems approach.* SPIE Physics of Medical Imaging 318:206–213, 1982.

Mann, S. *Cyborg seeks community.* Technology Review 102(3):36–42, 1999.

Mascarini, Ch et al. *In-house access to PACS images and related data through World Wide Web.* SPIE Physics of Medical Imaging 2711: 531–537, 1995.

MDIS Technical Development Team: *MDIS Medical Diagnostic Imaging Support System Acquisition Document.* Huntsville, US Army Engineer Division; 1991: C-23–C-57.

Motamedi, ME, Wu, MC, Pister, KSJ. *Micro-opto-electro-mechanical devices and on-chip optical processing.* Optical Engineering 36(5):1282–1297, 1997.

Perry, J, Prior, F. *Purchasing a PACS: An RFP toolkit.* In: Siegel, EL and Kolodner, RM (eds). Filmless Radiology. New York: Springer-Verlag, 1999:33–84.

Ravindra, H, Norman, RA, Baxter, B. *The effect of extraneous light on lesion detectability: A demonstration.* Invest Radiol 18:105, 1983.

Robb, RA. *Volume visualization and virtual reality in medicine and biology.* In: Lemke, HU, Vannier, MW, Inamura, K, and Farman, AG (eds), Proceedings of CAR '98: Computer Assisted Radiology and Surgery. Amsterdam, 1998; Elsevier: 131–142.

Rogers, DC, Johnston, RE. *Effect of ambient light on electronically displayed medical images as measured by luminance-discrimination thresholds.* J Opt Soc Am A4:976, 1984.

Ross, DT. *A personal view of the personal work station.* In: Goldberg, A (ed), A History of Personal Workstations, 54–111, ACM Press, New York, 1988.

Rossman, K. *Image quality.* Radiol Clin of North Amer 7(3):419–433, 1969.

Rostenberg, B. *The architecture of imaging.* Chicago; American Hospital Publishing: 1995.

Sampsell, JB. SID International Symposium Digest of Technical Papers. *An overview of the digital micromirror device and its application to projection displays.* 24:1012, 1993.

Say, DL et al. *Monochrome and color image-display devices.* In: Benson, KB (ed), Television Engineering Handbook. New York, McGraw-Hill, 1986: 12.1–12.53.

Sezan, MI, Yip, KL, Daly, SJ. *An investigation of the effects of uniform perceptual quantization in the context of digital radiography.* SPIE/Physics of Medical Imaging 767:622–630, 1987.

Scott Jr et al. *Interpretation of Emergency Department radiographs by radiologists and emergency medicine physicians: Teleradiology workstation versus radiograph readings.* Radiology 195:223–229, 1995.

Sherr, S. *Electronic Displays*, 2nd Edition. New York: John Wiley and Sons, 1993: Chapter 3: 201–340.

Shyankay, J. *Diamond films used in flat panel displays.* R&D Magazine, April 1995 44.

Slasky, BS et al. *Receiver operating characteristic analysis of chest image interpretation with conventional, laser printed, and high-resolution workstation images.* Radiology 174:775–780, 1990.

Spindt, CA et al. *Physical properties of thin-film field emission cathodes with molybdenum cones.* J Appl Physics 47(12):5248–5251, 1976.

Taira, RK et al. *Design of a graphical user interface for an intelligent multimedia information system for radiology research.* SPIE Physics of Medical Imaging 2435:11–23, 1995.

Taylor, JH. *Vision.* In: Parker, JF, West, VR (eds), Bioastronautics Data Book, 2nd Edition. Washington, DC, NASA:611–665, 1973.

ter Haar Romeny, BM et al. *The Dutch PACS project: Philosophy, design of a digital reading room and first observations in the Utrecht University Hospital in the Netherlands.* SPIE Physics of Medical Imaging 767:787–792, 1987.

Thacker, CP. *Personal distributed computing: The Alto and Ethernet hardware.* In: Goldberg, A (ed), A History of Personal Workstations, 267–289, ACM Press, New York, 1988.

van der Voorde, F et al. *Development of a physician-friendly digital image display console.* SPIE Physics of Medical Imaging 626:541–548, 1986.

Vannier, MW, Marsh, JL. *Three-dimensional imaging, surgical planning, and image-guided therapy.* Radiol Clin of North Amer 34(3):545–563, 1996.

Vining, DJ. *Virtual endoscopy: Is it reality?* Radiology 200:30–31, 1996.

Xu, XW et al. *Development of an improved CAD scheme for automated detection of lung nodules in digital chest images.* Med Phys 24(9):395–403, 1997.

STORAGE AND ARCHIVES

DOUGLAS TUCKER • AMIT MEHTA

The term "archive" has come to refer to a wide variety of storage and
preservation functions and systems. Traditionally, an archive is understood
to be a facility or organization that preserves records. It accomplishes this
task by taking ownership of the records, ensuring that they are understandable to the accessing community, and managing them to preserve their
information content and authenticity. Historically, these records have been
in such forms as books, papers, maps, photographs, and film, which can be
read directly by humans, or read with simple optical magnification and scanning aids. The major focus for preserving this information has been to ensure that they are on media with long-term stability and that access to this
media is carefully controlled.

The explosive growth of information in digital forms has posed a challenge not only for traditional archives and their information providers, but
also for organizations that have not traditionally thought of themselves as
archivists (Figure 9.1). Many different organizations are finding, or will find,
that they need to take on the information preservation functions typically
associated with traditional archives. Digital information is fragile; it can eas-

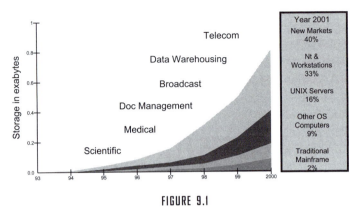

FIGURE 9.1

Storage requirements per industry.

ily be lost or corrupted. The pace of technology evolution is causing some hardware and software systems to become obsolete in a matter of a few years. These pressures are forcing many organizations to evaluate their role in the acquisition, storage, and management of digital data.

Long-term data storage is an important part of any PACS. The purpose of this chapter is to survey these data storage systems. The discussion will be kept generic and we will avoid in-depth discussions of specific technologies or their specific implementation challenges. The intent is to provide you with enough basic information to evaluate commercially available storage product designs and implementations by yourself.

ARCHIVE ROLES AND ARCHITECTURE

Figure 9.2 introduces the concept of the archive in a graphic form highlighting the main components, including both hardware and software. The role of this archive in the digital department is crucial, as shown in Figure 9.3.

As a common receiving location for all acquired images and as a source for all distribution of images, the archive is integral to a successful PACS implementation. Extrapolated further, the role of the archive can be perceived from the hospital level, as shown in Figure 9.4, and at the enterprise level, as shown in Figure 9.5.

In most instances the radiology PACS archive is independent from the central enterprise archive due to access issues and network bandwidth, but the concept can be extrapolated from the similar functionality of the two

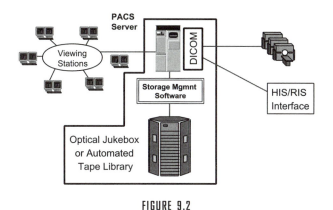

FIGURE 9.2

Architecture of a traditional archive.

systems. The archive is thus pivotal in a successful implementation. However, to better understand the archive concept, first must come an understanding of the terminology.

TERMINOLOGY

Throughout this chapter, a variety of terms are used to describe file and archive sizes, media capacity, speed, and data formats. A good understanding of these concepts is important to discuss archives and associated con-

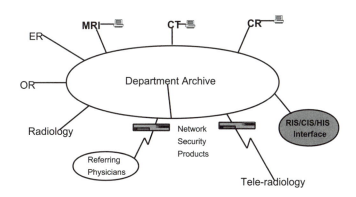

FIGURE 9.3

Architecture of a radiology department archive.

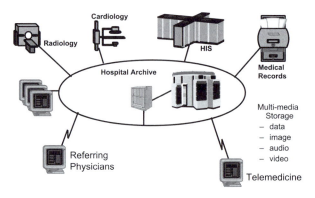

FIGURE 9.4

Architecture of a multidepartment archive and the enterprise level.

cepts. We will introduce few basic concepts and combine these concepts into more complex representations.

BITS AND BYTES

A *bit* is the simplest unit in data representation. A bit corresponds to a single unit of information, and can be thought of as a simple switch. Depending on the position of the switch, the bit can be used to represents either an "on" state or an "off" state, a "yes" or "no." The two

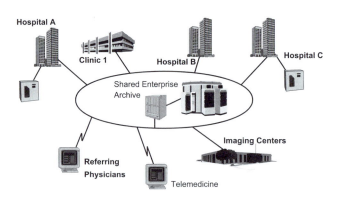

FIGURE 9.5

Architecture of an enterprise wide central archive.

possible states of a bit tie all computer systems to the binary numbering system.

Clearly, single independent bits of information are insufficient to represent complex ideas. Individual bits are grouped together and treated as a single unit in order to increase the number of possible representations. A *byte* is a common representation used in the computer industry. A byte consists of eight bits of information treated as a single entity. Since each bit of the byte can represent 2 possible states, a byte can represent: $2 \times 2 \times 2 \times 2 \times 2 \times 2 \times 2 \times 2$, or 2^8, or 256 different possible states. Commonly, the 256 states represent the values from 0 to 255 of the binary numbering system.

NUMBERS AND CHARACTERS, DATA REPRESENTATION

How do computers represent numbers and characters? The answer to this question is—in different ways. Characters, the "a," "B," "#" used to represent different sounds of a language, are encoded into single or multiple bytes of data. If you were to count the number of keys on a (now antique!) typewriter, you would find that there are less than 128 different characters. Computer scientists converted these typewriters for use as input devices to early computers. To represent each keystroke, each key was assigned a unique number. Because fewer than 256 different keystrokes were present, a single byte was used to encode the alphabet. Several different encoding schemes were used over time. Today, the American Standard Code for Information Interchange, or ASCII, coding system dominates. Extensions to the ASCII coding system allow for special computer symbols, as well as non-American character sets.

Numbers are represented in a different manner. As stated earlier, the bit is the basis of all modern computer systems. Because of this, it is understandable that essentially all modern computer systems are based on the binary counting system, as opposed to humans, who have 10 fingers and toes and operate on a base-10 (decimal) numbering system. Interestingly, some early computing systems were implemented using a base-10 numbering system. These efforts were soon abandoned in favor of the simpler binary system.

Integers are the simplest number to represent. We have already seen how a byte can be used to represent integers between 0 and 255. To increase the range of numbers represented, use more bits. For example, two bytes, or 16 bits, can represent 2^{16} or 65,536 different states, or the numbers 0 to 65,535. What about negative numbers? The most common method used to represent negative numbers is to reserve a single bit to indicate whether the number is positive or negative. This bit is referred to as the *sign-bit*. Returning to our two-byte example above, since one less bit is used to represent the number, there are 2^{15}, or 32,768 different positive numbers represented, and 32,767 negative numbers represented (no negative zeros, please!).

PIXELS

Digital imaging systems represent images as a mosaic of individual, uniform gray areas. Each area is referred to as a picture element, or *pixel* for short. The size of the pixel, or surface area it represents, is determined by a number of factors, including the total surface area of the image and the sampling frequency of the detector device (e.g., the resolution of a CR plate). More germane to this discussion, however, is the number of different "shades of gray" that each pixel can represent. Typically, pixels used in radiology range from one byte (8 bits) to two bytes (16 bits). Exceptions exist, most notably with color imaging systems. Color is represented in a number of different ways, including color coding (for PCs this is commonly refered to as palette mode, where a single byte is used to encode up to 256 different colors), or three bytes for RGB (where a single byte is assigned to each of the Red, Green and Blue content of a pixel). But for grayscale images, the number of bits per pixel determines the "grayscale resolution." Typically, the more bits used, the more shades of gray the imaging system can resolve (or represent).

PREFIXES

A bit is sufficient to represent the state of a binary system, and a byte is sufficient to encode systems with a limited number of possibilities (such as the alphabet). An image of a complex scene (such as your patient's chest) may require millions of pixels to represent accurately. Grouping several images together, such as a multi-slice CT examination, further increases the amount of data that is represented. We can quickly see that if we had to discuss the amount of data present in a medical record simply in terms of bits and bytes, we would be wasting a lot of paper with trailing zeros (e.g., a typical CT exam today is about 20,000,000 bytes in size!) There must be a better way, and there is.

To ease the discussions of large amounts of data, computer scientists

TABLE 9.1
Storage Terminology

Kilo	10^3	Kilobyte = 1000 bytes
Mega	10^6	Megabyte = 1000 Kilobytes
Giga	10^9	Gigabyte = 1000 Megabytes
Tera	10^{12}	Terabyte = 1000 Gigabytes
Peta	10^{15}	Petabyte = 1000 Terabytes
Exa	10^{18}	Exabyte = 1000 Petabytes
Zetta	10^{21}	Zettabyte = 1000 Exabytes
Yotta	10^{24}	Yottabyte = 1000 Zettabytes

have adopted simple rules. Prefixes are commonly used to represent three orders of magnitude differences. The prefix *kilo* is used to denote one thousand (10^3). One *kilobit* (Kb) equals one thousand bits and a *kilobyte* (KB) represents one thousand bytes. The next prefix, in order of magnitude, is *mega*. A *mega* denotes one million (10^6); a *megabit* (Mb) equals one million bits and a *megabyte* (MB) equals one million bytes. Similarly, a megabyte can be thought of as one thousand kilobytes. Table 9.1 lists commonly used prefixes.

ON-LINE, NEAR-LINE, OFF-LINE

Computer people frequently use hierarchies to classify different types of computer assets. For example, these hierarchies can be based on capacities, performance, or cost. Frequently these hierarchies are presented as triangles, and represent two different metrics, such as cost and capacity. The terms *on-line*, *near-line*, and *off-line* are an example of one such hierarchical representation used to discuss storage.

Many computer users are familiar with the message indicating that you have exceeded the capacity or performance of a particular computer asset. Many of us have witnessed the dreaded "out of memory" or "out of disk space" notice while editing documents. The memory involved in these interactions, whether solid-state or spinning magnetic disk, is referred to as *on-line* memory. On-line memory refers to nonremovable, high performance storage media that does not require human or robotic intervention. Due to the prohibitive costs associated with large amounts of on-line storage, the quantity is typically limited. On-line storage can be thought of as occupying the peak of our hierarchy.

Occupying the middle regions of our storage hierarchy is *near-line* storage. Near-line storage is removable storage media that requires a computer-controlled robot to quickly access vast amounts of data. Optical disk juke-boxes (ODJ) and automated cartridge system (ACS) are prime examples of near-line technology. Using these systems, the utility of an individual disk or tape drive is extended by the capacity of the library and the performance of the robot system. The capacity of the library (number of pieces of media housed) and performance of the robotic system (number of media exchanges per unit time) limit these systems.

Off-line storage rounds out this storage hierarchy. Once a particular library is full, or in many instances when no library exists, data written to a removable media is removed from the drive. Retrieval of data from the piece of media requires human intervention. Performance, in terms of access rate and reliability, is limited. However, off-line storage represents the highest (essentially unlimited!) capacity, typically at the lowest cost.

CURRENT STORAGE TECHNOLOGY

Data recording technology continues to enjoy significant progress in media capacity and price reduction. Storage prices continue to decline, with cost reductions of up to 30% per year not unprecedented. It is hard to think of many applications that are limited by physical storage capacities. In the following section we present several common storage technologies. The discussion is summarized in Table 9.2, which also highlights relative

TABLE 9.2
Differential Variables for Various Storage Options (in 2002)

Technology	Relative Cost per MB	Storage Capacity Range	Access Time (mS)
Solid-State Memory	$1.00–$100.00	MBs–GBs	.0001–2
Magnetic Disk	$0.09–$5.00	10's TBs	5–30
Optical Storage	$0.04	TBs	10000
Magnetic Tape Storage	$0.001–$0.01	TBs–PBs	10000–90000

hardware performance. We will avoid discussion of specific technologies and performance characteristics, as any specific discussion will become dated.

RANDOM ACCESS MEMORY (RAM)

RAM memory is the most expensive type of memory; it delivers the greatest speed for both reading and writing information. Physically, RAM memory is built on chips that reside on boards that are attached to the main computer board ("motherboard"). RAM today is usually measured in megabytes of capacity. Most RAM is volatile, meaning it is not permanent storage and must be constantly powered to retain the memory. When power is removed, data stored in RAM is lost. Nonvolatile RAM (NVRAM) does exist and is used in special applications, including portable computer systems. Typical personal computers for home use now routinely offer 128MB of RAM, with up to 256 MB not uncommon. It is not unusual nowadays to have special purpose UNIX workstations with gigabytes (thousands of megabytes) of RAM and PCs with hundreds of megabytes.

MAGNETIC DISK

Magnetic disk (or disk, for short) technology is a pervasive storage technology. The vast majority of on-line random access storage resides on magnetic disk. Magnetic disks provide fast, reliable access to data. Redundant Arrays of Inexpensive Disk (RAID) technology enhances both reliability and access. Much has been written about magnetic disk and RAID technology. Magnetic disk products come in many sizes, speeds, and capacities. It is not unusual to find disks in the 10 to 30 GB range with 50 and even 100 GB disks just around the corner.

All disk products have a few common characteristics. Disks have one or more read/write heads that are used to change the orientation of magnetic particles in a proscribed area on the disk's surface. The information stored in that area corresponds to a single bit. The number of bits per unit area on the storage medium's surface is referred to as *areal* density, and is a significant factor in the rapid evolution of storage technology. The disk platters (or surfaces) spin very fast, between 7200 and 10,000 RPM, and the read/write heads "fly" micrometers above the surface. Due to the fragile nature of this setup, and the devastating effects of the head touching the disk surface ("disk crash"), magnetic disks must stay within sealed, protected en-

TABLE 9.3
Description of Various Levels of RAID

RAID Level	Common Name	Number of Disks	Description
0	Disk Striping	N	No redundancy, Data distributed across N disks
1	Mirroring	2N, 3N, . . .	Data duplicated across multiple disks
3	RAID 3	N+1	Similar to RAID 0 with separate parity disk
5	RAID 5 "RAID"	N+1	Similar to RAID 3
6	RAID 6	N+2	Similar to RAID 5 with additional parity

vironments. For security, data should be maintained in multiple sites (i.e., backed-up) in case of disk failure.

RAID technology improves the reliability and performance of a single disk by spreading data between multiple disks. Using RAID technology, the failure of a single disk unit does not result in the total loss of data because a redundant data copy exists. To achieve this reliability, additional data (in the form of *parity* information) needs to be written to disk, and will adversely affect the total storage capacity of the RAID. The other major benefit of RAID technology is improved performance. With multiple disk drives available to read or write data, a RAID will simultaneously write in parallel across multiple data paths. Much greater read and write performance can be gained by this parallel operation. Several types of RAIDs, or RAID levels, exist. Table 9.3 briefly describes each of the common RAID levels.

OPTICAL AND MAGNETO-OPTICAL MEDIA

Medical imaging applications have used various optical storage technologies for many years, and several generations of optical storage devices have been used by the medical community. Optical technologies rely upon the reflective capacity of glass substrate to record information. Laser technology is used to selectively "burn" pits into the glass substrate. With older Write-Once, Read-Many (WORM) technology, recorded information cannot be altered once written. WORM technology provides a high level of security against nefarious data alteration. New magneto-optical disk (MOD) media use both magnetic and optical properties to both record and erase data.

Early PACS implementations used 14-inch WORM format products from Eastman Kodak (Rochester, NY) or 12-inch WORM formats from Philips (Best, Netherlands). More recently, 5-inch MOD products have been used. The large format platters provide large storage capacities (up to 14 GB) but have high media costs. Newer MOD platters, although providing less data storage per platter (latest technology at 5.2 GB) are significantly less expensive and provide better price per unit storage. These drives typically use small-computer system interfaces (SCSI) and provide sustained data rates of 3 to 4 MB/sec.

CD-R, DVD

Performance characteristics of CD-R (Compact Disk—Recordable, a write-once technology) and now CD-RW (Compact Disk—Rewritable) technologies have improved enough to consider them a viable medium for small to medium-sized radiology department archives. The capacity is approximately 600 MB, and write capabilities are approximately 0.6 MB/sec. The drives have become more robust and reliable. Drive and media costs have dropped significantly as the result of commercialization for the home personal computer marketplace.

DICOM has also fully embraced CD technology as a data *distribution* medium. Protocols exist to create device-independent file and file system structures on CD media. DICOM does not endorse CD as an archive medium, however.

DVD (Digital Versatile Disk) is an upcoming technology with video standards and a variety of commercial products existing today. Nonvideo formats are starting to appear. Unfortunately, no single standard dominates among several competing standards: DVD-R, DVD-RAM, DVD+RW, MMVF and ASMO. Some of these standards may be appropriate for medical data storage. DVD has the potential to improve upon shortcomings of CD technology. Most importantly, DVD will significantly improve storage capacity without significant read/write performance degradation. Existing formats offer approximately 5 GB media (double sided). Because of the commercial potential of DVD, it is expected that this technology will be significantly less expensive than competing technologies.

MAGNETIC TAPE

Magnetic tape products provide a low-cost removable storage medium. In the past 30 years, different tape products have been introduced and gone by the wayside. Performance limitations of early products relegated tape to the role of backup and disaster recovery purposes only. The intent of these backup schemes is to put "dead" data onto the lowest cost medium, and hope that one is never forced to read it again (affectionately known as WORN—write once, read never). Successive generations of tape products have provided newer technology with better price/performance ratios. Figure 9.6 demonstrates the difference in retrieval times for various storage modalities, including tape.

Tape media exist as either cartridges or cassette packages, and several different sizes exist in the marketplace. Cartridges contain a single spool of magnetic tape. During the read/write operations, the tape is unwound from the cartridge onto a take-up spool that exists within the tape drive mecha-

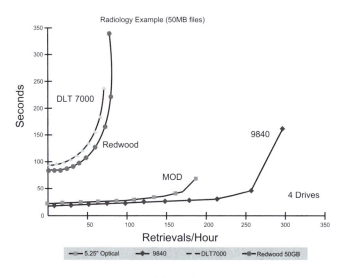

FIGURE 9.6

Times for average radiology ad-hoc retrieval.

nism. An example of cartridge technology is the digital linear tape (DLT) products offered by Quantum (Boulder, CO). Cassette packages, in contrast, have two spools. In a cassette, the tape does not physically leave the package. StorageTek's (Louisville, CO) 9840 product is an example of a cassette system offered in the same physical form-factor as the DLT cartridge. Advantages and disadvantages exist with both packaging technologies. Cartridge systems require pickup and threading mechanisms that are prone to failure. The tape leader strip, which contains information necessary to initialize and read the tape, is also subject to damage. Cassettes are less prone to loading problems. For a given package, however, cartridges are able to hold more recording medium than cassettes.

Three basic tape media types exist, with variations of each basic format:

▶ half-inch wide cartridge tape. Examples of this tape format include Storage Technology Corporation's 9840 and Redwood products, IBM's Magstar, and Quantum Corp's Digital Linear Tape (DLT).

▶ 8-mm wide cartridge tape. Exabyte and Sony manufacture products using this tape format.

▶ 4-mm wide cartridge. Hewlett Packard's Digital Audio Tape (DAT) is an example of this tape format.

Like film and optical media, tape devices have specific price, performance, capacity, and reliability characteristics. Individual products are designed and manufactured to address specific market needs, and 8-mm products typically target low price points and are therefore very applicable for desktop and small server or distributed archive applications. Half-inch tape products are designed for demanding environments such as large server, mainframe, and central archive applications. While more expensive, the half-inch products tend to be more robust and reliable.

High-capacity tape media has traditionally meant poor performance. In the last 5 years, magnetic tape has become a very robust, fast, and reliable method of storing "live" data. High capacity comes from long tapes combined with high-density data recording. These facts have adversely affected the usability of traditional tape products as "live" data storage products. Tape manufactures attempt to overcome this limitation in several ways, including the use of novel indexing techniques to facilitate rapid tape positioning. Newer tape products combine cassette packaging (reduced tape initialization time), mid-positioning of tape (first byte of data is now only $1/2$ the tape length away) and serpentine data tracks to significantly improve tape performance. Random retrievals of medical image studies (20 MB of data) can be performed, on average, within 20 sec.

ROBOTIC TECHNOLOGY

Individual media, whether magnetic disks, optical disks, or tape, have finite capacities. Tape and optical recording devices, fortunately, separate the read/write mechanism from the storage media, which allows multiple pieces of media to be serviced by one, or a few, readers. A manual procedure for replacing media, adequate for low-data demand environments, is inadequate for high-volume, high performance data archives.

Advanced robotic technology has been applied to this data storage problem. Automated library systems (ALS or "jukeboxes") consist of one or more readers, multiple shelves for media storage, and a robotic picker arm. The picker arm moves media to and from storage shelves and reader devices. The ALS attaches directly to a computer (usually an NT or UNIX server) via a SCSI interface (Small Computer Systems Interface) or serial port. Control of the ALS is separate from the control and data paths of the data drive. These two activities must be coordinated by software on the host computer for the complete system to function properly.

ALS for optical storage products are available from a number of manufacturers. Shelf capacities range from tens to hundreds of platters. Tape ALS are also available from a number of manufacturers. Products range from managing 10s to 1000s of tapes. High-end products enable multiple ALS to be physically connected, and tapes can be automatically passed between interconnected libraries. This feature extends the utility of both ALS and tape transports.

ARCHIVE CONSIDERATIONS

COSTS

Most radiology professionals are familiar with the direct cost of radiographic film. What is less well understood are the indirect costs associated with processing and personnel for handling, filing, and retrieving medical image data. Research performed at the Mayo Foundation indicated that the accumulated costs for acquisition, handling, and storage of film-based medical images ranged from 10s to 100s of dollars for 7 years per sheet of film. If you

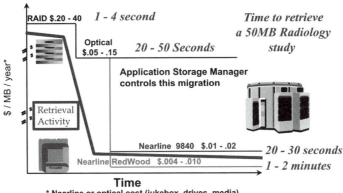

FIGURE 9.7

Storage cost matched with retrieval activity.

consider the total cost of ownership of an archive over a period of 5 or 7 years and divide that cost by the number of years, you can estimate the average cost of a given level of storage in dollars per MB per year. This cost can then be related to the level of archive featured and its role in the archive (Figure 9.7).

The cost of ownership should include the ALS, drives, media, and maintenance cost. Other operational costs, such as electrical power, cooling, and floor space (not insignificant if the device is located within a hospital), should not be overlooked.

CAPACITIES

It has been estimated that by the year 2003, 10% of the world's knowledge data will exist in digital format; the remaining 90% will remain on paper, microfiche, film or other nonmachine readable formats (Figure 9.8).

Healthcare is seeing a rapid transition from analog to digital information use and storage. The volume of data produced by an imaging department depends on the type, quantity and distribution of studies performed. The volume can be calculated easily by taking the number of each digital modality multiplied by the number of studies performed per year times the average study size. An average study size can be calculated by determining the number of bytes per image multiplied by the number of images per study. The number of bytes per images equals the number of pixels in the horizontal dimension multiplied by the number of pixels in the vertical di-

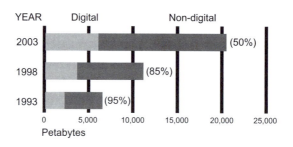

FIGURE 9.8

Trends in digital vs. nondigital storage.

mension multiplied by the number of bytes stored per pixel. For example, a CT image consists of 512 horizontal pixels $\times$ 512 vertical pixels $\times$ 2 bytes per pixel. If a study consists of 100 images, then 52.4 MB is required to store the study. Performing this calculation for each modality times the number of studies per year and tallying should provide the number of bytes produced per year. Table 9.4 lists storage requirements for common radiographic examinations, as well as other data storage for comparisons.

RELIABILITY

An extremely important aspect of any computer system is reliability and robustness. Most major companies that rely on data processing equipment for the daily operations fully understand the implications of what would happen if these systems were not available for even short periods of time. Financial institutions, mail order catalog companies, and insurance companies often measure their risk in the millions of dollars per hour that they are without their systems.

The reliability of an archive is often measured in terms of how often the system is "down" (unavailable) and therefore unable to retrieve requested data. Any number of reasons may lead to data being unavailable. Component failure, including individual media failure, ALS, computer, or even network failure can render the archive useless. In general, computer technology is very reliable, and metrics exist to help evaluate the reliability of individual pieces of technology. Unmanaged computer systems average approximately 90% uptime. Unfortunately, 90% uptime corresponds to 36 days/year when the system is not available. Implementing good management processes and procedures improves average uptime to greater than 99% (less

TABLE 9.4
Variable Size Considerations for Storage Options

Radiology	Size	Comments
CT Image	0.5 MB	(512 × 512) pixels × 2 bytes/pixel
MRI Image	0.03 MB	(128 × 128) pixels × 2 bytes/pixel
CR Image	7.67 MB	14" × 17" — (1760 × 2180) pixels × 2 bytes/pixel
Mammo Image	10.3 MB	8" × 10" — (2032 × 2540) pixels × 2 bytes/pixel
Departmental Archive	2 TB	100,000 exams/year (17.5% CT, 17.5% MR, 60% CR and 5% Mammography). Uncompressed
Printed Document		
Text page	2500 bytes	Single sided, ASCII
Printed Image	.9 MB	8" × 10" Black & White, 300 DPI
Novel	1 MB	400 pages
Library	10 TB	10 Million Volumes (Library of Congress)
Video		
Computer Screen	.31 MB	VGA, 256 colors
Video Frame	.9 MB	NTSC Studio quality
Movie	200 GB	120 minutes NTSC studio quality
Movie Library	10 PB	50,000 movies (nearly all?)
Audio		
Telephony	22 MB	One hour recording
CD	635 MB	One hour recording

than 3.6 down days/year). To improve reliability beyond this level requires specific design considerations, and plans can be developed to remove single points of failure and to mitigate the effects of technology failure.

Earthquakes, floods, fires (and related water damage), and tornadoes are all disasters that can destroy digital systems in a hospital and render PACS systems useless. Every radiology department that considers PACS for their facility should include disaster recovery (DR) planning in the purchase and implementation process of the system. The three main points regarding DR planning are:

❯ Have a plan,
❯ Test the plan, and
❯ Hope you never have to use the plan.

SCALABILITY AND ACCOMMODATING NEW TECHNOLOGY

The pace of technology evolution causes some hardware and software systems to become obsolete in a few years. The pace of change puts severe pressure on the ability of the related data structures or formats to continue to effectively represent information. This is not only a problem for traditional archives, but for many organizations that have never thought of themselves as performing an archival function. Although some archives may be temporary, some or all of their information may need to be preserved indefinitely. *Long-term* is long enough to be concerned with the impact of changing technologies, including support for new media and data formats, and with a changing user community. It extends indefinitely.

Analog forms of archiving (paper, film, or microfilm) require some sunlight, a magnifying glass and a good pair of eyes to read (assuming the medium is in good shape). The same cannot be said for digital media. Reading digital media is a complex undertaking requiring a specific "system." This system is composed of the media reader, a computer, and software, plus personnel trained to retrieve the data from the digital medium. If you are missing any one of these components the digital medium is useless. A manufacturer's assurances of 30 years of medium life is probably not the limiting factor when considering long-term digital data retrieval. It is important to understand that an organization's data represents one of its most valuable assets, and investment protection is very important.

Prudence is warranted when choosing technology (hardware, software and medium) for an archive. Choose a technology that meets your current needs as well as expected growth within a 5- to 7-year window. Consider financial, capacity, reliability, and performance variables carefully. Make sure that you understand the expected life of the technology you choose. You don't need to purchase 7 years' worth of storage up front, but do make sure that the system you buy can be easily upgraded by purchasing additional capacity. Buying the amount of storage you need for a year or so with the expectation of changing technology is wise only if you are assured that the storage you buy now will be easily upgraded (and not totally changed or swapped out).

If you choose to change to the latest and greatest storage device, it will most likely be very expensive and probably a painful process. There may, however, be reasons to change archive technology. As with any purchasing decision, you must carefully weigh the merits of moving to new technology. A few questions should be considered before investing in new technology. What is the financial life of your current system? Does it still meet the needs and requirements you defined before the implementation? When will your storage management software and computer operating system support the new hardware? What are the cost and benefits of changing to the new technology? Finally, how will data be migrated from existing technology to new technology? Poor planning can result in several technology changes, or possibly an archive requiring several types of media and devices for retrieval and reading.

FUTURE TECHNOLOGY AND TRENDS

OPTICAL STORAGE

Holographic storage today is an experimental technology. Holography relies upon the fact that certain inorganic crystals possess photorefractive properties. Data can be written to and read from the crystals using pairs of laser beams: one laser represents the object and the other represents a reference beam. The interference pattern created by the two beams is used to encode the data. Holographic storage devices have the potential to provide areal densities on the order of 800 Gb/in^2, far exceeding today's disk drives (approximately 1 Gb/in^2) and magnetic storage potential (approx. 20 Gb/in^2). Holography's low-cost, random access, and extremely high capacity represents the potential for a major breakthrough in data recording.

NETWORK ATTACHED STORAGE (NAS) AND STORAGE AREA NETWORKS (SAN)

Specialization is taking place as local area networks (LANs) become more common. Within the network infrastructure, general-purpose hubs are being replace by specialized routers and switches. This specialization is beginning to highlight looming storage and I/O bottlenecks that await broadly available network computing systems. Two storage trends are working to counteract the potential limitations. Network Attached Storage (NAS) devices are special purpose servers designed to perform one task—serving network files—very efficiently. Offloading storage and I/O function from application servers frees CPU cycles and bandwidth, resulting in improved application performance. An extension of the NAS is the Storage Area Network (SAN). SANs provide a physically separate network for storage traffic. In a SAN, storage devices form a pool that is externalized from individual servers, allowing large-scale storage systems to be shared between multiple host servers. By separating user and storage traffic, the number of application and storage servers can be scaled independently to meet user performance requirements. SANs are just beginning to gain momentum, and are being fueled primarily by advances in high-speed networks such as Fibre Channel and NAS.

REMOTE DATA VAULTS

Electronic data vaulting is an emerging strategy for off-site data storage. The market is being driven by the increasing number of natural disasters, terrorism, viruses, and widespread information and security exposures presented by the Internet. Electronic data vaulting provides off-site or geographically distant storage and retrieval of data. Alternative access to secondary data centers or backup hot-sites provides automated recovery in minutes instead of hours or days. Broadband transmission links, such as T3 and other optical fibers, between primary and secondary sites makes this an attractive alternative. The near-term prospect for reduced transmission costs from telecommunication companies, transportation, and utility companies offers further promise for this market.

IMAGE COMPRESSION

STEPHEN MANN

Modern medical practice has a need for storing enormous amounts of data. In addition, special applications like telemedicine place special constraints on bandwidth requirements, or more simply put, on the amount of information that can be sent in a given period of time. Telemedicine uses telecommunications—that is, the transmission of medical images over standard telephone lines, with satellite connections, or over a local area network (LAN)—to transfer medical services and information from one location to another. This includes not only data from information systems and teleconferencing, but also images from teleradiology. Whenever there are space or bandwidth limitations, image compression should be considered. Images usually make up the bulk of medical data, so compressing them can greatly reduce space requirements.

To introduce image compression, let's take a simple image and compress it. Suppose we have a small picture containing 8 rows of 12 dots (Figure 10.1). Each dot, called a *pixel* (zero picture element), represents 16 possible gray values ranging from 0 (completely black) to 15 (completely white). In this example picture, each row gets steadily lighter from left to right, and the last five rows get steadily darker from left to right starting from the fifth column. We wish to compress this image without loss. What do we do?

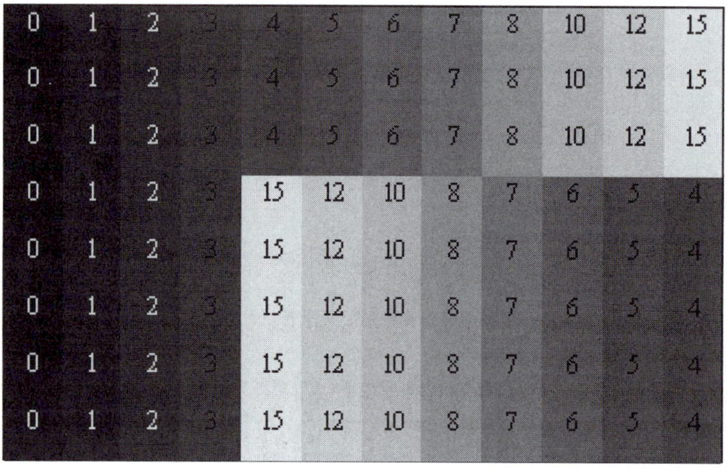

0	1	2	3	4	5	6	7	8	10	12	15
0	1	2	3	4	5	6	7	8	10	12	15
0	1	2	3	4	5	6	7	8	10	12	15
0	1	2	3	15	12	10	8	7	6	5	4
0	1	2	3	15	12	10	8	7	6	5	4
0	1	2	3	15	12	10	8	7	6	5	4
0	1	2	3	15	12	10	8	7	6	5	4
0	1	2	3	15	12	10	8	7	6	5	4

FIGURE 10.1

Small 8 × 12 example picture.

Since each pixel can be one of 16 possible gray values, it takes 4 bits to store each pixel value. There are 96 pixels, so 384 bits are needed to store this image in raw form: that is, without compression.

The first step is to choose a compression method. One simple method, which is supported in lossless JPEG, is difference encoding. In this model each gray pixel value is replaced by the difference between it and its prior value. Since the first pixel in each row has no prior pixel, the first pixel on the line above is used for differencing. However the first pixel of the first line has no pixel above, so the gray value of 8 (i.e., midway between black and white) is used for differencing. When this is done the image array shown in Figure 10.2 is created.

The first value is 0 minus 8 (the special case for the first pixel of the first line). The next pixel is 1 minus 0 or 1, the next pixel is 2 minus 1 or 1, and so on. The first 2 comes from 10 minus 8. The first pixel of the second line is 0 minus 0 (from the line above it).

A count of values can now be created and code values based on frequencies can be assigned (Table 10.1), where the value that occurs the most (1 occurs 39 times) is assigned the code value that requires the smallest number of bits (code 0 requires only 1 bit because it is only one bit long). These code values are called Huffman codes, and have these nice properties: (a) code lengths that are close to the minimum for the given frequencies and (b) each code is unique and unambiguous. This latter property means that the bits comprising the codes can be appended together, creating a sequence

-8	1	1	1	1	1	1	1	1	2	2	3
0	1	1	1	1	1	1	1	1	2	2	3
0	1	1	1	1	1	1	1	1	2	2	3
0	1	1	1	12	-3	-2	-2	-1	-1	-1	-1
0	1	1	1	12	-3	-2	-2	-1	-1	-1	-1
0	1	1	1	12	-3	-2	-2	-1	-1	-1	-1
0	1	1	1	12	-3	-2	-2	-1	-1	-1	-1
0	1	1	1	12	-3	-2	-2	-1	-1	-1	-1

FIGURE 10.2

Pixel differences from left.

of bits that can be uniquely parsed back into the original codes (during the decompression stage). Using the codes generated in Table 10.1, this bit stream begins:

111111 0 0 0 0 0 0 0 0 1101 1101 111110 1100 0 0 0 0 0 0 0 ...

TABLE 10.1

Pixel Frequencies and Codes (Left Differences)

Value	Frequency	Code	Code length
1	39	0	1
−1	20	100	3
−2	10	101	3
0	7	1100	4
2	6	1101	4
−3	5	1110	4
12	5	11110	5
3	3	111110	6
−8	1	111111	6

(The spaces have been inserted for clarity and visually delimit the next code value, or pixel.)

The total length of the code is:

$$39 \times 1 + 20 \times 3 + 10 \times 3 + 7 \times 4 + \ldots 1 \times 6 = 225$$

This is the number of bits required to represent the compressed image.

To see what happens with a different modeling of the image, consider a model in which each gray value is replaced by the difference between it and the pixel value *above* it (as opposed to the left of it as in the previous example). The first line will be treated as in the prior model. (This model is also supported in JPEG with selector-value set to 2.) We get the Figure 10.3 image array.

The first line is the same as above. The first pixel of the second line is 0 minus 0 or 0. The second pixel is 1minus 1 or 0, and so on for the rest of the line. The 11 comes from 15 minus 4, the 7 from 13 minus 6, etc.

A new count of values can be created and code values based on these new frequencies can be assigned (Table 10.2). As before, these code values are Huffman codes. Using the codes generated in Table 10.2, this bit stream begins:

11011 10 10 10 10 10 10 10 10 11000 11000 11001 0 0 0 0 0 0 0 0 0 0 0 0 0 0 . . .

-8	1	1	1	1	1	1	1	1	2	2	3
0	0	0	0	0	0	0	0	0	0	0	0
0	0	0	0	0	0	0	0	0	0	0	0
0	0	0	0	11	7	4	1	-1	-4	-7	-11
0	0	0	0	0	0	0	0	0	0	0	0
0	0	0	0	0	0	0	0	0	0	0	0
0	0	0	0	0	0	0	0	0	0	0	0
0	0	0	0	0	0	0	0	0	0	0	0

FIGURE 10.3

Pixel differences from above.

TABLE 10.2
Pixel Frequencies and Codes (Above Differences)

Value	Frequency	Code	Code length
0	76	0	1
1	9	10	2
2	2	11000	5
3	1	11001	5
−11	1	11010	5
−8	1	11011	5
−7	1	11100	5
−4	1	11101	5
−1	1	111100	6
4	1	111101	6
7	1	111110	6
11	1	111111	6

This is a different bit stream from than which we generated from Table 10.1. Also note that for decompression, the table must be included with the compressed data in order to properly interpret the code values. This overhead is usually negligible with medical images.

The total length of the code is:

$$76 \times 1 + 9 \times 2 + 2 \times 5 + 1 \times 5 + \ldots \; 1 \times 6 = 153$$

This is the number of bits required to represent the image.

A change in the method has changed the compression from 225 bits to 153 bits. This shows that the method used can have significant effect on the resulting compression.

IMAGE COMPRESSION BASICS

Image compression can be described using the diagram shown in Figure 10.4.

The encoding process converts a raw image into a coded image. The decoding process converts a coded image into a decoded image. The pur-

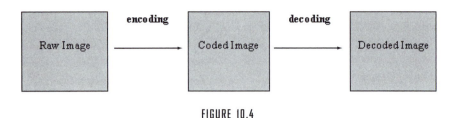

FIGURE 10.4

Compression/decompression.

pose of image compression is to make the coded image as small as possible, with the constraint that the decoded image has to be acceptably close to the raw image. Unfortunately, these goals are at odds with one another. Typically, the more compactly the image is compressed the worse the decoded image looks, and conversely, the better the decoded image looks the larger the coded image. Good compression techniques balance these two opposing goals and allow the user to trade compression for quality in any given image.

If the decoded image is identical to the raw image, we say that the method of encoding and decoding is *lossless*. If the decoded image differs from the raw image, we say that the method of encoding and decoding is *lossy*.

The coded image is saved in some standard interchange format, such as lossless JPEG or lossy JPEG. These standards are well defined and allow diverse applications to successfully decode an image.

All compression methods that we discuss can be described by the diagram shown in Figure 10.5. Decompression follows an analogous diagram where each process is effectively reversed. Together the modeling and entropy encoding processes make up the *compression method*. Likewise the entropy decoding and modeling processes make up the *decompression method*.

The *raw image* is represented by an array of width pixels per line by height lines per image. Each pixel represents a specific color or grayscale value, and there are width × height pixels per image. The *transformed image* is a conceptualization representing what happens to the raw image after the modeling process has been applied. The image may be physically represented as a separate image, but it is usually not explicitly created (typically no one needs to see this image). Values in the transformed image usually are directly entropy encoded (the process of storing pixel data more efficiently than is possible in the raw or transformed image) and placed in the coded image. The *coded image* holds the compressed data representing the

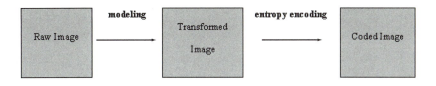

Decompression follows an analogous diagram where each process is effectively reversed:

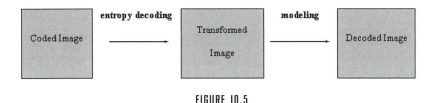

FIGURE 10.5

Compression and decompression methods.

original image. This data is typically in the form of a sequence of bits called a bit stream.

An image is characterized by the distribution of pixels in the image and the relationship between pixels. *Modeling* is a process based on this characterization, which converts a raw image into a transformed image. In addition, an appropriate modeling must be able to convert the transformed image back into a decoded image and should also have the property that the transformed image can be represented in less space than the raw image.

Many different models can be used to represent data; the trick is to find a good model with reasonable implementation. For example, a continuous-tone grayscale image such as an X-ray is represented by an array of pixels, where each pixel holds a value proportional to the brightness of the X-ray at that point. This representation is the raw image. In most such images a pixel's value tends to be close to the prior pixel's value. This leads to a modeling in which the *difference* between successive pixel values is stored rather than storing the pixel values directly. The transformed image is the array of differences rather than the original array of grayscale values. The justification for making this transformation is that the differences tend to be small, and the smaller values tend to be more frequent than the larger values. (We saw this tendency in the example in the introduction.) In the entropy encoding part of the compression, these small differences can be stored more compactly than the original grayscale values, thus giving a smaller coded image.

A model can be simple or complex; the model might introduce loss or it might be lossless. An appropriate choice of model depends on the class of the image. (More examples are given later.) Since the appearance of an image is very subjective, a good lossy model will take into account the human visual system when trying to find redundant or less significant information to discard. This is accomplished in JPEG by using the fact that the human eye is sensitive to certain image frequencies and not very sensitive to others. By setting up a frequency quantization table based on each image, JPEG can take advantage of the eye's sensitivity by reducing the precision of certain frequencies yet maintaining an image that is visually close to the original.

Entropy encoding is lossless. The amount of data is reduced by removing redundant information, but there is no loss of information in that the original data can be re-created. Thus, the transformed image prior to entropy encoding is the same as the transformed image after entropy decoding.

For additional information on general image compression, the link: *http://compression-pointers.com* points to most other references of interest on the Net. The link *http://cctpwww.cityu.edu.hk/public/graphics/ g_std.htm* refers to general graphics and multimedia standards. Also see Kay and Levine (1992) for various file interchange formats.

CLASSIFICATION OF IMAGES AND COMPRESSION STANDARDS

There are a number of different types of images; each type has a different pixel distribution and therefore a different apparent model for transforming the data. For medical imaging we are concerned with the following types of images:

1. Continuous-tone grayscale images, such as X-rays, MRI scans, or PET scans.
2. Continuous-tone color images, such as those used in plastic surgery, dental reconstruction, or microscope slides.
3. Continuous-tone grayscale motion video, such as those made during CAT scans or ultrasounds.
4. Continuous-tone color motion video, such as Doppler ultrasound or thermal imaging.
5. Discrete grayscale or color-palletized images such as graphs, EKGs, or other recorder output.
6. Bilevel documents, such as lab reports and patient histories.

Compression methods for medical images have been defined by the Digital Imaging and Communications in Medicine (DICOM) committee. This committee has created a standard that is a set of rules allowing medical images to be exchanged between instruments, computers, and hospitals. The standard establishes a common language that guarantees a medical image produced on one vendor's machine will be displayable on a workstation from another vendor. The DICOM standard evolved from a long series of meetings between software engineers from all major imaging and computer companies (representing the National Electrical Manufacturers' Association, NEMA) and physician representatives from major professional societies, such as the American College of Radiology, the American Society of Echocardiography, and the American College of Cardiology. The DICOM committee has deemed lossless JPEG and lossy JPEG to be acceptable image compression techniques for use on medical images.

JPEG (Joint Photographic Experts Group) is an ISO/IEC international standard for compression and coding of continuous-tone still images. MPEG (Motion Picture Expert Group) is an ISO/IEC international standard for compression and coding of continuous-tone motion video and audio. G3/G4 (Recommendation T.4: *Standardization of Group 3 Facsimile Apparatus for Document Transmission* / Recommendation T.6: *Facsimile Coding Schemes and Coding Control Functions for Group 4 Facsimile Apparatus*) are international standards for lossless compression used to save and store bilevel images (e.g., black and white images such as documents).

Image types 1 and 2 in the foregoing list are candidates for lossy JPEG compression; image types 3 and 4 are candidates for MPEG compression or motion JPEG; image types 1 and 5 are candidates for lossless JPEG compression; and image type 6 is a candidate for G3/G4 compression or more likely for storage in ASCII (that is, as text instead of as a picture) as part of the DICOM record. For medicine, JPEG provides a good general-purpose method for a wide variety of images. This is one reason why JPEG is used in the DICOM standard.

Image types 1 and 2 are candidates for wavelet compression and are supported in the latest version of JPEG called JPEG 2000.

ERROR

How faithful to the original raw image is the decompressed image? If the compression/decompression method is lossless, you can be sure that there is no loss and that no more faithful image can be created. However, lossless compression gives only two to three times reduction on most images. Usually this is not enough for reasonable storage or transmission requirements. To gain significantly more compression, lossy compression must be used. How can this loss be measured?

This is a tough problem because the appearance of an image is very subjective. Further, in medical applications, the features that are of interest, such as irregularities in texture, small fractures, and subtle shadows, are often the first elements of the image discarded. There are standard statistical analyses, such as Root Mean Square Deviation (RMSD), which can compare the raw image with the decoded image on a pixel-by-pixel basis to give a number, but this statistic is not very satisfactory. For example, suppose the decoded image is identical to the raw image shifted right by one pixel. Comparing the raw image with the decoded image will give a very high RMSD, but the images will appear identical.

Conversely, suppose the raw image is a picture of a smiling face and the decoded image is identical to the raw image except that one front tooth is blackened. Comparing the raw image with the decoded image will give a very low RMSD, but the decoded image will be unacceptable. The RMSD statistic is used only because no better statistic has been universally accepted.

How, then, should lossy compression be used? One answer is to not use lossy compression at all! This is a very conservative answer based partly on the reasoning that "you can't be sure that information discarded is not significant," and on the legal argument that a doctor should not make a decision based on partial information if more complete information is available.

This answer is not supported in a practical sense. Usually the image contains diagnostic features that readily support a doctor's diagnosis; these features are not so subtle that they are lost by the compression method. Second, some loss is inevitable because the scanning process introduces error. The low-order bits of a 10-bit or 12-bit scan are usually noise. Attempting to preserve this noise is not only a waste of compression space but also gives a false sense of accuracy. Third, the compression method and parameters should be "tuned" to the particular application. This means that an image set that represents the range of images of interest should be compressed using various quality/compression settings of the compression method. A conservative setting that gives satisfactory quality for all the decompressed images can be used with reasonable confidence. In most cases a 10- to 15-fold reduction in image size can be obtained with this conservative setting. This is significantly better than the two- to three-fold reduction that lossless compression gives.

Other medical uses for imaging can compress much further. Images used for training and other nondiagnostic purposes can usually be compressed 20-fold or more without visual loss. Also, the proportional amount of redundant information in an image tends to grow with image size. A 256×256 scan of a tooth X-ray might be compressed satisfactorily at 10:1. A 4000×8000 scan of a chest X-ray might be compressed satisfactorily at 60:1. Such examples reinforce the point that tests should be made prior to selecting a compression level for a particular application.

RUN-LENGTH COMPRESSION

A simple compression technique that is especially good for computer-generated charts and graphs, in which many pixels have the same value, is run-length compression. The idea is quite simple. Instead of storing each pixel as it occurs, the method stores a pixel and the number of times it is repeated.

For example, let's take the differences from our first example image in Figure 10.2. We compute the run-length counts and values in Table 10.3.

TABLE 10.3
Run-length Counts

Count	Value
1	−8
8	1
2	2
1	3
28	0
1	11
1	7
1	4
1	1
1	−1
1	−4
1	−7
1	−11
48	0

Let us assume the counts range from 1 to 16 so that the value count − 1 may be stored in 4 bits. (This means that the count of 8 will be stored as 7 = 8 − 1, and 28 will be stored as 15 = 16 − 1 plus 11 = 12 − 1.) If we then apply the code values found in Table 10.3, we get the bit stream shown in Figure 10.6.

We have reduced the bit stream to 63 bits plus bits required to represent Table 10.3 in the bit stream for decompression. While this is pretty good for our simple example, continuous-tone grayscale images do not usually have such large repetitions. This method should be reserved for discrete grayscale or color-paletized images, such as graphs, EKGs, or other recorder output.

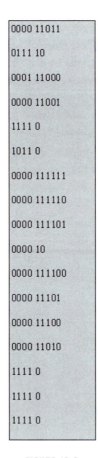

FIGURE 10.6

Run-length bit streams.

G3/G4 COMPRESSION (FAX)

G3 is no more than a run-length encoding of the white and black spaces in a line. Each run-length is stored as a predetermined Huffman code, and since the white and black runs must alternate, there is no need to store the actual pixel value. Therefore a coded line consists of the Huffman code for the number of initial white spaces followed by the Huffman code for the number of successive black spaces followed by the Huffman code for the number of successive white spaces, and so on until the end of the line is reached. G4 is similar to G3, using the same Huffman table but taking advantage of the previous line's pixels to position successive runs of white and black pixels.

See *www.ncs.gov/n6/content/standard/html/ftr1062.htm* to acquire the standard.

This method is most appropriate for bilevel documents such as lab reports and patient histories.

JPEG COMPRESSION

JPEG compression is designed for continuous-tone grayscale images, such as X-rays or MRI scans, and for continuous-tone color images, such as color photographs or stained slides.

Both lossless and lossy JPEG compression share a common file representation. This representation is flexible and easy to extend for adding new image components if needed. The file is nothing more than a sequence of marker segments. Each such segment contains a marker code that indicates the type of segment optionally followed by length and data fields. The length field indicates how long the length-data field is, and the data field holds the information corresponding to the segment type.

The exact format of the marker codes and the values they must contain is specified in the ISO document: *Digital Compression and Coding of Continuous-tone Still Images.* This chapter describes both the lossy and lossless methods of JPEG compression (see Pennebaker and Mitchell, 1993). To obtain an actual program to perform lossless and lossy JPEG compression and decompression, see the companion CD or go to the Web site *www.jpg.com.* This Web site also has a number of JPEG utilities and a program called Viewmed for viewing medical images.

All JPEG files begin with a Start Of Image (SOI) marker. This marker has no length or data field and is used only to indicate the start of the image. The next marker segments hold table information, such as the Define Quantization Table (DQT) marker and the Define Huffman Table (DHT) marker. Next comes the Start Of Frame (SOF) marker. This marker contains such information as the sample precision (typically 8 for 256 levels of gray), the number of lines in the image, the number of pixels per line, the number of image components in the image (typically 1 for grayscale or 3 for color), the various quantization tables to use, and other information. Additional tables can follow this marker. Then comes the Start Of Scan (SOS) marker. This marker indicates the number of image components and indicates which of the Huffman tables to use. Additional information, depending on whether the compression is lossy or lossless, is also included in this marker. Immediately following this marker comes the entropy-coded segments that hold the actual compressed data. The data is so constructed that any marker codes that might be embedded in the data can be easily recognized. Additional markers may follow the entropy-coded segments. The last marker is an End Of Image (EOI) marker. It denotes the end of the image data and can be used as a check that the proper number of pixels have been decompressed.

All the code from the SOI up to and including the EOI comprise the JPEG interchange format for compressed image data. Any application that purports to read JPEG must be able to recognize this code. Additional markers can be included in the compressed image, such as a comment marker and general application markers holding arbitrary information, but these markers can be ignored by an application. For medical applications, it is best to use the DICOM structures for comments and image descriptions rather than the JPEG internal comments, since other medical applications have access to the DICOM data but not necessarily to the JPEG data.

LOSSLESS JPEG

In this modeling of the image, each pixel value x is predicted from previously decoded pixel values. The difference of the predicted value from the actual value is stored in the transformed image. If the prediction is good, the differences will be small and good compression can be achieved.

In Figure 10.7, let a be the value of the pixel to the left of the target pixel value x, let b be the value of the pixel above the target pixel x, and let c be the value of the pixel above-left of the target pixel value x. Various predictions using a, b, and c can be used to compute x' which is an estimate for x.

Lossless JPEG provides seven different predictions denoted by a selection-value (Table 10.4). The standard DICOM selector-value is 1; that

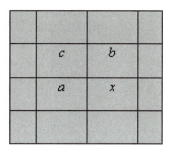

FIGURE 10.7

Neighbors of x.

is, the prediction for x is simply the value of the pixel preceding x. Of course the boundary cases have to be handled. The first pixel in a row of pixels has no preceding x; for this case the first pixel in the prior row is used. For the first line, the first pixel is simply estimated as midway between the possible gray values; thus, if there are 256 possible gray levels, the value 128 is used as the estimate of the first pixel of the first row. The rest of the first row uses the prior pixel value to predict the next pixel value. In this manner there is a prediction for all possible pixel values. Once a prediction x' is made, it is subtracted from the actual pixel value x. This difference $(x - x')$ is the value in the transformed image, which is subsequently entropy encoded. For lossless JPEG, the entropy encoding is simply Huffman encoding using a

TABLE 10.4

JPEG Predictors

Selection-value	Prediction
1	$x' = a$
2	$x' = b$
3	$x' = c$
4	$x' = a + b - c$
5	$x' = a + (b - c)/2$
6	$x' = b + (a - c)/2$
7	$x' = (a + b)/2$

TABLE 10.5
Typical Huffman Codes

Difference	Huffman value
. . .	. . .
−3	01100
−2	01101
−1	0100
0	00
+1	0101
+2	01110
+3	01111
. . .	. . .

table optimized for the particular image. For example, Table 10.5 might be generated. If the original pixel values were 8 bits, replacing these values by differences that average 4 bits would give a reduction in code size by 2:1. The Huffman values in the table must be included in the coded image to allow proper decompression. This overhead, although small, must be included in the size of the compressed image.

LOSSY JPEG

This discussion treats grayscale images; the extensions to color are discussed later. In this modeling of the image, shown in Figure 10.8, the image is broken up into blocks of pixels 8 pixels wide × 8 pixels high. Except for the first coefficient, each of these blocks is then compressed independently of one another.

Each 8 × 8 block of pixel values is transformed into an 8 × 8 block of DCT coefficients using what is known as the Forward Discrete Cosine Transform (FDCT). This transform converts the block from the spatial domain to the frequency domain. The reason for this transform is apparent in the next step.

So far there has been no significant loss in the image. The FDCT transformation may have introduced some round-off error, but this is usu-

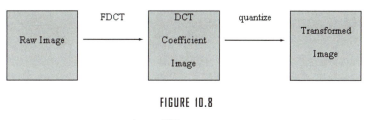

FIGURE 10.8

Lossy JPEG compression.

ally within a bit of being correct. Next we purposely introduce loss to further reduce the compressed image size.

The eye is more sensitive to certain frequencies than others. To gain significant compression without apparent visual loss, certain of the block's frequencies can be "quantized"; that is, their values can be represented with less precision than usual. To take an example, suppose a certain frequency has a value in the range 0, 1, 2, 3, . . . 15. We can quantize this frequency value by dividing the value by 3 and throwing away any remainder. The values are then 0, 0, 0, 1, 1, 1, 2, . . . 5. We can then store a value in the range 0 to 5 instead of a value in the range 0 to 15, thus gaining a reduction in size. The loss arises when we decompress the block. The only possible decompression values are 0, 3, 6, 9, 12, and 15. If the original value had been 1 or 2, its decompressed value is approximated by 0. If the original value had been 7 or 8, its decompressed value is approximated by 6, and so on. The divisor (3 in the above case) needs to be chosen so that the loss due to quantization for that frequency is not visually apparent. There are 64 such divisors, one for each possible frequency. This set of divisors makes up the quantization table, which is stored in the DQT marker segment at the start of the image. (If the image is in color, there may be one or two more quantization tables corresponding to the frequencies for other components: red, blue, and green for example.) Changing the table produces different levels of compression with a corresponding change in the quality of the resulting image. If you use JPEG to change the quality/size parameter, you are actually changing the quantization table.

After quantization, the transformed image goes through entropy encoding as usual. This encoding takes advantage of the fact that many (most) of the new quantized values are 0. By cleverly arranging the coefficients (in what is called the zig-zag order), most of the 0 coefficients come at the end of the sequence of coefficients. When all remaining coefficients are 0, an end-of-block symbol can be used to significantly shorten the number of codes sent, which reduces the compressed image size. As in lossless JPEG, an optimized Huffman table is generated, which gives good compression for the runs of 0, the coded quantized coefficients, and the end-of-block. This table is stored in the DHT marker segment.

COLOR COMPRESSION FOR JPEG

Up to this point we have avoided the issue of color. Color images are usually captured as three images, corresponding to red, green, and blue, which correspond to the three colors to which the eye is sensitive. Other colors are admixtures of these three colors with varying intensities. Because the eye is much less sensitive to color information than it is to brightness information, an opportunity for compressing color arises. This is done by first converting the RGB colors into YC_bC_r colors. YC_bC_r colors use the Y component to hold the luminance value (to which the eye is sensitive) and the C_b and C_r components to hold the color information (to which the eye is less sensitive). JPEG has provisions to subsample the C_b and C_r components with respect to the Y component. For example, suppose we have the 6×4 raw pixel values (in color, each pixel contains a red, green, and blue value) (see Figure 10.9).

We first compute Y, C_b, and C_r from R, G, and B for each pixel using an appropriate algorithm. Then we subsample C_b and C_r by averaging groups of C_b and C_r pixel values both horizontally and vertically. We get the results shown in Figure 10.10.

Only one quarter of the C_b and C_r values are used and the total number of pixels has been cut in half. When we decompress the image, the missing values of C_b and C_r are interpolated from the given values. Since the eye is not very sensitive to the color values, the reconstructed image appears almost the same as the original.

R_{11} G_{11} B_{11}	R_{12} G_{12} B_{12}	R_{13} G_{13} B_{13}	R_{14} G_{14} B_{14}	R_{15} G_{15} B_{15}	R_{16} G_{16} B_{16}
R_{21} G_{21} B_{21}	R_{22} G_{22} B_{22}	R_{23} G_{23} B_{23}	R_{24} G_{24} B_{24}	R_{25} G_{25} B_{25}	R_{26} G_{26} B_{26}
R_{31} G_{31} B_{31}	R_{32} G_{32} B_{32}	R_{33} G_{33} B_{33}	R_{34} G_{34} B_{34}	R_{35} G_{35} B_{35}	R_{36} G_{36} B_{36}
R_{41} G_{41} B_{41}	R_{42} G_{42} B_{42}	R_{41} G_{43} B_{43}	R_{44} G_{44} B_{44}	R_{45} G_{45} B_{45}	R_{46} G_{46} B_{46}

FIGURE 10.9

Raw color pixel values.

Y_{11}	Y_{12}	Y_{13}	Y_{14}	Y_{15}	Y_{16}
Y_{21}	Y_{22}	Y_{23}	Y_{24}	Y_{25}	Y_{26}
Y_{31}	Y_{32}	Y_{33}	Y_{34}	Y_{35}	Y_{36}
Y_{41}	Y_{42}	Y_{43}	Y_{44}	Y_{45}	Y_{46}

C_{b11}	C_{b13}	C_{b15}
C_{b31}	C_{b33}	C_{b35}
C_{r11}	C_{r13}	C_{r15}
C_{r31}	C_{r33}	C_{r35}

FIGURE 10.10

Subsampled color pixel values.

Since loss is incurred both in converting the RGB values to YC_bC_r values and in subsampling, the foregoing method is mostly applicable to lossy JPEG compression. Lossless JPEG compression of color images usually treats the RGB image as three separate images—a red, green, and blue image, each of which is compressed separately. On decompression these three images are re-created and merged to get the reconstructed image.

WAVELET COMPRESSION

Raw pixels are localized in space but are not localized in frequency. Thus, it is not easy to take advantage of the eye's insensitivity to certain frequencies by quantizing in the spatial domain. JPEG solves this problem by transforming the spatial coefficients into frequency coefficients using the cosine transform. The cosine transform is not localized in space but is localized in frequency. This allows frequency quantization but, because the cosine is not localized in space, blocks are required to limit the frequencies to a small spatial range. Because the image is broken into blocks that are compressed independently, sometimes, especially under high compression, the boundaries between blocks are visible. In addition, the quantization error can cause objectionable "ringing" around sharp edges, especially text.

To solve these problems, wavelet compression has been proposed. Individual wavelet functions can be localized both in space and in frequency. There are different sets of wavelets; the different sets make trade-offs between spatial localization, frequency localization, and smoothness. The advantage of using wavelets is that no block boundaries arise because the image is not broken into blocks. In addition, by choosing an appropriate "basis function," wavelet coefficients are often better than cosine coefficients in preserving relevant details and in reducing ringing.

The image is transformed into a wavelet domain using a wavelet transform similar to the FDCT. Then bits are allocated to the wavelet coefficients to minimize code size while taking into account the eye's sensitivity to certain frequencies. As in JPEG, the coefficients are quantized using a quantization table, and the table can be adjusted to provide trade-offs between compression and quality. Next, these quantized coefficients are entropy encoded. Unlike JPEG, the JPEG 2000 entropy encoding allows the code bits to be ordered in such a fashion that the image can be progressively decompressed. (JPEG does provide a progressive mode, but that is not quite the same thing.) The idea is that for a given number of bytes from the coded image, some decoded image can be created. As more and more bytes are received, the decoded image gets better and better until all the coefficients from the coded image have been received. The advantage of this process is that judiciously truncating the coded image produces an image with reduced resolution quickly. This reduced resolution image can be dynamically created and displayed in a variety of resolutions—say as a thumbnail—or displayed full-sized but with reduced resolution image in teleradiology applications. As more information is transmitted, a higher resolution image can be displayed.

JPEG 2000 is under final committee review. See the Web site *www.jpg.org*. DICOM has indicated that it will incorporate JPEG 2000 into its standard once the new JPEG 2000 standard has been accepted.

To find out more about wavelets, see the wavelet page at *www.iso.ch/cate/d18902.html* or the paper *What is wavelet theory?* by Kirk. The Web page *www.fmah.com* gives examples of medical images and video images.

MOTION JPEG AND MPEG COMPRESSION

Some applications use continuous-tone motion video, such as videos made during CAT scans, ultrasounds, Doppler ultrasounds, or thermal imaging. These videos can be grayscale or color. To compress these types of images, Motion JPEG and MPEG can be used.

Motion compression can be achieved by successively compressing still images at a high rate. When 10 frames (images) a second are displayed motion is perceived, although the motion may appear jerky until 24 to 30 frames/sec are reached. This method is known as *Motion JPEG*. Both lossless and lossy JPEG can be decompressed fast enough on modern machines to give smooth motion.

Motion JPEG is not very good from a compression standpoint because a lot of information is redundant from frame to frame. *MPEG* attempts to compress the images by reducing this redundancy. To do so, MPEG starts off with an I-frame (Intradependent or Independent frame), which is basically a standard JPEG still image. The next image is differenced from the prior image and the change is then compressed. As we have seen for still images, the differences can usually be compressed much more than the original pixels can. At a scene change or at other times, new I-frames are inserted. This gives up some compression but allows the application to skip forward or backward to another I-frame without having to determine intermediate frames.

MPEG is actually more complex than this. Moving from one frame to another can shift the placement of certain features on the second frame from their position on the first frame. As a simple example, Figure 10.11 shows the image of a person walking in front of a tree. The background (the tree) is stationary while the person shifts position from frame to frame. MPEG attempts to capture this motion by searching for blocks that are similar (except for position) from frame to frame. A vector indicating the block's motion is stored as part of the compressed frame. When compressing, a block on the first frame is moved according to the vector and placed on the second frame. These adjusted frames are then differenced and that difference is actually what is stored in the transformed image.

Decompression works as you would expect—almost. From a given frame any regions are extracted and positioned on the next frame with the appropriate vector. The frame difference is then added to produce the next frame. However, frames may be skipped. This may be necessary

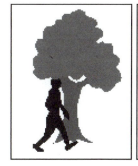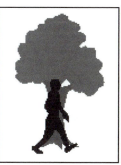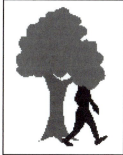

FIGURE 10.11

Example of motion.

because the machine is slow or busy doing other things. Usually there is an audio stream that must be decompressed and played at the same time. It is important to synchronize audio and video, so that if the video lags behind, frames may be skipped to speed up the video and help keep it synchronized.

THE FUTURE OF IMAGE COMPRESSION

Image compression is constantly improving. Shortly there will be JPEG 2000, which is based on wavelets. It will give better image quality for a given compressed size or the same quality for a smaller compressed size. Wavelets are also more naturally suited for telemedicine applications than the DCTs as used in the current JPEG. See *www.jpeg.org* for a summary of JPEG 2000 features.

WHAT ELSE CAN BE DONE?

One research avenue is template compression. In this compression, certain reference images are used as a starting point for difference or motion-type compression. Let's take the image of a kidney, for example. There are many standard variants of a kidney and many diseases of the kidney. Suppose we have images for this large collection of kidneys. These images are called templates. Then, given an arbitrary kidney, the closest template match can be found and oriented to it. The difference can then be found using MPEG-like "motion vectors." This template number and region/difference information is then stored as the transformed image. This method not only would give very small compressed images, but also allow valuable diagnostic information to be obtained.

In the far future computers might be able to determine the condition of an organ from parameters derived from genetic material or direct scanning. Compression in that case would be no more than storing these parameters. Because images usually make up the bulk of medical information storage, it is worthwhile to reduce this storage by compressing the images. Lossless image compression has been accepted for some time in the medical community, but advances in compression technology now allow DICOM to promote JPEG as an acceptable lossy compression method. In the future other compression methods will enhance image storage and transmission even further.

CONCLUSION

▶ Encoding is the process of taking a raw image and making a coded image.

▶ Decoding is the process of taking a coded image and making a decoded image.

▶ Lossless compression happens when the raw image is the same as the decoded image.

▶ Lossy compression happens when the raw image differs from the decoded image.

▶ Encoding (decoding) has two parts: modeling and entropy encoding (decoding).

▶ The choice of model significantly affects the type of encoding (decoding).

▶ The class of image determines the appropriate modeling or compression technique.

▶ Errors in the decoded image are very subjective and only experiment will give proper compression/quality settings.

▶ JPEG is DICOM's current compression technique of choice for medical images both lossy and lossless.

▶ JPEG has two distinct compression methods: lossless and lossy.

▶ JPEG 2000 will use wavelets to improve quality and reduce the size of the compressed image.

▶ There is much more that can be done in image compression.

▶ REFERENCES

General

www.compression-pointers.com—Link to almost all other compression links.
cctpwww.cityu.edu.hk/public/graphics/g_std.htm—Graphics and multimedia standards and related information.
Kay D, Levine J. *Graphics File Formats*. Windcrest/McGraw-Hill. New York 1992.

Sonka M, Hlavac V, Boyle R. *Image Processing, Analysis and Machine Vision.* Chapman & Hill. London 1994.

DICOM

www.nema.org/nema/medical/dicom—DICOM home Web page.

FAX

www.ncs.gov/n6/content/standard/html/ftr1062.htm—URL to purchase the standard.
18.ITU-T T.4 (1993.03) AMD2 08/95. *Standardization of Group 3 Facsimile Apparatus for Document Transmission.* AMD2 08/95.

JPEG

www.lib.ox.ac.uk/internet/news/faq/archive/jpeg-faq.part1.html—August 10, 1995.
www.jpg.com—A program demonstration of JPEG (lossless and lossy) and wavelet compression.
ISO/IEC 10918-1. *Information technology—Digital compression and coding of continuous-tone still images: Requirements and guidelines.* Geneva. 1994.
Pennebaker J, Mitchell J. *JPEG Still Image Data Compression Standard.* Van Nostrand Reinhold. New York 1993.

MPEG

www.cselt.stet.it/mpeg—The MPEG home Web page.
www.mpeg1.de/mplinks.html—Further MPEG links.

WAVELET

www.iso.ch/cate/d18902.html—Wavelet links.
www.fmah.com—Examples of medical images and video images.
www.cis.ohio-state.edu/text/faq/usenet/compression-faq/top.html—Kirk R. *What is wavelet theory?* July 27, 1995.

CHAPTER 11

VOICE RECOGNITION

AMIT MEHTA

As computer technology continues to streamline the radiology practice with more data becoming digital, new technologies are becoming largely ubiquitous. The impetus to utilize technologies is two-fold. Firstly, despite constraints on healthcare spending, the past several years have experienced a continuing increase in use of the healthcare dollar for radiology services. With this continual increase, there has been a demand for improved performance sheerly due to volume. This has forced the radiologist to deal with the task of providing increased services more efficiently in terms of both time and cost. In the analysis of steps of image workflow that can be modified, dictation and transcription represent key bottlenecks.

Voice recognition technology represents a solution within an area of radiology practice that allows radiologists to achieve efficiency goals and become more competitive in this new environment. It serves as a link that can improve the speed of communcation between radiologists and their referring physicians (Figure 11.1).

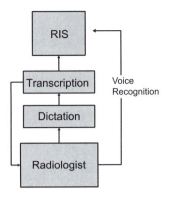

FIGURE 11.1

Role of voice recognition in radiology workflow.

HISTORY

The use of computers to recognize human speech has a long history within medicine and more recently in the commercial arena. In the late 1980s, radiologists and other medical subspecialists started to use expensive dedicated hardware systems that employed specialized vocabulary to recognize reports dictated in a discrete speaking style. After several years of use, it was deemed that voice recognition technology was not mature enough to handle the high-volume demand for the transcription requirements of most radiology practices. The late 1980s and early 1990s were plagued with limited usage and general nonacceptance of the voice recognition technology for commercial application. However, despite the lack of widespread use, development and distribution continued, and by 1994, speech recognition systems in American English had progressed to the point where speech recognition engines had vastly improved in addition to increased computer processing power. This combination of improvements led to accuracy rates that became acceptable for commercial applications, especially medicine. At this time, with the burden of limited computer processing power eliminated, vendors were also able to focus on more specific markets, namely radiology. It became apparent once development began in full swing that no specialty was better suited to voice recognition applications than radiology.

The mid-1990s saw the introduction of speech recognition systems into mainstream large radiology departments in the USA. Although these sites were alpha- or beta-testing facilities, the implementations proved that voice recognition technology was ready for mainstream usage. For the last three to four years, there have been over 300 installations throughout the U.S. with continued interest throughout the world. The technology has encountered both acceptance and rejection based on several ergonomic factors. Overall, the benefits greatly outweigh the negatives, and as hardware and software continue to improve, recognition accuracy rates continue to increase and the acceptance of early adopters becomes visionary.

ACCEPTANCE AND CONTINUED INTEREST

Speech recognition software packages offer many factors that work in its favor for its adoption by medical practitioners. First, continuous speech recognition systems require limited amounts of learning and adaptation compared to other transcription systems and methods. The systems are designed to conform to people's most natural way of communicating and essentially do not require the user to alter this method. Second, the ability of the software package to integrate almost seamlessly into existing radiology and hospital information workflow makes transition effortless (Figure 11.2). The disadvantages are always those of resistance to change and fear of technology. As these are overcome, the vast benefits become apparent and user acceptance increases. As user acceptance increases, developers are encouraged to continue development. Currently several factors drive the interest in speech recognition. First, continued development coupled with increasing processing power lead to improved accuracy rates and the easier use of natural

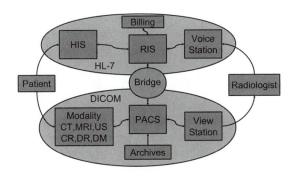

FIGURE 11.2

Radiology departmental workflow.

speech. Second, a shortage of medical transcriptionists is occurring in most medical markets; this forces healthcare institutions and practice groups to seek alternative strategies to foster growth and maintain services. Third, there is an immediate return on investment, with decreased operating costs and improved services. Finally, when thoroughly analyzed, this technique does not require physicians to drastically change their practice in terms of transcription, a feature setting it far apart from competing technologies.

RESISTANCE TO ADOPTION

Despite the bright future for this technology, several factors delay its widespread implementation. As mentioned, physicians have an inherent resistance to adopt new technologies. As the next generation of medical practitioners who have been trained on computer systems begin to practice, we will see a change in the dissemination of new technologies; however, most current practitioners were not initially trained to use computer systems and resistance is apparent. Second, the common experience of even those physicians who embrace change and technology has been that of poorly functioning voice recognition systems from the early 1990s. Accuracy rates are always an area of contention; although accuracy rates in the 60 to 70% range were clearly unacceptable, achievable accuracy rates of 90 to 97% remain unacceptable for many physicians. Lastly, there has been limited development of specialized vocabulary for medical subspecialties—vocabularies that would enhance widespread application into existing markets.

CURRENT OFFERINGS

Solutions on the market have several components, as shown in Figure 11.3.

First is a speech recognition engine; currently engines are offered by several vendors including, Dragon Systems, IBM, Philips, Microsoft, Verbex, Command, and L&H. Differences between recognition agents are minor and accuracy rates are similar. The core engine is packaged in a solution that focuses on the needs of the client. These needs include an interface for the user with necessary elements such as areas to entire accession and medical record numbers, sign buttons, and other key features (Figure 11.4).

In addition, there is a user-specific and medical subspecialty-specific vocabulary database, or "Language Model," with terms commonly used in dictation. Lastly are the tools necessary to integrate the voice recognition

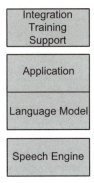

FIGURE 11.3

Levels of application support for voice recognition solutions.

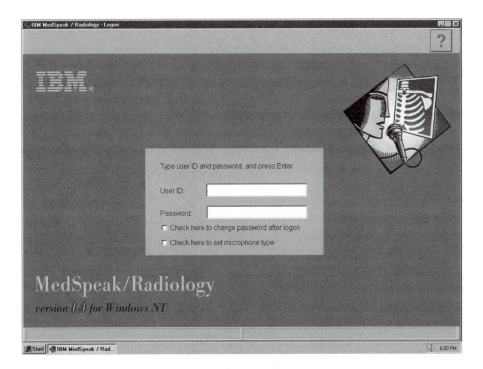

FIGURE 11.4

Sample validation interface screen.

package seamlessly into the existing practice by ensuring well-planned training and support. The use of third-party support vendors by the creators of the voice recognition engines allows dedicated sales forces to focus on sectors of the medical marketplace and better serve the needs of the user.

TECHNOLOGY

Voice recognition software at the human interface level comprises four core technologies: the recognition of the spoken human speech; the synthesis of the spoken speech into readable characters; the identification of the speaker and often verification; and understanding of the recognized word. These technologies are often referred to as to speech recognition or speech-to-text; speech synthesis or text-to-speech; speaker identification and verification; and natural language understanding.

These four core technologies do not occur in all software packages, depending on the niche the software solution serves. Speech recognition or speech-to-text operates in two distinct functions. First is command recognition or command control operation. This type of voice recognition handles the recognition of single words or short phrases spoken with discrete breaks in speech in a staccato style. Conventionally, this type of speech recognition has been used for use in navigation in computer control—for example, "Open file" or "Exit application." This form of dictation requires low processing requirements and requires the user to enunciate each spoken word with a discrete gap between commands. The second and more computer-processor intensive is continuous speech recognition. This type of speech recognition is used in medical applications. This type of recognition does not carry the limitation of requiring short pauses between words and allows users to speak in their natural style. With this added benefit, there is the cost of higher processing power requirements in the workstations used. As continuous speech recognition is most applicable to the radiology implementation, this chapter will focus on an explanation of its uses and requirements.

The second core component of speech recognition products for radiology is speech synthesis or text-to-speech. This component enables the computer to produce the phonemes that a human would make when the text dictated is read aloud, akin to the replay button on a conventional tape dictation system. With the addition of this option, the radiologist is able to listen to a report via audio playback as well as review individual points of a dictation during the generation of a report.

Third is the identification and verification component of the software package. Prior to full-scale use of a speech recognition system, the user is often required to perform a short enrollment procedure during which the system acquires the nuances in the individual voice components for over 200 to 300 dictated words. These nuances in voice are stored in a speech file for that user on a central server. To achieve high accuracy rates, the system requires that this speech file be loaded each time the user logs onto a workstation to dictate. This is accomplished by user identification and verification (Figure 11.4). There are various methods of performing this task, but the simplest and easiest is a user name and password entry prior to the dictation session. This step in the dictation process is similar to push-button entry of an identification code number on a conventional dictation system.

The fourth and least used component in a speech recognition system is a natural language understanding module. This technology makes it possible for the computer to understand what the user is trying to say in the string of words used. Natural language understanding allows the user to interact with the workstation in the native language format and allows the computer to perform the queried task. Although the first iteration of this technology involves the execution of simple commands, the possibilities are enormous. For example, the user may wish to know what possible commands it (the computer) can understand and execute, in which case the user would say, "What can I say?" This feature is found in most speech recognition packages today. In the future, this technology will allow the execution of tasks specific to radiology. For example, with the phrase, "Display a list of all unread CT scans from three days ago," the system will query the radiology information system (RIS), acquire all studies that meet the defined criteria (CTs in this case), and potentially relay this information to the PACS system, which will transfer these studies to the local workstation being used. Although this technology requires further development, it will make the use of speech recognition packages more widespread and functional.

HARDWARE

Each software recognition package states selected hardware requirements with their purchase. Commonly, most systems identify a minimum specific processor and speed, usually a Pentium 200 MHz chip as well as an operating system, usually the Windows NT platform. In addition to individual workstations, the system requires integration into a network for two reasons.

First, by integrating workstations into a network, a user can dictate at any terminal within the intranet and not be restricted to certain systems. Second, the network link allows integration with the RIS through the voice recogni-

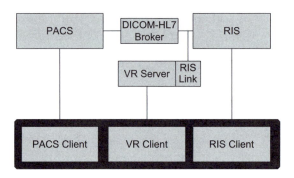

FIGURE 11.5

Integration of voice recognition client into the digital department.

tion server and ultimately into the HIS and PACS (Figure 11.5). Most systems also require the use of high-quality microphones and sound cards to achieve high accuracy rates. This often results in the purchase of a noise-canceling microphone (Figure 11.6) and an upgraded sound card for factory-purchased computers. The commitment to upgrade hardware for this reason inevitably leads to improved recognition rates. Future hardware technologies include improvements in both raw power as well as ancillary devices. A recent announcement has shown a commitment by the consumer computer industry to voice recognition by the development of a processor chip with integrated and

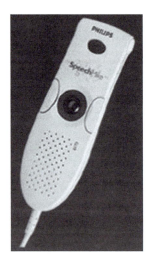

FIGURE 11.6

Sample ergonomic integrated input microphone device.

dedicated speech recognition components. With circuitry dedicated to the speech recognition engine, there is less taxation on the main CPU and hence improved overall performance over the entire system. Second, the continual development of integrated microphone, bar code, and trackball systems allow all the day-to-day functions of the radiologist to be at the fingertips.

SOFTWARE

The key to the integration of speech recognition systems into the radiology department is seamless deployment with the existing system (Figure 11.5). Based on the experiences of alpha- and beta-testers, the integration of a voice recognition system into the radiology department is not a trivial process. Several key factors are required for successful implementation of a voice recognition system. Most voice recognition systems currently available on the market for radiology offer these key features (most of these features are shown in Figure 11.7).

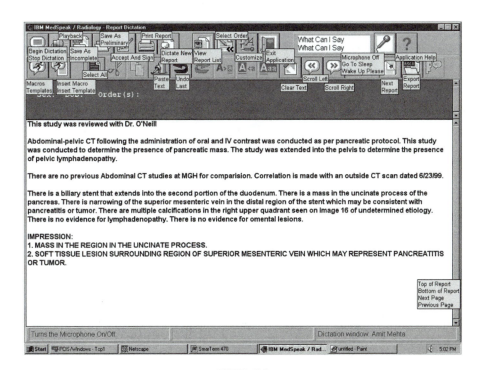

FIGURE 11.7

Sample radiologist dictation edit screen.

RIS/HIS INTERFACE

Any new dictation system needs to provide links to the existing infrastructure, allowing seamless integration with the RIS, HIS, PACS, and billing system. Most software packages incorporate backend transparent interfaces that allow the speech recognition system to query the RIS for demographic data as well as report status (Figure 11.8). In addition, the system allows the upload of dictated reports to the RIS and ultimately to the HIS. To achieve this task, most software packages contain HL7-compliant application programming interfaces that use standard formats and protocols. More robust speech recognition systems contain an open HL7 interface that allows the recognition of dictations created by other dictation systems. Depending on the level of HL7 interface, most systems allow the radiologist to create a work list by modality, date, or wild-card categories.

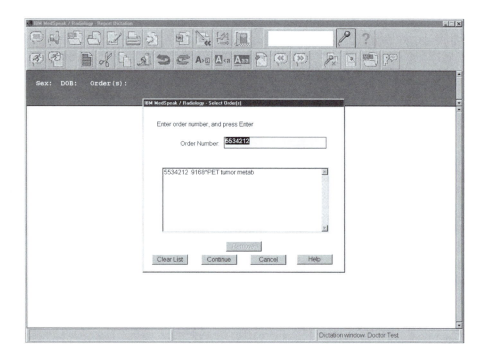

FIGURE 11.8

Sample RIS interface screen.

STANDARD REPORTS

A speech recognition system should allow members of the radiology department to create predefined reports for individual radiologists or the institution. These predefined reports may be categorized for normal studies or commonly performed studies. For example, a predefined report may be represented by the normal chest radiograph, which would describe the cardiomediastinal silhouette and the clear lungs. To invoke these predefined dictations, some systems use a single-command order, such as macro-chest, others use more complicated systems.

TEMPLATES/MACROS

As an extension of the standard report function, many systems allow the creation of standard reports with customizable templates and fields. The template capability gives the radiologist the flexibility to create a form with blank areas that vary with each dictation. For items such as procedures, the radiologist is able to dictate the necessary components to fill in the blanks. This feature has great value when describing different dosages or instruments. Most systems contain a feature-filled macro/template creation/editing utility. Using this function during report generation greatly improves the efficiency the radiologist and decreases the time required to dictate reports (Figure 11.9).

CUSTOMIZABLE FIELDS

Most packages permit custom definitions by the institution of multiple fields associated with a report. These fields may include ICD-9, CPT, BI-RADS, ACR/NEMA codes, or ACR pathology identifiers. The data entered into these fields may be shared with other information systems, such as the HIS-RIS integration interface. The integration of these fields into a speech recognition solution allows many adjunctive benefits. For example, an institution may generate a database that can be used for research and education purposes. By defining cases by ACR codes, trainees can retrospectively review cases with selected words. By employing ICD-9 codes, the radiology billing services are greatly facilitated. The various uses of these fields is innumerable.

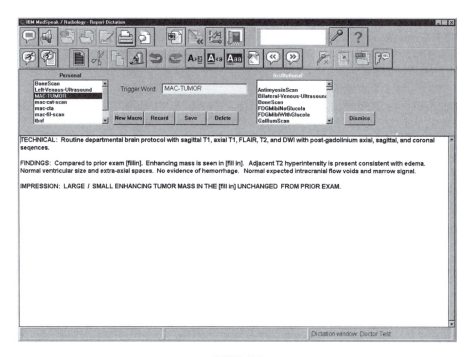

FIGURE 11.9

Sample predefined report edit screen.

BAR CODES

Bar code interfaces exist in most legacy dictation systems. Most voice recognition software packages support the use of a bar code laser reader or integrated microphone laser reader into the system (Figure 11.6). The user has the option of using the bar code reader or manually entering the accession or medical record number to identify cases. A bar code reader is especially useful when the radiologist is reading radiographs in batch mode.

SYSTEM SECURITY

The voice recognition software package must ensure that security is maintained by requiring each radiologist to enter a user identification code and password to sign on and begin dictation (Figure 11.4). This is also a utility in the speaker identification and verification function to ensure high accuracy rates. In addition, most systems require the radiologist to enter the same password or another predefined password in order to sign off on the dictated report and allow its transfer to the RIS and HIS. This second password feature ensures that the user is the designated physician identified by the system as dictating the report. Further security measures include the inability to log onto multiple workstations within a facility, which ensures that user workstations are not left unattended.

IMPLEMENTATION

The experience at Massachusetts General Hospital in phasing in the conversion of the dictation system to speech recognition highlighted several issues; timely solutions made the transition process a success. Prospective knowledge of ultimately imperative operational issues will improve the process for centers considering the installation of voice recognition dictation.

The first key issue that we realized over the 3-year implementation period was that the technology continues to mature. Over the course of phasing in, we experienced both the progression of hardware coupled with a decrease in the cost of the technology. This only helped: the use of more sophisticated and powerful systems in turn led to improved accuracy rates of the voice recognition engines. We will continue to realize improvements in both operation and use of the speech recognition system over the life of the product, whereas most legacy dictation systems are static. This prospect allowed senior management to convince radiologists that newness of the technology should not be a deterrent to its acceptance.

Once this fact was accepted, what did become apparent was that inadequate training and attention to details within day-to-day operations constituted our most serious drawback. We quickly realized that if these issues were not addressed early in the integration process, the entire effort would become misguided and acceptance by users would be lost. It became apparent that the implementation team's focus should be on two areas: training and operation.

KEY STEPS DURING DEPLOYMENT

The training of radiologists to use voice recognition software and workstations must occur prior to its wide-scale use in a department. Radiologists must first be able to navigate the basic functions of the conventional operating systems; secondly, they must be versed in the use of computer input devices such as a keyboard, mouse, microphone—whether head mounted or a hand style—and bar code reader. Then the radiologist must become familiar with the software interface of the voice recognition package. Many packages offer navigation by voice, which requires the user to remember the names of each function, such as "Accept and sign" or "Save as preliminary." Other packages require mouse clicks to perform these same functions.

Usually, the championing of the conversion by a key radiologist who facilitates learning eases the implementation. Such an individual can be instrumental in promoting acceptance and training colleagues in the use of the new system. For departments without an individual who can assume this role, vendors offer hired training specialists who conduct sessions tailored to individual radiologists prior to deployment. In our experience, owing to the size of our department (conducting over 450,000 studies annually with 80 users—both radiologists and residents) the solution was to hire training specialists who later became support personnel for the system in its day-to-day operation. Once completed several times, training becomes routine and can be extrapolated and utilized by other departments considering similar strategies.

BASICS OF TRAINING THE USER

The key steps in training for voice recognition technology is to first identify the key audience. By knowing who will be learning the necessary skill set, training specialists are able to tailor classes to work at the level of the user. Many of our radiologists needed assistance in navigating through the speech recognition application, but once versed in performing this task, could dictate reports within minutes; others could navigate without difficulty but needed to get used to returning to the report to correct dictation errors.

Secondly, our training specialists determined the training goals for most users. They created training materials and tools that simplified both learning and using the software by the end user. This not only made it easier for users during the initial process, but also aided the technical support staff in providing education on specific topics on demand. Lastly, the training process was completed with users completing a survey evaluation of the program. With over 80 individuals to train, we were able to improve the training procedures continually, thereby tailoring them to the needs of our classes.

IDENTIFYING THE AUDIENCE

The first decision in developing proper training involved determining what the target audience should be. We had to consider whether the most efficient training schedule would be to train individual radiologists, divisions as a whole, an entire department in a single sitting, or simply key individuals who could then assist in training the remaining radiologists whether in their section or the entire department. The final decision was settled upon largely due to time constraints and the organizational task of allocating the large number of people that required training. We chose to train individual radiologists in their own environment and on their own time schedules. This eased the process of adopting new technology by the users and also allowed different levels of expertise to be taken into account. The specialists did choose group sessions conducive to (including residents by year and staff at departmental meetings) when training could be targeted toward these groups. After all the radiologists were trained, it was evident that training radiologists on an individual basis not only accommodated varied levels of computer experience, but also allowed users to learn at their own pace. This only served to encourage acceptance of the technology.

DETERMINING TRAINING GOALS

The second key step in planning a successful training procedure was to ensure that the training specialists understood what knowledge our radiologists both required and desired. Due to the varied levels of computer expertise, certain users only wanted to gain a basic understanding of functions from a focused training session. Once they had learned these basic functions, skills they would build through their own experience. The opposite group was a large number of users whom had little computer experience and required intensive training with navigational functions and operating system nuances. The attention paid to this detail with dedicated training time later helped gain acceptance of the system.

CREATING MATERIALS AND TOOLS

Providing the user with a written review of the steps they have performed serves to reinforce computer-based training. Our training specialists devised written material that was graphically intensive and later helped the users after the training session. The manual was a well organized spiral-bound color-coded training manual that covered all aspects of the speech recognition product as well as the contact numbers of the training specialists and the technical support individuals. By having easy access to these individuals, radiologists were assured that support was available around the clock. We further created learning aids such as laminated cards and posters placed adjacent to workstations, which provided users with shortcuts and enhancements to make the experience more productive. These additions reinforced the department's commitment to the success of the system, and also allowed many radiologists to solve their own problems without using the technical support personnel, who could then devote time to making other enhancements throughout the system.

TECHNICAL SUPPORT

All machines stop working at times. This is obvious to all users and inherent in all computers despite precautions taken to prevent downtime. The size of our operation and the number of users demanded that a single "champion" of the system clearly could not provide technical support to such a huge undertaking. Thus, we chose to hire a full-time technical support individual who understood not only the technical operation of our network infrastructure but the ins and outs of the voice recognition product. Within our department, this individual was available by pager during working hours, and a well-documented off-hour technical support system was first arranged through off-hours operations managers.

SURVEYS

Once the first training session had been completed, all radiologists were asked to fill in surveys that probed key areas within the program. Using this feedback, we were able to alter and focus subsequent training sessions, which made them be more effective. Combined with well-documented training material, the training sessions soon became efficient and effective and able to target issues for each user.

OPERATIONS

From the initial thought of employing a voice recognition system to all stages during the deployment, close attention to operational planning is necessary. This attention must be generated both departmentally as well as individually. In general, the overall operational plan must touch upon several factors, including understanding by those who will provide the leadership during the effort.

The first impressions of voice recognition systems are that they are slow and often cause significant delays with large volumes. It is always difficult to foster change in a department, especially when the ultimate benefits of improved report turnaround times and departmental cost savings seem to occur at the expense of the radiologist's time. To successfully overcome these hurdles, there must be a general understanding of the impact a system shift of this magnitude will have on the radiologists' daily workflow, especially by those who champion such an effort. Only upon acknowledgment of these general concepts by the designated leadership will it be feasible to achieve milestones and communicate these steps to the members of the department. Beyond these operational issues, specific issues must be addressed during the integration of voice recognition into a department.

SPECIFIC DELIVERY

During the installation of our system, its four operational issues needed to be considered prior to its full-time use in the practice. We first needed a firm grasp of the hardware and infrastructure requirements necessary to create the support systems that would allow seamless integration into the department. Secondly, individuals who could assist radiologists with technical issues promptly and effectively needed to be certified. Thirdly, timely operational checks with close follow-up were necessary to balance and monitor that users were productive with the new system. By ensuring that individual users were effectively operating with the new system, enterprise benefits could be realized. The final operational issue that we required was a plan for the removal of our legacy dictation system so that we could guarantee penetration and use within the department.

PHYSICAL/HARDWARE PLANNING

Beyond understanding the software package, the voice recognition implementation team needs to be well-versed in the different hardware requirements of conventional voice recognition systems. If the technical support individuals understand these requirements and their effects on performance from both a server and workstation perspective, they can better help the end user when issues arise. Performance differences may result from various machine configurations due to the machines themselves or the users and their use of the system. Ideally, if the technical support team has this understanding, solving problems that radiologists encounter in day-to-day operations will be fixed easily.

We also found that the minimum requirements for both the server and the client workstations are carefully defined for each vendor. Although such requirements should be closely adhered to, installing more powerful machines whenever the budget allows or in high-volume areas helps achieve maximum performance and maximum accuracy. The peripheral hardware involved in voice recognition systems including sound cards, microphones and bar code readers also affect the overall performance of the system and the accuracy of recognition. All support staff must be cognizant of these facts. Finally, the installation of networks and limitations in the existing infrastructure must be addressed by senior management in conjunction with information systems personnel for the institution, who perform routine maintenance.

CERTIFICATION

With an operation as large as ours, it is important that individuals who will be responsible for both implementing and supporting the new dictation system possess a certain level of certification. Usually, such certification is established internally; it allows the department to maintain quality control and to designate higher-level problems to those who possess larger skill sets. This usually involves the designation of an individual who understands the integration of the system into the radiology information system from the standpoints of its specification, implementation, and functionality. These "certified" personnel should understand all elements of the inbound link, the outbound link, electronic signing options, teaching options, as well as vendor-specific software options—all technical factors beyond the scope of the senior management championing the effort.

OPERATIONAL CHECKS

For continued success in voice recognition system implementation, the department must make a commitment to guarantee continued support and use. First and foremost, technical support must be quick, knowledgeable, and courteous. The time that lapses between the response to a "distressed" user should be monitored, because once fully implemented, a nonfunctioning voice recognition system is costly to both the productivity and morale of the department. A workstation that crashes usually results in the complete cessation of workflow because of its absolute necessity, especially once 100% penetration has been achieved. Often, users will resort to using legacy dictation systems if they are available, but this further hampers the operational benefits of the system. Secondly, the support team must follow up on all outstanding events to prevent recurrence of common problems. There should be a well-documented contingency plan in the event of system failure and a means of communicating this to both radiologists and other users of the system.

REMOVAL OF OLDER DICTATION SYSTEMS

During the phase-in of the voice recognition system, a point is reached where a well organized and timely removal of legacy dictation systems must occur. The removal of these alternate dictation systems ensures both primarily use of the voice recognition system as well as a commitment on the part of the department to the radiologists. It also demonstrates that a well-planned contingency structure is in place in the event of failure. Experience has demonstrated that every department has users who resist change and will continue to use legacy systems if they are available (and in some cases even if they are not readily available!). However, the removal of older dictation systems once the voice recognition system is in place, coupled with encouragement from department heads and senior management, allows usage to steadily increase and goals to be reached.

GOAL FULFILLMENT

Once our training and operational issues were clearly defined, the process of deploying voice recognition technology in our department led to the installation of 60 workstations. This complement of workstations totaled a 70% penetration mark and served to generate nearly 900 reports per day (Figure 11.10).

Following the installation of the voice recognition system, our report turnaround time has greatly decreased (Figure 11.11).

COST SAVINGS

Several areas of cost savings are associated with the implementation of a voice recognition system. The obvious and most apparent in the radiology

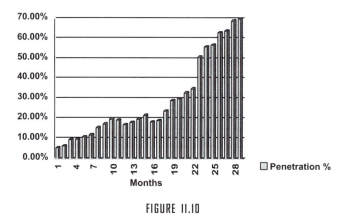

FIGURE 11.10

Rate of penetration percentage in a major academic teaching institution.

practice is the transcription cost. With the direct dictation and transcription of the report, the number of personnel can be decreased who previously handled the transcription process. The cost savings are not only realized in terms of salaries and benefits, but in the host of other costs associated with personnel.

The indirect cost savings are realized through the use of computer systems. Although this may appear as an added cost due to the purchase of hardware, the actual savings come from the multiple uses of a desktop PC. With the integration of the medical record to include radiology, pathology and other image based specialties, the practice of radiology is undergoing drastic changes in the availability of information to the radiologist. Hous-

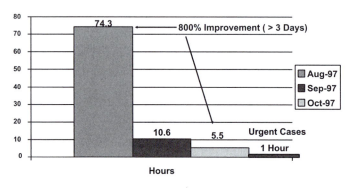

FIGURE 11.11

Changes in hospital practice report turnaround with voice recognition and PACS.

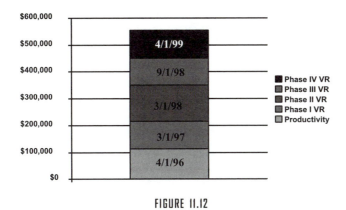

FIGURE 11.12

Cumulative cost savings with voice recognition.

ing the voice recognition system on a conventional desktop PC allows other information agents, including references, paging systems, and HIS-RIS applications to be coupled to this system. Adding these services to a unifying system saves both time and physical space.

The phase-in process of our voice recognition installation spanned three years due to our alpha- and beta-site status. Currently in the fourth of five phases, we have realized a cost savings in our transcription budget of over $500,000 (Figure 11.12). This does not take into account the intangible costs from having an integrated PC workstation.

REPORT TURNAROUND

During the installation of our voice recognition system, our dictation practices have remained relatively constant. Prior to the automation of this process, we would dictate our reports using a commercially available dictation system. These reports would then be typed by transcriptionists and returned to our radiologists for review. Once edits and addendums had been completed, the report was signed and finalized becoming available on the radiology and ultimately hospital information systems. In the event a resident had dictated a report, the edited version would enter a preliminary status pending approval of a staff radiologist. This entire process on average took 3.4 days to complete. The introduction of the voice recognition system eliminates the transcription and correction steps and a report by a staff radiologist becomes final immediately after being dictated and edited. In the

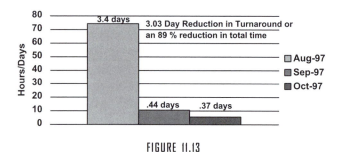

FIGURE 11.13

Improved report turnaround time at remote ER healthcare offices.

case of a resident, the final report again is preliminary pending approval of the staff. After several months of usage in our department and growing familiarity with the system by our radiologists, the report turnaround time had drastically dropped to 0.4 days (Figure 11.11). Time to finalization is instantaneous for staff radiologists dictating reports and usually for private practices. At our satellite clinic without the aid of resident radiologists, our imporvement in report turnaround time has been upwards of 800%, or a reduction from 74.3 hours to less than 1 hour (Figure 11.13).

CONCLUSION

Our institution served as an alpha- and beta-test site for the MedSpeak IBM product. Our experiences to date not only centered around fostering an understanding for speech recognition technology, but also to gain a sense of pitfalls and challenges that might occur during implementation as well as a realization for operational issues. We also set out to allow our radiologists to be on the cutting edge of technology and help embrace advances that were being made in the field. We solicited their advice on these evolutions and potentially shaped a market to create solutions and further meet our needs.

CHAPTER 12

ENTERPRISE IMAGING

KEITH J. DREYER

A t the heart of the digital radiology department exist two main computational systems, RIS and PACS (Figure 12.1). While the RIS encompasses many text-based computing functions including transcription, reporting, ordering, scheduling, tracking, and billing, PACS deals with image-based computing functions such as acquisition, interpretation, storage, and local image distribution. The proper use of these automated systems dramatically reduces the use of film and paper within a radiology department. However, removing film and paper removes the conventional method for distributing radiology information throughout the hospital. Because the goal of any radiology department is to deliver timely and accurate interpretations to requesting clinicians, the digital department needs a digital method to deliver its results. Enter the Internet.

THE INTERNET

An introduction to the emerging world of enterprise image distribution requires a basic understanding of the terminology and jargon associated with

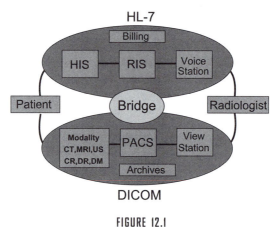

FIGURE 12.1

The digital radiology department.

the Internet and the World Wide Web. For some, this is new and funda-mental information for others; a review.

The Internet (Figure 12.2) is a collection of computers (i.e., a network) communicating over a variety of transmission lines throughout the world, us-ing a single common protocol known as TCP/IP. TCP/IP, or Transfer Com-munication Protocol/Internet Protocol, essentially allows all of the computers in the world to communicate. This low-level protocol allows computer users and programs to communicate with each other using higher-level protocols such as SMTP (Simple Mail Transport Protocol, i.e., e-mail) (Figure 12.3).

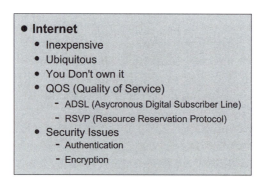

FIGURE 12.2

Advantages of the Internet.

- **E-Mail**
  - SMTP - Simple Mail Transport Protocol
- **File Transfer**
  - FTP - File Transport Protocol
- **The World Wide Web**
  - HTTP - Hpertext Transport Protocol
    - HTML - HyperText Markup Language
    - XML - Extensible Markup Language

FIGURE 12.3

Common protocols available over the Internet.

HTTP (HyperText Transport Protocol) allows the distribution of text and images (and a variety of other media types) and is commonly referred to as the World Wide Web (or the Web for short). It is easy to see why the idea of using a universally common way to transmit and receive text and images—the Web—to distribute radiologic information is becoming so universally accepted. Essentially, it is the process of turning your digital radiology department into a Web site. And, like all successful Web businesses, the Web doesn't change your business (radiology) or your customers (clinicians), it just changes the way you deliver your business to your customers. If done correctly, Web distribution can offer great efficiencies to you and your clinicians.

Of note, on top of the HTTP protocol sits several languages that are used to define the details of the Web pages. HTML (HyperText Mark-up Language) is the Web's basic language and has been in place since 1994. XML (eXtensible Mark-up Language) is a newer language gaining steam in the Web world due to its ability to separate data from display parameters, thus preserving the structure of all data fields. What does this mean? It means, for example, that even if a patient's medical record number is deeply buried in the middle of a Web page, written in XML, a computer program reading that page (yes, they can read Web pages too) could find it easily and use it to get more information on the patient from a different Web site.

HOSPITAL-WIDE IMAGE DISTRIBUTION

With the installation of PACS into many institutions around the United States, the task of distributing images to referring clinicians becomes apparent. In the legacy system, physicians who wish to view their images rely

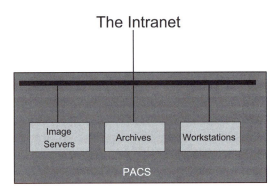

FIGURE 12.4

Typical components of a PACS intranet.

on obtaining their films from the radiology department's film library. Often, these films are used to communicate with patients, family members, and consultants for patient education and patient management. The advent of PACS eliminates this classic film-based workflow. The use of pre-existing intranet to distribute images is gaining momentum and acceptance within hospitals due to its ubiquity, portability, and cost (Figure 12.4). (The intranet is the part of the Internet that's behind your hospital's firewall—and see Chapter 4, "Networks," for more details.) The Internet, and associated hospital intranets, have increasingly become the technological basis for both image management within the radiology department and image distribution to the enterprise (Figure 12.5). Despite the fact that current PACS instal-

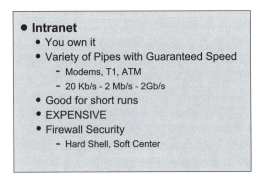

FIGURE 12.5

Advantages and disadvantages of an intranet.

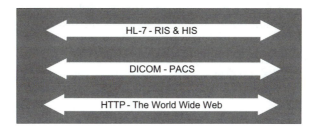

FIGURE 12.6

Common hospital intranet protocols.

lations have not been designed around Web technology, vendors are able to add Web-based solutions with relative ease. Central to the appeal of Web-based distribution is the ability for any physician, anywhere, whether at home or within the clinical setting, to use a personal computer as a virtual light box and view radiologic images and reports.

Early in the process, visionaries in the PACS arena predicted that the problem of image management and distribution should be approached from an enterprise point of view—creating a parallel structure in radiology with respect to the development of the electronic medical record. The guiding principle in system design should be that images go wherever alphanumeric medical information goes, a task best achieved by a flexible, integrated Web-based solution. The various protocols available allow this flow of information with guaranteed connectivity (Figure 12.6).

COSTS

The cost of primary interpretation workstations on current PACS hardware and software platforms can reach up to $100,000 each and thus do not offer a viable alternative for each referring physician who needs to review his or her ordered examinations. The current ubiquity of the desktop PC is a resource that obviates the need for custom-designed distribution channels. For example, Partners HealthCare System Inc., Boston, the parent corporation of Massachusetts General Hospital and the Brigham and Women's Hospital, has more than 20,000 PCs currently on its intranet. Utilizing this resource for image distribution comes at essentially no additional cost.

There remains a confusion of pricing of web solutions within the industry. The alternatives include cost per user, cost per view (or click), cost per maximum users, cost per concurrent users, cost per studies stored, and a one-time cost in annual licensing. This range of pricing structures often creates confusion when comparing products using a price performance analysis, but generally these systems result in a one-time capital expense between $10,000 and $100,000, and an equally wide range of recurring annual operating expenses. These estimated expenditures include hardware and software for the Web server component and software only for the viewing clients.

INFRASTRUCTURE

Inherent to standard Web protocol is a client/server relationship. Whereas the Web server is a computer that contains the images to be distributed for viewing, the client, in this example, is basically the clinician's PC. The following paragraphs describe the requirements for both the server and client systems of a typical radiology distribution system.

SERVER

A Web server used for radiology image distribution needs to perform several functions. Theses are listed below.

- Accept images from a variety of DICOM sources.
- Compress images in either a lossy or lossless format (or both).
- Store compressed images in a local, fast access device (e.g., RAID).
- Act as an HTTP server waiting for Web requests over TCP/IP.

Typically, Web servers for radiology are either NT-based PCs or Solaris-based Sun Microsystem computers. We feel that either system is adequate for this function and that several factors need to be weighed against each other for optimum performance in the enterprise. These factors include: cost, speed, number of concurrent users, reliability, and support. If the hospital distribution workflow calls for more than one Web server, it should be determined whether each server should have its own archive or if one archive should be shared between all servers. In most circumstances, a single archive should be shared, with each Web server accessing a common, compressed RAID. As demand increases from clinicians for Web access, more powerful servers may be needed to maintain performance. One way to accommodate these growing needs is by increasing the server's processing power and RAM. Another way is by simply increasing the number of servers available to the task.

CLIENT

The client device is quite variable (i.e., it can be any form of computer with access to the Internet). In fact, possibly the only commonality necessary among clients is that they contain an HTTP browser to access the server. Further, the browser can be from a variety of manufacturers (Netscape Navigator and Microsoft Explorer are among the most common). Because of the large file sizes and video requirements for display of medical images, and because the most common client in the hospital setting is an IBM-compatible PC, *minimum* configurations for PC-based client machines accessing radiology images can be defined and are listed below.

- 200 MHz Pentium class processor
- 64 MB system RAM
- 4 MB video RAM with 1024 x 768 resolution @ 16.7M colors
- 1GB Hard Drive Space
- 10 Mb Ethernet Card
- 17" Monitor (Dependent upon purpose and image type to be viewed)

This is not to say that a client system will not perform without these minimums, but it will probably do so with some degree of unacceptability. In fact, this is one of the most challenging aspects of ubiquitous Web distribution. Because any computer on the intranet can access the radiology Web server, it is often difficult to enforce a minimum client requirement. Therefore performance is unpredictable. For a new institution it is simple to recommend the purchase of a certain level of PC. But for most of us, there is an existing fleet of PCs throughout our institutions that would probably require upgrades to meet these core requirements. For a large institutional deployment of clients, it is best to evaluate users' needs individually to assess the intent of specific clinical access. Typically, some client computers are dedicated to specific clinicians while other systems are common and available to several users (ideally with individual logons and passwords).

EXAMPLE: THE WEB EXPERIENCE AT MASSACHUSETTS GENERAL HOSPITAL (MGH)

Prior to full PACS deployment, a Web-based solution was installed in 1995 for image distribution (Figure 12.7), as we believed this was a film alternative that would allow the hospital to cost-effectively distribute radiology images to all clinicians. The growing popularity of the Web over the past five years guaranteed a degree of familiarity with the client software (i.e., a browser) and was additionally easy to use and install with low support costs from the hospital Information Services department. It was felt that a Web server solution would layer onto any basic security system, such as firewalls, token delivered coded access numbers, passwords and usernames, secure socket layers (SSL), and virtual private networks (VPN) (Figure 12.8), and that these technologies, as they evolved, would enable the radiology department to ensure security and patient confidentiality regardless of the referring physician's access method and location.

Four NT-based, Web/Intranet Image Servers, each with 23 GB of RAID, were installed as a DICOM destination for 12 existing digital modalities (five CTs, four MRs, two CRs, and one digital fluoroscopy unit). Each of the Web servers was designed to include a Java-based interface to the RIS, database storage of DICOM image files, and future connectivity to a then-undetermined DICOM PACS. Incorporated into the Web-based so-

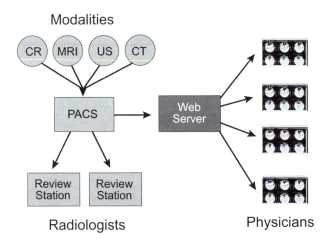

FIGURE 12.7

Web-based enterprise solution.

- **PCT** - Private Communication Technology

- **SET** - Secure Electronic Transaction

- **S-HTTP** - Secure Hypertext Transfer Protocol

- **SSL** - Secure Sockets Layer

- **VPN** - Virtual Private Networks

FIGURE 12.8

Internet security options.

lution was the use of a wavelet image compressor/decompressor that rapidly distributes images throughout the enterprise while preserving compatibility with DICOM workstations.

Upon purchase of a departmental PACS in 1996, integration of the existing Web distribution system offered access to a deeper archive of ever-expanding medical image data.

Currently, the MGH web server farm has grown to nine NT devices and provides real-time (1 to 2 sec), on-demand image distribution for images obtained within the most recent months, without any impact on PACS resources. (The Web server's compressed archives are designed to maintain several months of image data locally.) Requests for older examinations are automatically fetched from the PACS archives and are available for Web viewing in approximately 1 to 2 minutes. The threshold of time necessary when this fetching occurs (weeks, months, years) is a product of three things:

▶ Web server RAID size,

▶ Web server image compression factor, and

▶ image volume directed toward the Web servers.

Although the client system is under continual development, several key features are available (Figure 12.9):

1. Because multiple concurrent requests of prior examinations might be needed for conferences or patient chart reviews, a Web inter-

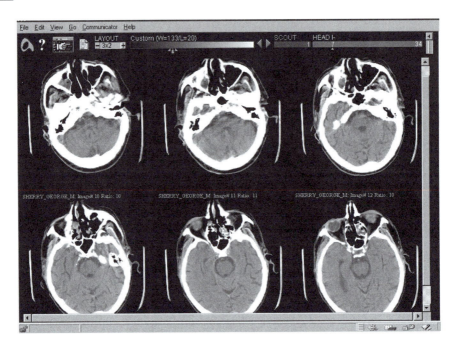

FIGURE 12.9

Sample client Web image viewer for computed tomography with selected features from text depicted.

face to the hospital paging system allows automatic notification of Web delivery of all request images, if desired.

2. Preservation of the 12-bit data provides the client with interactive window/level and magnification control within the Web browser environment.

3. A pixel recruitment algorithm provides auto-layout capability for CR and DR at initially reduced resolution to desktops with smaller screens, while full resolution is available on demand.

4. Local printing and image file export to the client's floppy or hard drive.

5. Simultaneous comparison of prior examinations.

CONCLUSION

Converting from film-based radiology to filmless radiology is challenging, to say the least. Surprisingly, most of the challenges exist outside of the department of radiology. To clinicians, replacing film means providing them with another distribution mechanism. While there is great momentum within hospitals to keep the status quo, Web distribution offers many advantages over film. The successful deployment of Web servers and client viewers throughout our hospital enterprise has proven critical for the conversion to a truly digital radiology environment.

THE FUTURE

Although Web distribution of radiologic images has in general proven essential to clinical decision making, most clinicians prefer viewing medical information in a more patient-oriented approach. When radiologic information can be combined with all other known information about a patient (e.g., orders, results, documentation, demographics, and medical history) and presented to the clinician in a patient-centric form, it serves as a rudimentary electronic medical record (EMR), offering the clinician greater decision-making power. If the EMR is the future of medical care, in the past five years we have seen the rapid advancement of radiology to where it is now ready for this future.

CHAPTER 13

TELERADIOLOGY

JAMES H. THRALL • GILES BOLAND

Telemedicine can be defined as the "delivery of healthcare and sharing of medical knowledge over a distance using telecommunications systems." This simple definition is rapidly evolving into a rich and diverse set of clinical, educational, and research applications underwritten by an equally diverse set of technologies. However, there is now enough collective experience with telemedicine to look at the challenges facing the field from the point of view of healthcare quality and cost rather than from a technological point of view. Telemedicine and teleradiology will become important in clinical practice to the extent that they solve real unmet medical needs to improve quality, and do so in a cost-effective way. Technical innovation will create more and more opportunities for telemedicine applications, but technology must be thought of as part of the enabling infrastructure and not an end in itself. This is a lesson learned repeatedly in the world of medical imaging. As noted by one reviewer of telemedicine, "The literature is characterized by an array of approaches and technologies, with no replications or cross validation studies" (Grisley et al. 1995).

From a historical perspective, the telephone was the first medium for long-distance medical consultation, and it is the most enduring medium. The first recorded use of the telephone in 1880 by its inventor, Alexander Graham Bell, was to summon his assistant for help with a medical problem occasioned by an accident in his laboratory. After the telephone, the first serious attempts at telemedicine in the United States took place in the late 1950s and throughout the 1960s, in which closed-circuit television was used to bring doctors and patients together and to transmit images of radiological and pathological specimens. Interactive television for psychiatric consultations was first used in 1959, and teleradiology was accomplished in the same year using coaxial cable to transmit video fluoroscopy (Wittson et al. 1961; Jutra 1959; Peredinia and Allen 1995).

In the late 1960s, Dr. Kenneth T. Bird of Massachusetts General Hospital established a telemedicine practice using interactive television via a direct microwave link between the hospital and Logan airport in Boston. Its purpose was to offer multi-specialty consultations with patients seen in a travel clinic at the airport. Bird also studied the transmission of radiographs, pathology slides, and dermatology examinations (Andrus and Bird, 1972; Bird 1972; Murphy et al. 1972; Murphy and Bird 1974). This early project was partially funded by the U.S. Public Health Service and provided the seminal data for many subsequent undertakings that explored a wide variety of applications.

Another early program sponsored by the government was optimistically entitled "Space Technology Applied to Rural Papago Advanced Health Care" (STARPAHC). This project was funded by NASA to exploit monitoring systems developed for use in space and served the Papago Reservation. The project demonstrated the feasibility of telemedicine in a rural setting but received mixed reviews for cost and practicality (Fuchs 1979).

The collective early experience with telemedicine was conceptually encouraging but it suffered from inadequate technology. The systems were inconvenient and expensive, and communications bandwidth was limited. The shortcomings in the technological infrastructure led to a quiet period during the 1970s and early 1980s, during which very little advancement was made in either the concept or implementation of telemedicine. Outside of the space program, which has consistently used telemetry of medical data, there are few enduring projects from the first round of activity. The program serving areas in Newfoundland at Memorial University in Canada is a notable exception (Grigsby et al. 1995; Perednia and Allen 1995).

Interest in telemedicine has exploded in the 1990s, fueled by the simultaneous development of medical devices suited to capturing images and other data in digital electronic form and the development and installation of increasingly high-speed, high-bandwidth telecommunication systems around the world (Grigsby et al. 1995; Perednia and Allen 1995). Interactive video conferencing, including the use of inexpensive desktop computers, is making face-to-face telecommunication between doctors and patients widely available in the United States and internationally. These systems—coupled with digital acquisition devices for X-ray images, digitally modified microscopes, and special attachments for stethoscopes, EKG machines, and cameras—allow specialists to provide consultations for patients in remote locations. These include both direct interaction with the patient and the ability to review substantial amounts of medical data almost as if the patient were immediately at hand. Via landline or satellite, an electronic link can be created between any two locations on earth. It is now possible to offer a wide range of services to patients in remote locations that would not otherwise be available.

CLINICAL APPLICATIONS OF TELEMEDICINE

Table 13.1 provides examples of clinical applications of telemedicine by the type of data being transmitted and the mode in which the data is used (Calcagni et al. 1996; Cawthon et al. 1991; Dakins 1997; Elam et al. 1992;

TABLE 13.1
Current Applications of Telemedicine

High-Resolution Images (Store and Forward)	Telemetry of Data (Store and Forward)	Interactive Video (Real Time)
▶ Teleradiology	▶ Electonic "house call"	▶ Clinical consultation
▶ Telepathology		
▶ Teledermatology	▶ ECG, BP, HR, Pulse, oximetry	▶ Physical examination
▶ Tele cardiology		
▶ Telegastroenterology		▶ Endoscopy
▶ Other	▶ Electonic medical record	▶ Telepresence surgery-robotics
		▶ Tele-education

*Tele-education can also be done as one-way noninteractive video.

Fosberg 1995; Franken et al. 1995; Franken, Harkens, and Berbaum 1997; Fuchs 1979; Gagner et al. 1994; Goldberg et al. 1993; Goldberg et al. 1994; Goldberg et al. 1997). In practice, real-time applications are more expensive and logistically demanding because they require coordination of scheduling between participants in multiple locations. Interactive video is the most common real-time technology used in telemedicine and is most suited to direct patient consultations and tele-education.

Using data in a store-and-forward mode has the advantage of being less logistically demanding and substantially less expensive, both in telecommunications costs and personnel costs. The store-and-forward model is useful for both high-resolution images and alphanumeric data. Note that all of the applications listed under the store-and-forward headings can also be delivered in real-time, but this is not the dominant mode in current clinical practice.

Data from a recent survey indicate that teleradiology is the most common clinical application in telemedicine, with 57% of respondents reporting a teleradiology program at their institution. Teleradiology is followed by telecardiology (46%), teledermatology (44%), telepsychiatry (43%), emergency medicine (40%), home healthcare (23%), telepathology (21%), and oncology (20%) (Dakins 1997).

TELERADIOLOGY

In many respects teleradiology, including telenuclear medicine, is the best-defined telemedicine service. As noted above, teleradiology is the most commonly deployed telemedicine service, and the rapid conversion in the medical imaging world from analog methods to digital methods has simply facilitated the practice of teleradiology (Goldberg 1996). In fact, many of the technical challenges in teleradiology relate to legacy systems that are not compatible with contemporary standards, and for this reason each teleradiology system must be tailored for the local conditions. The following discussion summarizes some of the key issues in image acquisition, transmission, interpretation, and clinical practice of teleradiology. A pictorial representation of a typical teleradiology system is illustrated in Figures 13.1 and 13.2.

IMAGE ACQUISITION AND IMAGE DIGITIZATION

Although any type of medical image may be transmitted by teleradiology, all images must be in a digital form before transmission can occur. Con-

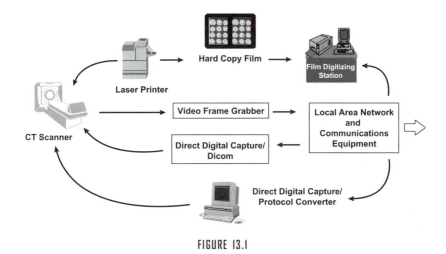

FIGURE 13.1

Schematic diagram of different approaches to image acquisiton in teleradiology.

ventional hard copy images from any modality can be digitized by special high-resolution laser or charge-coupled device (CCD) scanners (Figure 13.1). Simplistically, film scanners for teleradiology function similarly to fax machines by scanning analog data and converting it into digital form. CCD scanners using the same technology as video cameras have tiny photocells

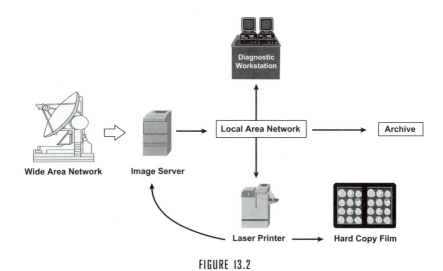

FIGURE 13.2

Schematic layout of a teleradiology interpretation site.

that acquire data from a transilluminated film. Laser scanners offer better signal-to-noise ratios than CCD scanners, leading to superior contrast resolution (Frosberg 1995). They are however, more expensive. Additional studies are required to determine if the superior contrast resolution offered by laser scanners is diagnostically significant.

Another alternative to image digitization of hard copy films is the use of a video camera to view a film on a light box. The analog video signal can then be converted into a digital format. This approach was very common in the early days of teleradiology but has been largely abandoned due to inadequate image quality.

Many images are inherently digital: computed tomography, magnetic resonance, ultrasound, nuclear medicine, computed radiography, and digital fluoroscopy. All can be directly linked to a teleradiology system if they are in a standard format (Figure 13.1). Fortunately, more and more imaging devices are complying with the ACR-NEMA (American College of Radiology and National Electronics Manufacturer's Association) DICOM-3 standard (Digital Image Communication in Medicine—version 3). DICOM-3 is important to teleradiology because a direct digital connection can be made from the image source to the teleradiology server and then from the teleradiology-receiving computer to a diagnostic workstation. Furthermore, DICOM-3 offers no loss of the full 12-bit data set (2056 grayscales) generated from digitally acquired images, no image degradation, and has full capability to adjust image window and level settings. DICOM-3 is a great step forward, although implementation of the standard is still not uniform. Some manufacturers may be DICOM-compliant, but the standard allows for enough flexibility that implementations can vary from one manufacturer to another. However, these incompatibilities are usually resolved with the cooperation of the respective vendor.

In practice, many digitally acquired images cannot be directly linked to teleradiology systems because they are acquired on older equipment that is not DICOM-compliant. Different manufacturers of imaging equipment historically used proprietary file formats and communications protocols, which prevent direct interfacing to communications networks. These digitally acquired data need to be converted into the standard DICOM-3 format before image transmission can occur (Figure 13.1).

Various solutions are available to convert proprietary digital data into an acceptable form for transmission over a teleradiology network. One of the most commonly used methods is to simply take the hard copy rendition of a digital modality and digitize the image with a laser or CCD digitizer. Although this is not scientifically elegant, it overcomes a number of problems. Another alternative is to use a video frame grabber wherein the video signal output that is sent to an imaging console is converted to digital form (Figure 13.1). It is also possible to use a protocol converter, which is a special computing device that converts proprietary image data to the DICOM-3 compliant format.

IMAGE COMPRESSION

File sizes for typical digitized medical images are large (Table 13.2). Transmission of this volume of data requires significant bandwidth (the capacity of a communication medium to carry data). Therefore these file sizes may be too large for teleradiology to be effective, both practically and economically. To reduce the amount of digital data to be transmitted, the digital data can be compressed prior to transmission.

Table 13.3 illustrates the potential benefits of compression. Using the example of a typical radiographic exam with four images, the table shows that it takes 231.5 minutes to transmit at 14.4 Kb/sec, the bandwidth of most older standard phone lines and modems. This is completely impractical, and teleradiology systems use both compression and access to higher bandwidths (Table 13.4) to reduce transmission times to manageable levels.

Compression can be "lossless" (reversible), with compression ratios typically in the range of 3:1 and the original data set can be fully regenerated, or "lossy" (irreversible), where much higher compression ratios are

TABLE 13.2
File Sizes for Digital Medical Images (Megabytes)

Modality	Image Matrix	Study	Images/File size (Mb)
Mammography	$4096 \times 5120 \times 12$	4	125.0
Plain radiographs	$2048 \times 2048 \times 12$	4	25.0
Fluoroscopy	$1024 \times 1024 \times 8$	18	19.0
CT	$512 \times 512 \times 12$	30	12.0
MRI	$256 \times 256 \times 12$	100	10.0
US	$256 \times 256 \times 8$	24	1.6
Nuclear Medicine	$128 \times 128 \times 8$	24	0.4

TABLE 13.3

Effect on Transmission Times (minutes) of Compression for Digitized Radiographs (25 MB)

Compression Ratio	Bandwidth				
	14.4 Kbps†	28.8 Kbps	56 Kbps	1.455 Mbps(TI)	155 Mbps(ATM)
1:1	231.5*	115.7	58.8	2.2	0.02
2:1	115.7	57.8	29.4	1.1	0.01
10:1	3.1	11.5	5.9	0.22	0.002
20:1	11.5	5.7	3.0	0.11	0.001
30:1	7.7	3.8	2.0	0.07	0.0006
60:1	3.8	1.9	1.0	0.04	0.0003

†Kilobits per second.

possible. Compression ratios of at least 10:1 are generally required before data compression can have a significant economic effect. Although lossy compression requires some loss from the original data set, several studies have shown that compression ratios of 20:1 or higher can be achieved without sacrificing diagnostic image content (Goldberg et al. 1997; Goldberg et al. 1994; Aberle et al. 1993).

TABLE 13.4

Effect of Bandwidth on the Transmission Times (minutes) of Medical Images

Modality	Bandwidth				
	14.4 Kbps†	28.8 Kbps	56 Kbps	1.544 Mbps(TI)	155 Mbps(ATM)
Plain Radiographs	231.5*	115.7	58.8	2.2	0.02
Fluoroscopy	176	88	44	1.6	0.02
CT	111	55.5	27.8	1.0	0.04
MRI	94	47.5	23.5	0.9	0.01
Nuclear Medicine	6.4	3.2	1.6	0.03	0.0003

*All transmission times in minutes.
†Kilobits per second.

The Joint Photographics Experts Group (JPEG) standard is the most commonly employed technique, but a number of alternatives exist, including wavelets, which have proven to be a practical and powerful compression tool. Both JPEG and wavelets can be used in either a lossy or lossless mode. JPEG compression is the only technique currently supported by the DICOM-3 standard. JPEG's principal advantages are that it is inexpensive, is widely acceptable to most computing platforms and is implemented in both hardware and software. It does, however, suffer from "block artifacts" (artificial edges created between pixel blocks to which the human eye is sensitive), particularly at higher compression ratios (Ho et al. 1993). Wavelet compression may be advantageous at higher compression ratios, which may be required for implementation of a teleradiology system that is both practical and economical. The DICOM working group on compression (Group 4) is evaluating alternative compression techniques such as wavelets for inclusion in the standard.

A major advantage of wavelet compression over JPEG compression is that it permits substantially higher compression ratios while maintaining image quality. This has practical implications for high-volume teleradiology, particularly from international sites, where the cost of data transmission becomes a significant factor in the overall cost of the teleradiology system. Several studies have now confirmed that compression ratios of up to 20:1 are diagnostically acceptable (Goldberg et al. 1994, 1997). Film transmission times can therefore be significantly reduced, thereby permitting images to reach the referral site within a fraction of the time at significantly reduced costs (Table 13.3). "Real-time" teleradiology therefore becomes a reality, enabling remote consultations while the patient is still in the doctor's office or emergency room at the remote site.

Wavelet compression algorithms consist of three basic functions: (1) transformation, (2) quantization, and (3) lossless coding (Goldberg et al. 1997). Once discrete wavelet transformation has occurred, the image is processed using quantitization, which is the lossy step in the compression algorithm. Care must be taken at this stage not to lose image quality because of the lossy step in the process. Finally, lossless coding is performed, which removes redundant information from the data set. Once compressed, the image is transferred to the remote site where it requires decompression before it can be interpreted. The lossless step that was performed as the last step in image compression is reversed. Quantization cannot be reversed as it is a lossy function. Finally, the image is reconstructed using an inverse transformation process, which is then available for image interpretation.

Although image degradation occurs at higher compression ratios using wavelet compression, these artifacts produce less image degradation than

JPEG artifacts at similar compression ratios. Practical image quality is maintained up to compression ratios of 20:1 and even higher.

IMAGE TRANSMISSION

Several forms of transmission media exist with different bandwidths (Table 13.4) including: conventional dial-up telephone lines (9.6 to 28.8 kilobits/second—Kb/s), switched digital service (56 Kb/s), frame relay (up to T1), Integrated Services Digital Network or ISDN (128 Kb/s), T1 lines (1.544 Mb/s), DS-3 (44.736 Mb/s), and Asynchronous Transfer Mode or ATM (typically 155 Mb/s). Although ATM can be extremely fast, it is expensive. T1 and ISDN lines are variably deployed, and may be expensive for small-volume teleradiology. Many teleradiology requirements can be satisfied with conventional telephone lines, providing compression ratios of at least 10:1 along with high-speed modems (28 or 56 Kb/sec). Ultimately, the choice of line depends on the customer's needs, the volume of studies to be transmitted, the types of studies, turnaround times, and expected peak activity. If all the images are transmitted during one period of the day, then higher bandwidth may be required. As indicated in Table 13.4, if sufficient bandwidth is available, transmission times become quite short even for uncompressed large image files.

Transmission of digitized data requires communication equipment. The nature of the equipment depends on the communication medium being used. This may be a modem for conventional telephone lines, a terminal adapter for an ISDN line, or a channel service unit (CSU) for a T1 line.

IMAGE INTERPRETATION

Once images are received from the wide area network (WAN) at the interpretation site, they can be sent directly to an interpretation workstation or to an image server that permits distribution within the institution (Figure 13.2). Archiving or storing the images for long periods may not be required, as is necessary for PACS. Provided images are on-line for several days to handle delays in processing (i.e., weekends and holidays) or to respond to clinical questions pertinent to the case, longer-term storage usually is not necessary because the images are typically archived in the department of origin.

The type of monitor used to read the studies depends on whether full primary readings are being performed or whether the system is being used for "on-call emergencies." The American College of Radiology (ACR) recommends that a minimum resolution of 2000×2000 pixels $\times 12$ bits for image acquisition and display is required for conventional radiographs (Ho et al. 1993). Monitors capable of this degree of resolution are expensive and impractical for general home use when "on-call." For lower resolution images (CT, MRI, ultrasound, and nuclear medicine), 512×512 pixels $\times$ 8-bit resolution is adequate, for which most monitors used for home personal computers suffice.

ACCURACY OF TELERADIOLOGY

Improvements in teleradiology systems and the imperatives of contemporary medical practice have led to the widespread use of teleradiology. Two of the major concerns by early adopters have been whether radiologists would accept "softcopy" review of images on computer workstation screens vs. traditional hardcopy, and whether the accuracy of interpretation was sufficient to justify deployment of clinical teleradiology. Both questions have now been answered to variable degrees. First, radiologists have readily adapted to computer viewing to the point that many departments are using it not only for teleradiology cases but also for routine work. At Massachusetts General Hospital, substantially all modalities, including plain radiography, fluoroscopy, angiography, CT, MRI, ultrasound, and nuclear medicine, are routinely acquired, viewed, interpreted, and managed in a digital electronic environment. In most cases, hardcopy films are no longer printed, and there is a growing consensus that in many applications the ability to optimize image contrast and intensity greatly facilitates the radiologist's practice.

With respect to accuracy of interpretation of softcopy vs. hardcopy, the issues are more complex. For the relatively low-resolution cross-sectional modalities, including CT, MRI, ultrasound, and nuclear medicine, the accuracy of softcopy interpretation has, for all practical purposes, not been an issue. It has not been the subject of intense clinical research investigation. Radiologists have simply switched with a collective subjective impression of equal or superior interpretive accuracy. The relatively low resolution of these studies is easily encompassed by the resolution of commonly available monitors. The ability to use flexible viewing formats, such as "stack mode," which allows the radiologist to move quickly back and forth through a series of tomographic sections, has supported the change in practice from hardcopy to softcopy viewing of these modalities. In the teleradiology application, softcopy viewing of these modalities is no different remotely than locally, once acquisition of the original digital data sets has been accomplished.

With respect to conventional radiographic images, the question of accuracy is less clear (Gorden, Knapp, and Sanders 1991; Grigsby et al. 1995; Ho et al. 1993; Hubble et al. 1993; Jutra 1959; Kvedar et al. 1997; Larson et al. 1998; Mullick, Fontelo, and Pemble 1996; Murphy and Bird 1974; Murphy et al. 1972; Perednia and Allen 1995; Rajavi et al. 1992; Rayman 1992; Sanders and Tedesco 1993). A significant body of literature compares accuracy of interpretation of original hardcopy radiographs with digitized radiographs viewed in softcopy mode. As pointed out by Larson et al. (1998) among others, there is an inevitable loss of spatial and contrast resolution in the digitization process, with some subjective decrease in image quality (Ho et al. 1993). However, in their study of the sensitivity for detecting nodules, pneumothoraces, interstitial lung disease, and fractures, there were no statistically significant differences between the original hardcopy analog radiographs and the digitized images viewed on a 1280×1024 pixel matrix monitor equipped with an 8 bit/pixel grayscale display. An important point in Larson's study is that the overall accuracy for detection of conditions such as nodules and pneumothoraces is less than optimal in the first place, averaging 60% and 77%, respectively. These numbers are in keeping with the literature and indicate that the real issue is finding more accurate ways of detecting subtle abnormalities regardless of viewing method. Computer-assisted diagnostic techniques will probably be required to boost detection of subtle nodules and pneumothoraces from historic levels.

Another problem in assessing the accuracy of softcopy interpretation of radiographs is the low resolution and low quality of much of the equipment, including digitizers and workstations used for these analyses. For example, papers by Ackerman (1993) and Scott (1993, 1995) demonstrated statistically lower detection rates for digitized radiographs vs. analog radiographs for pneumonia and fractures (Kvedar et al. 1997; Larson et al. 1998; Murphy and Bird 1974). However, the digitizer used in their studies had a spot size of 210 μm compared with the 100 μm spot size used in Larson's work. Also, the monitor resolution was either 1280×1024 or 1200×1600 pixels. Each of these is lower than the minimum standard recommended by the American College of Radiology of 2.5 lp/mm at a 10-bit depth (Hubble et al. 1993). This line pair resolution requires a equates to a roughly 2000×2500 resolution matrix for a 14" $\times$ 17" radiograph.

Optimistically, some studies with high resolution monitors have demonstrated substantial equivalency between hardcopy vs. softcopy interpretation. Goldberg's prospective study (1993) of 685 cases of double-read softcopy and hardcopy produced overall agreement in 97% of cases without a statistical advantage for either approach (Perednia and Allen 1995). Ten cases were judged to be false negative by softcopy interpretation, three cases were judged to be hardcopy interpretation errors, and one case was unresolved as observer variation. In Rajavi's series of 239 pediatric cases (1992), no significant difference was found between hardcopy interpretation and use of high resolution 2000×2000 pixel softcopy images on a CRT monitor. The clearly agreed-upon exception to softcopy viewing is mammography, which requires higher spatial resolution than is available on current monitors.

The major problem in sorting through the literature on the accuracy of softcopy interpretation of radiographs is the lack of standardization. Digitizers of widely varying spot size and workstations with different spatial resolutions, luminosities, and functional characteristics have been used, and there is no widespread use of standard sets of reference images, making true comparisons between observers difficult. Work on defining the necessary parameters for optimal softcopy viewing continues. In the meantime, the practice of softcopy interpretation of radiographs is rapidly becoming widespread as departments of radiology become increasingly digital. There is also no question that the quality of radiographs obtained by computed radiography or direct digital capture are superior to radiographs obtained in original analog hardcopy format and secondarily digitized by a CCD or laser digitizer. The optimal configuration for teleradiology of all modalities is direct digital capture with transmission of the full digital data set.

APPLICATIONS OF TELERADIOLOGY

Table 13.5 summarizes current clinical, research, and educational uses of teleradiology. Although exact numbers are not available, several thousand teleradiology systems are deployed in the United States. Many of these, if not the majority, are "lower end" or entry-level systems used by radiologists to provide emergency or on-call coverage for their practices. The home workstation is often a personal computer, so that CT, MRI, ultrasound, and nuclear medicine images up to 512×512 pixels or somewhat more can be displayed at full resolution. These systems often allow image magnification so that plain films may be viewed at nominal full resolution according to the American College of Radiology standards, as noted. Full resolution is equivalent to roughly 2000×2500 pixels.

On-call applications are proving extremely valuable in the clinical practice of radiology. Radiologists are able to provide more rapid consultations than would be possible if physical travel to the hospital were required. Radiologists

TABLE 13.5

Applications of Teleradiology

1. On-call coverage—Emergency/24 hr.
   — Hospital to home
   — Inter- and intrainstitutional
2. Primary Interpretations
   — Free-standing imaging centers
   — Rural hospitals and clinics
   — Imaging centers within regional delivery systems
   — Nursing homes, other special care facilities
3. "Reverse" teleradiology
4. Second opinions/consultations
5. Access to subspecialty expertise at academic medical centers
   Domestic and international consultations
6. Image processing
7. Utilization management
8. Quality assurance
9. Overreads by second radiologist
10. Research
11. Image data collection and management
    Image analysis
12. Teaching files
13. Care presentations
14. On-line journals

can cover multiple institutions simultaneously, and subspecialists within a group can provide on-call coverage more flexibly. Interinstitutional on-call coverage is also beginning. This will be invaluable as radiologists are challenged to provide 24-hour-per-day emergency interpretation services. Round-the-clock service is impractical for solo practitioners or small groups. However, teleradiology offers the opportunity for individual radiologists and small groups to come together in coverage consortia. By doing so they can stand on the same competitive turf to provide contemporaneous interpretation without having to be on-call an undue or impractical percentage of the time.

One of the best-documented teleradiology programs in the United States providing services to rural hospitals and clinics is at the University of Iowa (Rayman 1992; Sanders and Tedesco 1993). Franken et al. (1995) have studied patterns of use and have tried to determine what value is added by radiologists' consultation vs. having studies reviewed by nonradiologists. They have confirmed that higher accuracy is achieved by radiologists. For example, in one of their teleradiology series, radiologists demonstrated a 92% vs. 86% sensitivity compared with family practitioners in interpreting studies of the chest and extremities.

Another growing application of teleradiology is coverage for free-standing imaging centers, outpatient clinics, nursing homes, and smaller hospitals. In these applications, common themes are improved coverage, improved access to subspecialist radiologists, and lower cost of service provided. Using the experience with the Massachusetts General Hospital (MGH) as an example, teleradiology is used for all of the purposes cited. Prior to teleradiology, if a clinician in a neighborhood health center needed an immediate interpretation, films were put into a taxicab and taken to the MGH main campus. This cumbersome and expensive solution was never satisfactory and is being replaced by teleradiology, with essentially real-time, On-line interpretative services becoming available throughout the MGH service region. Routine interpretations from the affiliated imaging centers had been available only through batch reading of cases brought twice a day to the MGH main campus or one of the larger satellite centers. Now, every case can be read immediately by a subspecialist radiologist. The MGH experience highlights the observation that teleradiology will be used extensively by regional integrated delivery systems to improve radiology coverage.

The rapid growth in freestanding imaging centers, often dedicated to cross-sectional imaging, has provided another impetus for teleradiology. Hundreds of these centers across the country have been established by nonradiologist entrepreneurs, who then approach the radiology community for professional interpretation support. Teleradiology is an efficient way for groups of radiologists to work with these imaging centers to expand their practices and benefit from the growth in demand for imaging studies without unduly disrupting the logistics of their practices, especially in the case of hospital-based radiology groups.

A number of institutions, including MGH as well as the U.S. military (Satava 1992; Satava 1993; Satava and Jones 1996; Scott et al. 1993; Scott et al. 1995; Slasky et al. 1990; U.S. Department of Commerce 1997), are exploring the concept of "reverse teleradiology" by sending cases from larger centers to smaller centers. In some situations, small departments require a radiologist to do procedures or to meet requirements for direct supervision but do not generate enough work to keep them busy or justify their cost. By sending cases from busier departments, the presence of the on-site radiologist can be cost-justified, with the added benefit of improving the quality of care offered at the smaller location. At MGH, this model provides coverage for a series of high-tech imaging centers that the department has established in the community surrounding Boston. This allows the department to place a staff radiologist at each location without loss of productivity.

Teleradiology also provides access to subspecialty expertise at academic medical centers or to second opinions and consultations among larger radiology groups. This practice is growing both domestically and internationally and is being highly influenced by the Internet. Patients, physicians, third-party payers, and government agencies all need second opinions from time to time. Web sites on the Internet are being established to solicit and accommodate these opinions. In other cases, academic practices, larger radiology groups, and commercial enterprises dedicated to teleradiology are making their services available for second opinions and consultations.

The increasing importance of image postprocessing suggests another application of teleradiology that has been used in the early days of CT and may become common. Smaller facilities without on-site access to 3-D rendering software or personnel with image-processing expertise can readily access both via teleradiology. Multi-site institutions send image sets to central processing.

The possibility for radiology groups to help each other in their quality assurance programs is another potential use of teleradiology. In this model, a statistical sampling of cases from one group can be sent to another group via teleradiology for a quality assurance overread. This model is also useful for helping radiology groups initiate services in a new modality. For example, if a group that has not provided MRI services begins doing so, as they come up to speed they can use teleradiology to send cases to a more experienced group for an overreading function. This was a common practice in the early days of MRI, although the cases were often sent as hardcopy.

Research and educational applications of teleradiology are less well-publicized than direct clinical applications. The department at MGH has used teleradiology to manage clinical trials in which imaging is an important part of the data collection. This application is likely to grow dramatically with the increased use of imaging-based surrogate endpoints in drug trials and the establishment of the ACRIN (American College of Radiology Imaging Network) by the American College of Radiology for the purpose of organizing clinical trials aimed at assessing the efficacy of imaging technologies.

Educational applications of teleradiology are burgeoning over the Internet. Many academic departments have Web sites with extensive teaching files. These files are often augmented by case presentations. The American Board of Radiology is exploring the possibility of administering its certifying examinations electronically. Major journals have extensive Web sites providing a range of services for their subscribers and even for non-subscribers, and it is likely that the applications of remote education will become among the most prevalent uses of teleradiology.

WHAT WE HAVE LEARNED ABOUT THE PRACTICE OF TELERADIOLOGY

Table 13.6 summarizes some of the practical dicta learned over the last decade from the day-to-day practice of teleradiology. These do not fall into the realm of science or technology, and most are not covered by the ACR standards. For example, we have learned that there is still a need to communicate directly with referring physicians. Even though the consultation can be provided for a patient and physician who are hundreds or even thousands miles away, there is no substitute for direct person-to-person discussion of complex and difficult cases, especially when the diagnosis is not clearcut. A corollary point is that, being remote carries a greater responsibility because there is a greater risk of losing track of a particular case during follow-up.

TABLE 13.6
Pragmatic Issues in Teleradiology Practice

1. There is still a need for physician-to-physician communication

2. If anything, being remote from the patient carries a greater responsibility

3. The technology must be affordable and user friendly

4. Contingency plans must be in place for system down-time

5. Management of a high volume multi-site practice requires organization and well designed standards for operation

6. Ideally, both the sending and receiving sites should use a common radiology information system

7. Good image quality is a sine qua non for acceptance by radiologists

8. Billing by the sending (remote) entity is generally more efficient

9. Speech recognition for reporting is a useful adjunct to teleradiology

Teleradiology systems are subject to downtime just like any other device. Therefore, to the extent that a practice depends on teleradiology, there is greater exposure to equipment failure. Redundancy and backup contingency plans are highly desirable.

In the early days of teleradiology, people were fascinated by the technical tour de force of being able to capture images digitally and send them to another location. This, of course, is not the point of teleradiology. Rather, the purpose of teleradiology is to provide a clinical service, and therefore the technology must be user-friendly to all involved, especially the radiologists. Nothing kills a teleradiology practice faster than clumsy equipment that slows everyone down. An important corollary here is that good original image quality is a sine qua non for acceptance by radiologists. In some sense, there is a greater imperative to deal with a substandard image when it arrives from some faraway place, but expecting radiologists to constantly deal with images of lower quality than they would accept in their own practice is not sustainable over the long run. Trying to improve image quality actually offers a great opportunity for a teleradiology center to work with the sending location on imaging protocols and to provide feedback on image quality.

The management of high-volume teleradiology practice is qualitatively different from the management of a small-volume practice. The occasional case can be dealt with in an ad-hoc manner. As volumes go up and more people are involved, especially in a practice that distributes cases to different subspecialists, a high level of organization is required. MGH has several teleradiology coordinators who help with case distribution and who oversee the quality control of reports, including report demographics, as they are returned to the sending location. Ideally, a common radiology information system would be used on both sides of the teleradiology practice. Generally, this is not possible when services are provided to outside entities. This creates an extra burden and responsibility to make sure that images are matched up with the right patient and right sending location. The technology for electronic connectivity for the images per se is now way ahead of the information system infrastructure necessary to sustain large-volume teleradiology practices.

From a practical standpoint, billing by the sending entity that deals directly with the patient is generally more efficient than trying to bill for teleradiology services remotely. This is especially true when the service is in another state and the provider entity has no physical presence in the service area. One interesting exception is Medicare; the local intermediary can be billed for a service provided outside its service region because Medicare patients are covered everywhere in the country.

Billing arrangements are handled in a myriad of ways that can accomplish this objective. For example, the originating hospital or imaging center can effectively make the teleradiology provider part of its practice and credential the individuals involved as though they were members of the remote group. Alternatively, the teleradiology interpretation can be considered a consultation to the radiologist at a remote site, in which case that individual would bill the patient under his or her name and remit the consultation fee to the teleradiology provider. Some freestanding imaging centers prefer to bill globally, with the teleradiology provider executing an assignment agreement and receiving a per case amount. In other arrangements, the billing can be split between technical and professional, except when this becomes problematic at a distance because of the need to collect detailed insurance information from the patient, as discussed previously.

The essence of teleradiology is speed. The incorporation of speech recognition dictation into the process is a useful adjunct to teleradiology to reduce turnaround time and enhance the overall service provided to the remote site. At MGH, voice recognition dictation has also reduced the number of "pending" cases, greatly simplifying the management of the teleradiology operation.

LEGAL AND SOCIOECONOMIC ISSUES

Table 13.7 lists legal and socioeconomic issues affecting telemedicine. Most of these are still unresolved to variable degrees.

TABLE 13.7
Legal and Socioeconomic Issues

1. Medical licensure and credentialling
2. Malpractice insurance coverage
3. Jurisdictional control over malpractice suits
4. Confidentiality of medical records
5. Physician-patient relationship
6. Technical and clinical practice standards
7. Reimbursement by third parties
8. Turf issues between radiologists

LICENSURE AND CREDENTIALLING

A conflict between, on the one hand, the ability of teleradiology and other telemedicine services to transcend geographic barriers technologically and, on the other, the legal responsibilities of medical licensing authorities within individual states has increased. Both the American Medical Association and the American College of Radiology have adopted policies that recommend full licensure in states were teleradiology or other forms of telemedicine are practiced (Wilson and Hodge 1995; Wittson, Affleck, and Johnson 1961). The ACR policy says: "states and their Medical Board should require a full and unrestricted medical license in the state in which the examination originates, with no differentiation by specialty, for physicians who wish to regularly practice telemedicine." This means that a physician must be licensed in both the state of his or her residence and in the other state where the image originated. Many states have either passed legislation or implemented rulings by state medical boards to this effect. These laws and rulings are summarized in Chapter 14. Requirements for full licensure are pending in several additional states, and a number of states are considering a limited license or registration program, with the proviso that the provider physician be licensed in another state. The Federation of State Medical Boards favors special-purpose licensure providing telemedicine services.

The ultimate outcome of the licensure issue will have a dramatic impact on how teleradiology is deployed in the United States. If the country is balkanized through excessive state-level protectionism, the full benefit to patients and the health system will not be realized. On the other hand, legitimate concerns about quality control and accountability that must be addressed.

In addition to licensure, some hospitals may require teleradiology providers to apply for staff credentials. It is not clear how widespread this practice is, but the question of whether credentials are necessary or desirable should be addressed on a case-by-case basis.

MALPRACTICE INSURANCE COVERAGE

It behooves all radiologists providing teleradiology services outside of their states, even if they are licensed in other states, to determine prospectively the willingness of their insurance providers to extend coverage for teleradiology. Although, as noted by Leonard Berlin (1998) no lawsuits have alleged malpractice related to teleradiology or telemedicine as of mid-1998 (Zajtchuk and Zajtchuk 1996), it is inevitable that this will happen some day.

Moreover, as Berlin points out, it is an established legal principle that the state in which the injury occurs and that has the greatest connection to the injury possesses jurisdiction over the lawsuit. Thus, a physician and his or her insurance company may face the prospect of defending themselves in a remote location, which can be expensive and time-consuming, and carry the added disadvantage of having the teleradiology provider be looked upon as an outsider. Moreover, some states have capped malpractice awards, and plaintiffs can shop elsewhere for the most favorable jurisdiction.

PATIENT CONFIDENTIALITY

The issue of patient confidentiality is addressed in the American College of Radiology guidelines, but there is no assurance in practice that this standard is being achieved (Hubble et al. 1993). Computer networks, including the Internet, have historically suffered major lapses in security. For teleradiology, the image-compression process encrypts the image in a way that prevents casual theft, but much more work needs to be done to ensure patient privacy. Failure to take appropriate steps to protect the medical record against unapproved access and to protect it from inappropriate or unauthorized alteration can in itself result in malpractice litigation. The issue of patient privacy has been exacerbated by the increasing intrusion of third-party insurance companies into the lives of patients through their medical records and has raised the issue of patient privacy and confidentiality to a high profile nationally.

STANDARDS

As noted in the telemedicine report to Congress from the U.S. Department of Commerce (1997), there are no specialty-generated technical standards, protocols, or clinical guidelines for telemedicine (Wittson, Affleck, and Johnson 1961), with the exception of the American College of Radiology (ACR), which has developed practice guidelines for teleradiology. The American Medical Association, the American Telemedicine Association, and a number of other professional societies are currently developing practice standards for telemedicine. The Department of Commerce report also notes that the FDA is the lead federal agency with responsibility for ensuring the safety and effectiveness of telemedicine devices marketed in the United States.

The ACR has deemed that several criteria in the teleradiology process should meet minimum standards. (The ACR guidelines are included as an appendix to this chapter.) It would be prudent for anyone providing teleradiology services to review the ACR standards. Highlights from the guide-lines include:

▶ For small matrix studies (e.g., CT, MRI, ultrasound, nuclear medi-cine, digital fluorography, and digital angiography), $512 \times 512 \times$ 8-bit acquisition data sets should be used; for large matrix images (e.g., conventional radiographs), data sets should be a minimum of 2.5 1p/mm at a minimum 10-bit depth.

▶ Minimum display resolution is not specified, although the display device should be capable of displaying all acquired data. In practice this means a 512×512 monitor for small matrix studies and a 2000×2500 monitor for large matrix studies.

▶ Image annotation (patient demographics and examination informa-tion) should be included.

▶ Image display stations should provide functionality for window width and level settings, inverting contrast, image rotation, measurement function, and magnification.

▶ Cathode ray tube (CRT) brightness of at least 50 ft-lamberts should be achieved (conventional view-boxes are 300 to 400 ft-lamberts).

▶ Compression ratios should be displayed with the image (no specifi-cation for what type or level of compression).

▶ Reasonable measures must be taken to protect patient confidentiality.

REIMBURSEMENT

Many private insurance companies and government programs have been re-luctant to pay for general telemedicine services. Teleradiology has been an exception, with fairly uniform recognition by third parties. Medicare and Medicaid have provided coverage for teleradiology but not for services such as video consultations between doctors and patients. The key issue for Medicare is whether face-to-face contact would ordinarily be required be-tween patient and physician. One interesting initiative cited in the Telemed-icine Report to Congress is a law passed in Louisiana that mandates reim-bursement rates for physicians involved in telemedicine and specifically prohibits insurance carriers from discriminating against telemedicine as a medium for delivering health care services (Wittson, Affleck, and Johnson 1961). California has also passed legislation requiring private managed care plans to cover telemedicine services.

Teleradiology is clearly an advantaged service when it comes to reimbursement because face-to-face contact is not ordinarily required for most radiology services. However, Medicare does not recognize teleradiology coverage as sufficient to meet its requirements for direct supervision. In addition, for safety reasons as well as prudence, on-site physician coverage should be present for administration of contrast media.

TURF ISSUES

The radiology community is divided on the issue of teleradiology. Although the general concept has been widely embraced throughout different practice settings—from the largest academic institutions to solo practitioners in private practice—the practice of teleradiology continues to create controversy. Some people in the radiology community have expressed concern that larger groups, including academic medical centers, will use their financial resources, prestige, and clout to invade the turf of smaller groups who regard their geographic service area as inviolable. In defending this view, the point is made that it is important for radiologists to provide more than just interpretations and to take part in the medical life of the respective hospital or health care community. Counterarguments include the view that teleradiology provides patients and their attending physicians the opportunity to access more highly subspecialized experts than may be available in the local community, and that it is not appropriate for individual radiologists to stand between the patient and such expert opinions.

It is far from clear how the issues of mistrust and suspicion on the part of community radiologists vs. the desire of larger subspecialist groups to offer their expertise more broadly will be resolved. However, one opportunity open to community radiologists is to come together among themselves to form larger networks in which individuals can begin to subspecialize and, as discussed above, where smaller groups can provide coverage to each other for a variety of purposes. The one thing abundantly obvious in the Internet age is that patients will increasingly expect electronic access when they see it as beneficial to their interests and needs. Doctors, including radiologists, will be ill-served to stand in the way of that new and increasing imperative.

CONCLUSION

Teleradiology has transitioned from its infancy and is no longer a technological curiosity. It is already part of daily practice. It is here, it works, and it will have an enduring role in shaping the future of radiology. It is likely that, in less than a decade, the term "teleradiology" will be obsolete for the simple reason that remote interpretations and consultations will be such an integral part of radiology practice that referring to them will neither require nor occasion a special term.

ACKNOWLEDGMENT   Portions of this chapter were published as Thrall JH, Boland G. *Telemedicine in Practice.* Seminars in Nuclear Medicine. 28: 142–157 1998 (with permission).

▶ REFERENCES

Aberle DR, Gleeson F, Sayre JW et al. *The effect of irreversible image compression on diagnostic accuracy in thoracic imaging.* Invest Radiol 28:398–403, 1993.

Ackerman S et al. *Receives operating characteristic analysis of fracture and pneumonia detection: Comparison laser-digitized workstation images and conventional analog radiographs.* Radiology 186:263–268, 1993.

ACR Bulletin 53:13, 1997.

ACR Standard for Teleradiology. American College of Radiology, Reston, VA 1994.

Andrus WS, Bird KT. *Teleradiology: Evolution through bias to reality.* Chest 62:655–657, 1972.

Baer L et al. *Pilot studies of telemedicine for patients with obsessive-compulsive disorder.* American Journal of Psychiatry 152:1383–1385.

Baer L et al. *Automated telephone screening survey for depression.* JAMA 273:1943–1944, 1995.

Berlin L. *Malpractice issues in radiology: Telereadiology.* AJR 170:1417–1422, 1998.

Bird KT. *Cardiopulmonary frontiers: Quality health care via interactive television.* Chest 61: 204–207, 1972.

Black-Schaffer S, Flotte TJ. *Current issues in telepathology.* Telemedicine Journal 1:95–106.

Calcagni DE et al. *Operation Joint Endeavor in Bosnia: Telemedicine systems and case reports.* Telemedicine Journal 2:211–224, 1996.

Cawthon MA et al. *Preliminary assessment of `computed tomography and satellite teleradiology from Operation Desert Storm.* Investigative Radiology 26:854–857, 1991.

Dakins D. *Market targets 1997.* Telemedicine and Telehealth Networks 3:25–29, 1997.

Elam EA et al. *Efficacy of digital radiography for detection of pneumothorax: Comparison with conventional chest radiography.* AJR 158:509–514, 1992.

Fosberg DA. *Quality assurance in teleradiology.* Telemedicine Journal 1:38–44, 1995.

Franken EA et al. *Added value of radiologist consultation to family practitioners in the outpatient setting.* Radiology 197:759–762, 1995.

Franken EA, Harkens KL, Berbaum KS. *Teleradiology consultation for a rural hospital: Patterns of use.* Academic Radiology 14:492–496, 1997.

Fuchs M. *Provider attitudes toward STARPAHC, a telemedicine project on the Papago Reservation.* Medical Care 17:59–68, 1979.

Gagner M et al. *Robotic interactive soporoscopic cholecystectomy.* Lancet 343:596–597, 1994.

Goldberg MA. *Teleradiology and telemedicine.* Radiologic Clinics of North America 43:647–665, 1996.

Goldberg MA et al. *New high resolution teleradiology system: Prospective study of diagnostic accurracy in 685 transmitted clinical cases.* Radiology 186:429–434, 1993.

Goldberg MA et al. *Application of wavelet compression to digitized radiographs.* AJR 163:463–468, 1994.

Goldberg MA et al. *Effect of 3-D wavelet compression on the detection of focal hepatic lesions at CT.* Radiology 202:159–165, 1997.

Gomez E et al. *Tertiary telemedicine support during global military humanitarian missions.* Telemedicine Journal 2:201–210, 1996.

Gorden JW, Knapp CF, Sanders JH. *Ophthalmologic electronic imaging and data transfer.* Journal of the Kentucky Medical Association 89:115–117, 1991.

Grigsby J et al. *Effects and effectiveness of telemedicine.* Health Care Financing Review 17:115–131, 1995.

Ho BKT et al. *A mathematical model to quantify JPEG block artifacts.* SPIE Physics of Medical Imaging 1987:169–274, 1993.

Hubble JP et al. *Interactive videoconferencing: A means of providing interim care to Parkinson's disease patients.* Movement Disorders 8:380–382, 1993.

Jutra A. *Teleroentgen diagnosis by means of videotape recording.* AJR 82:1099–1102, 1959.

Kvedar JC et al. The substitution of digital images for dermatologic physical examination. Archives of Dermatology 133:161–167, 1997.

Larson A et al. *Accuracy of diagnosis of subtle chest disease and subtle fractures with a teleradiology system.* AJR 170:19–22, 1998.

Mullick FG, Fontelo P, Pemble C. *Telemedicine and telepathology at the Armed Forces Institute of Pathology: History and current mission.* Telemedicine Journal 2:187–194, 1996.

Murphy RLH, Bird KT. *Telediagnosis: A new community health resource.* American Journal of Public Health 64:113–119, 1974.

Murphy RLH et al. *Accuracy of dermatologic diagnosis by television.* Archives of Dermatology 105:833–835, 1972.

Perednia DA, Allen, A. *Telemedicine technology and clinical applications.* JAMA 273:483–488, 1995.

Rajavi M et al. *Receiver-operating-characteristic study of chest radiographs in children: Digital hard-copy film versus 2K × 2K soft copy images.* AJR 158:443–448, 1992.

Rayman BR. *Telemedicine: Military applications.* Aviation and Space Environment Medicine 63:135–137, 1992.

Sanders JH, Tedesco FJ. *Telemedicine: Bringing medical care to isolated communitites.* Journal of the Medical Association of Georgia 82:237–241, 1993.

Satava RM. *Robotics, telepresence and virtual reality: A critical analysis of the future of surgery.* Minimally Invasive Therapy 1:357–363, 1992.

Satava RM. *Virtual reality surgery simulator: The first steps.* Surgical Endoscopy 7:203–205, 1993.

Satava RM, Jones SB. *Virtual reality and telemedicine: Exploring advanced concepts.* Telemedicine Journal 2:195–200, 1996.

Scott WW et al. *Subtle orthopedic fractures: Teleradiology workstation versus film interpretation.* Radiology 187:811–815, 1993.

Scott WW et al. *Interpretation of emergency department radiographs by radiologists and emergency physicians: Teleradiology workstation versus radiographic readings.* Radiology 195:223–229, 1995.

Slasky BS et al. *Receiver operating characteristic analysis of chest image interpretation with conventional, laser printed and high-resolution workstation images.* Radiology 174:775–780, 1990.

U.S. Department of Commerce. *Telemedicine Report to Congress.* January 31, 1997.

Wilson AJ, Hodge JC. *Digitized radiographs in skeletal trauma: A performance comparison between a digital workstation and the original film images.* Radiology 196:565–568, 1995.

Wittson CL, Affleck DC, Johnson V. *Two-way television group therapy.* Mental Hospital 12:22–23, 1961.

Zajtchuk JT, Zajtchuk, R. *Strategy for medical readiness: Transition to the digital age.* Telemedicine Journal 2:179–186, 1996.

▶ APPENDIX

ACR STANDARD FOR TELERADIOLOGY

(Reprinted with permission of the American College of Radiology. No other representation of this article is authorized without express written permission of the American College of Radiology.)

I. INTRODUCTION AND DEFINITION

Teleradiology is the electronic transmission of radiological images from one location to another for the purpose of interpretation and/or consultation. Teleradiology may allow more timely interpretation of radiological images and give greater access to secondary consultations and to improved continuing education. Users in different locations may simultaneously view images. Appropriately utilized, teleradiology may improve access to radiological interpretations and thus significantly improve patient care.

Teleradiology is not appropriate if the available teleradiology system does not provide images of sufficient quality to perform the indicated task.

When a teleradiology system is used to produce the official interpretation, there should not be a clinically significant loss of spatial or contrast resolution from image acquisition through transmission to final image display. For transmission of images for display use only, the image quality should be sufficient to satisfy the needs of the clinical circumstance.

This standard defines goal, qualifications of personnel, equipment guidelines, licensing, credentialing, liability, communication, quality control, and quality improvement for teleradiology. While not all-inclusive, the standard should serve as a model for all physicians and health care workers who utilize teleradiology. A glossary of commonly used terminology (Appendix A) and a reference list are included.

II. GOALS

Teleradiology is an evolving technology. New goals will continue to emerge. The current goals of teleradiology include:

A. Providing consultative and interpretative radiological services in areas of demonstrated need;

B. Making radiologic consultations available in medical facilities without on-site radiologic support;

C. Providing timely availability of radiological images and radiological image interpretation in emergent and non-emergent clinical care areas;

D. Facilitating radiological interpretations in on-call situations;

E. Providing subspecialty radiological support as needed;

F. Enhancing educational opportunities for practicing radiologists;

G. Promoting efficiency and quality improvement;

H. Sending interpreted images to referring providers;

I. Supporting telemedicine; and

J. Providing direct supervision of off-site imaging studies.

III. QUALIFICATIONS OF PERSONNEL

The radiological examination at the transmitting site must be performed by qualified personnel trained in the examination to be performed. In all cases this means a licensed and/or registered radiologic technologist, nuclear medicine technologist, or sonography technologist/sonographer. This technologist must be under the supervision of a qualified licensed physician licensed physician.

It is desirable to have a physicist and/or image management specialist on site or as consultants.

A. PHYSICIAN

The official interpretation[1] of images must be done by a physician who has:

1. An understanding of the basic technology of teleradiology, its strengths and weaknesses (as well as limitations), and who is trained in the use of the teleradiology equipment.
2. Demonstrated qualifications as delineated in the appropriate American College of Radiology (ACR) standard for the particular diagnostic modality being transmitted through teleradiology.

B. TECHNOLOGIST

The technologist or sonographer should be:

1. Certified by the appropriate registry and/or possess unrestricted state licensure.
2. Trained to properly operate and supervise the teleradiology system.

C. PHYSICIST

A qualified medical physicist is an individual who is competent to practice independently one or more of the subfields in medical physics. The American College of Radiology considers that certification and continuing education in the appropriate subfield(s) demonstrate that an individual is competent to practice one or more of the subfields in medical physics and to be a qualified medical physicist. The ACR recommends that the individual be certified in the appropriate subfield(s) by the American Board of Radiology (ABR).

---

[1]ACR Medical Legal Committee defines official interpretation as that written report (and any supplements or amendments thereto) that attach to the patient's permanent record. In healthcare facilities with a privilege delineation system, such a written report is prepared only by a qualified physician who has been granted specific delineated clinical privileges for that purpose by the facility's governing body upon the recommendation of the medical staff.

The subfields of medical physics are Therapeutic Radiological Physics, Diagnostic Radiological Physics, Medical Nuclear Physics, and Radiological Physics.

Continuing education for a qualified medical physicist should be in accordance with the ACR Standard for Continuing Medical Education (CME) (Res. 27, 1996).

D. IMAGE MANAGEMENT SPECIALIST

1. The image management specialist should be an individual who is qualified by virtue of education and experience to assess and provide problem-solving input, initiate repair, and coordinate system-wide maintenance programs to assure sustainable high-image quality and system function. This individual would also be directly involved with any system variances and expansion programs.

2. This specialist should be available in a timely manner in case of malfunction to facilitate return to optiimal system functionality.

IV. EQUIPMENT SPECIFICATIONS

Specifications for equipment utilized in teleradiology will vary depending on the individual facility's needs but, in all cases, should provide image quality and availability appropriate to the clinical need.

Compliance with the ACR/NEMA (National Electrical Manufacturers Association) Digital Imaging and Communication in Medicine Standard (DICOM) is strongly recommended for all new equipment acquisitions and consideration of periodic upgrades incorporating the expanding features of that standard should be part of the ongoing quality-control program.

Equipment guidelines cover two basic categories of teleradiology when used for rendering the official interpretation: small matrix size (e.g., computed tomography (CT), magnetic resonance imaging (MR), ultrasound, nuclear medicine, digital fluorography, and digital angiography) and large matrix size (e.g., computed radiography and digitized radiographic films).

Small matrix: A data sot should provide full-resolution data (typically 512×512 resolution at minimum 8-bit depth) for processing, manipulation, and subsequent display.

Large matrix: A data set allowing a minimum of 2.5 lp/mm spatial resolution at minimum 10-bit depth should be acquired.

A. ACQUISITION OR DIGITIZATION

Initial image acquisition should be performed in accordance with the appropriate ACR modality or examination standard.

1. Direct image capture

The image data set produced by the digital modality both in terms of image matrix size and pixel bit depth should be transferred to the teleradiology system. It is recommended that the DICOM standard be used. This is the most desirable mode of digital image acquisition for primary diagnosis.

2. Secondary image capture

a. Small matrix images. Each individual image should be digitized to a matrix size as large or larger than that of the original image by the imaging modality. The images should be digitized to a bit depth of 8 bits per pixel or greater. Film digitization or video frame grab systems conforming to the above specifications are acceptable.

b. Large matrix images. These images should be digitized to a matrix size corresponding to 2.5 lp/mm or greater, measured in the original detector plane. These images should be digitized to a bit depth of 10 bits per pixel or greater. Film digitizers will generally be required to produce these digital images.

3. General requirements

At the time of acquisition (small or large matrix), the system must include:

Annotation capabilities including patient name, identification number, date and time of examination, name of facility or institution of acquisition, type of examination, patient or anatomic part orientation (e.g., right, left, superior, inferior, etc.), amount and method of data compression. The capability to record a brief patient history is desirable.

B. COMPRESSION

Data compression may be performed to facilitate transmission and storage. Several methods including both reversible and irreversible techniques, may be used, under the direction of a qualified physician, with no reduction in clinically diagnostic image quality. The types and ratios of compression used for different imaging studies transmitted and stored by the system should be selected and periodically reviewed by the responsible physician to ensure appropriate clinical image quality.

C. TRANSMISSION

The type and specifications of the transmission devices used will be dictated by the environment of the studies to be transmitted. In all cases for, official interpretation, the digital data received at the receiving end of any transmission must have no loss of clinically significant information. The transmission system shall have adequate error-checking capability.

D. DISPLAY CAPABILITIES

General: Display workstations used for official interpretation and employed for small matrix and large matrix systems should provide the following characteristics:

1. Luminance of the gray-scale monitors should be at least 50 footlamberts;
2. Care should be taken to control the lighting in the reading room to to eliminate reflections in the monitor and to lower the ambient lighting level as much as is feasible;
3. Provide capability for selection of image sequence;
4. Capable of accurately associating the patient and study demographic characterization with one study images;
5. Capable of window and level adjustment, if those data are available;
6. Capable of pan functions and zoom (magnification) function;
7. Capable of meeting guidelines for display of all acquired data;
8. Capable of rotating or flipping the images, provided correct labeling of patient orientation is preserved;
9. Capable of calculating and displaying accurate linear measurements and pixel value determinations in appropriate values for the modality (e.g., Hounsfield units for CT images), if those data are available;
10. Capable of displaying prior image compression ratio, processing, or cropping; and

11. Elements of display that should be available include:
   a. Matrix size;
   b. Bit depth; and
   c. Total number of images acquired in the study.

There may be less stringent guidelines for display systems when these display systems are not used for the official interpretation.

E.   ARCHIVING AND RETRIEVAL

If electronic archiving is to be employed, the guidelines listed below should be followed:

1. Teleradiology systems should provide storage capacity capable of complying with all facility, state, and federal regulations regarding medical record retention. Images stored at either site should meet the jurisdictional requirements of the transmitting site. Images interpreted off-site need not be stored at the receiving facility, provided they are stored at the transmitting site. However, if the images are retained at the receiving site, the retention period of that jurisdiction must be met as well. The policy on record retention should be in writing.

2. Each exam data file must have an accurate corresponding patient and examination database record, which includes patient name, identification number, exam date, type of examination, facility at which examination was performed. It is desirable that space be available for a brief clinical history.

3. Prior examinations should be retrievable from archives in a time frame appropriate to the clinical needs of the facility and medical staff.

4. Each facility should have policies and procedures for archiving and storage of digital image data equivalent to the policies that currently exist for the protection of hard-copy storage media to preserve imaging records.

F.   SECURITY

Teleradiology systems should provide network and software security protocols to protect the confidentiality of patients' identification and imaging data. There should be measures to safeguard the data and to ensure data integrity against intentional or unintentional corruption of the data.

G. RELIABILITY AND REDUNDANCY

Quality patient care depends on availability of the teleradiology system. Written policies and procedures should be in place to ensure continuity of care at a level consistent with those for hard-copy imaging studies and medical records within a facility or institution. This should include internal redundancy systems, backup telecommunication links, and a disaster plan.

V. LICENSING, CREDENTIALING, AND LIABILITY

Physicians who provide the official interpretation[2] of images transmitted by teleradiology should maintain licensure appropriate to delivery of radiologic service at both the transmitting and receiving sites. When providing the official interpretation of images from a hospital, the physician should be credentialed and obtain appropriate privileges at that institution. These physicians should consult with their professional liability carrier to ensure coverage in both the sending and receiving sites (state or jurisdiction).

The physician performing the official interpretations must he responsible for the quality of the images being reviewed.[3]

Images stored at either site should meet the jurisdictional requirements of the transmitting site. Images interpreted off-site need not be stored at the receiving facility, provided they are stored at the transmitting site. However, if images are retained at the receiving site, the retention period of that jurisdiction must be met as well. The policy on record retention should be in writing.

The physicians who are involved in practicing teleradiology will conduct their practice in a manner consistent with the bylaws, rules, and regulations for patient care at the transmitting site.

---

[2]ACR Medical Legal Committee defines official interpretation as that written report (and any supplements or amendments thereto) that attach to the patient's permanent record. In healthcare facilities with a privilege delineation system, such a written report is prepared only by a qualified physician who has been granted specific delineated clinical privileges for that purpose by the facility's governing body upon the recommendation of the medical staff.

[3]The ACR Rules of Ethics state: "it is proper for a diagnostic radiologist to provide a consultative opinion on radiographs and other images regardless of their origin. A diagnostic radiologist should regularly interpret radiographs and other images only when the radiologist reasonably participates in the quality of medical imaging, utilization review, anti matters of policy which affect the quality of patient care."

VI. DOCUMENTATION

Communication is a critical competent of teleradiology. Physicians interpreting teleradiology examinations should render reports in accordance with the ACR Standard for Communication.

VII. QUALITY CONTROL AND IMPROVEMENT, SAFETY, INFECTION CONTROL, AND PATIENT EDUCATION CONCERNS

Policies and procedures related to quality, patient education, infection control and safety should be developed and implemented in accordance with the ACR Policy on Quality Control and Improvement, Safety, Infection Control, and Patient Education Concerns.

Any facility using a teleradiology system must have documented policies and procedures for monitoring and evaluating the effective management, safety, and proper performance of acquisition, digitization, compression, transmission archiving, and retrieval functions of the system. The quality control program should be designed to maximize the quality and accessibility of diagnostic information.

A test image, such as the SMPTE test pattern[4] should be captured, transmitted, archived, retrieved, and displayed at appropriate intervals, but at least monthly, to test the overall operation of the system under conditions that simulate the normal operation of the system. As a spatial resolution test, at least 512×512 resolution be confirmed for small matrix official interpretation, and 2.5 lp/mm resolution for large-matrix official interpretation.

As a test of the display, SMPTE pattern data files sized to occupy the full area used to display images on the monitor should be displayed. The overall SMPTE image appearance should be inspected to assure the absence of gross artifacts (e.g., blurring or bleeding of bright display areas into dark areas or aliasing of spatial resolution patterns). Display monitors used for primary interpretation should be tested at least monthly. As a dynamic range test, both the 5% and the 95% areas should be seen as distinct from the respective adjacent 0% and 100% areas.

The use of teleradiology does not reduce the responsibilities for the management and supervision of radiologic medicine.

---

[4]SMPTE test pattern RP 133-1991. Gray JF, Lisk KG, Haddick DH, Harshberger JH, Oosetehof A, Schwenker R. Test pattern for video displays and hard copy cameras. Radiology 1985; 154:519–527.

IV

FUTURE OPPORTUNITIES

LEGAL ISSUES AND FORMAL POLICIES

JOHN J. SMITH • HARRY ZIBNERS

The past decade has brought explosive growth in PACS technology, making large scale teleradiology an integral part of many radiology practices. This reality has left legislatures, the courts, and a wide variety of organizations that formulate healthcare policy scrambling to keep pace with an ever-changing practice environment. The result as a new century dawns is a patchwork of laws, courts decisions, and formal policies formulated by the American College of Radiology (ACR) and others that address a wide variety of issues relating to teleradiology. Some issues, such as the medical licensure and institutional credentials necessary to practice teleradiology in a given jurisdiction, are fairly well defined. However, the majority of legal and policy issues that confront this increasingly important aspect of radiology practice are unsettled or not even addressed, leaving a broad range of unanswered questions.

THE CURRENT SITUATION

Society is currently in the midst of an era of rapid technical innovation and change that is probably unequalled in recorded history. Computing power that required whole rooms a few short decades ago can now be conveniently carried. The cost of this computing power has fallen dramatically, making possible the widespread use of powerful computing platforms. There has been accompanying dramatic innovation in communications technology, allowing the inexpensive transfer of large volumes of data over long distances.

These innovations have combined to make teleradiology and PACS technology an everyday reality in many medical settings. Digital images are acquired, transmitted, displayed, and stored in a wide variety of settings. These range from purely local exercises, such as the interpretation of CT images at a scanner's dedicated workstation, to transmission of images over hundreds or thousands of miles for official interpretation and storage. The activities currently possible through available technology are in many ways limited only by the creativity of those who use it.

Like most activities with the potential to impact the health of the population, teleradiology and PACS technology are subject to controls established by the law and policies developed by various organizations. Laws are developed by Congress at the national level and by the various legislatures at the state level. After being finalized by the signature of the president or governor, laws are implemented by the executive branch though administrative agencies. These agencies draft regulations that define the day-to-day operation of the legislation, providing detail that is often absent from the law itself. The Food and Drug Administration (FDA) and the Health Care Financing Administration (HCFA) are well-known examples of federal agencies; a variety of state administrative agencies perform similar functions for state laws.

The content, meaning, or appropriateness of laws and regulations is often subject to dispute. Parties may contend that administrative agencies misinterpreted the law when drafting regulations, or perhaps overstepped the discretion that the law allowed them. In extreme cases, there may be questions as to whether Congress or the legislatures possessed the authority to pass the law itself. In any such dispute, it is the courts at the federal, state, and local level that serve as the final arbiter of the law. In this role, they shape the final enforcement of any legislation.

Another source of control are policies, guidelines, and standards developed by private organizations with interests in a field. In teleradiology and PACS, the American College of Radiology (ACR) has played a key role in developing standards for both the equipment employed and the role of radiologists and other personnel in applying the technology. While these standards lack the force of law, they serve an important function in defining teleradiology and PACS for those both in and outside of the radiology. In this context, similar standards have been used by courts in examining disputes involving medical practice.

The various sources of law and policy do not ordinarily prospectively address issues. Rather, it is typical for legislatures, administrative agencies, and professional organizations to develop law and policy after problems have developed that demand resolution. This means that a conflict or problem must first occur and be identified before any action is taken.

Even when the need for a new law or policy is recognized, developing that law or policy is not a quick or easy process. Congress and the state legislatures may take years to draft and enact legislation, and administrative agencies years to define the new law with regulations. Courts may be even slower to resolve new legal problems, as a number of decisions on similar disputes are typically needed to form a body of law. Even professional organizations with vested interests in areas like teleradiology and PACS, such as the ACR, generally have in place a complex mechanism to develop standards or guidelines, a process that may take years after the need for action is identified.

The result—in rapidly changing, technologically driven fields such as teleradiology and PACS—is a definite disparity between the capabilities of the technology and the institution of laws and policies to govern its use. Today, only a fraction of pertinent teleradiology and PACS issues have been addressed. Although almost every state has explicit or implied licensure requirements for radiologists interpreting teleradiology images from inside its borders, there is a dearth of court decisions addressing the various legal issues that are sure to affect its everyday practice. Furthermore, new laws are passed and new policies established on an ongoing basis, with the pace of these new controls bound to increase as the technology matures and its use becomes even more widespread.

This chapter attempts to outline current law and policy as it pertains to teleradiology and PACS. It also outlines issues with the potential to affect the fields in the near future. It is not a substitute for qualified legal advice, and radiologists engaging in these activities are urged to consult qualified legal counsel prior embarking into practice employing these technologies.

STANDARDS AND POLICIES OF PROFESSIONAL ORGANIZATIONS

The provision of medical services has been a long-standing focus of professional societies, and the activities made possible by the development of teleradiology and PACS technology are no exception. Given the technology's pronounced impact on the practice of radiology, the American College of Radiology (ACR) has taken a leading role in defining what constitutes professionally acceptable teleradiology and PACS services, developing a variety of standards and other policies. The American Medical Association (AMA) has also examined the practice of teleradiology and telemedicine. The standards and policies developed by such organizations do not have the force of law, but they do represent a detailed consensus of expert opinion in the field. As such, they may serve as important indicators regarding what constitutes the professional standard of medical practice in teleradiology and PACS.

AMERICAN COLLEGE OF RADIOLOGY (ACR)

The ACR is a leading professional society in radiology, with a membership composed of radiologists, radiation oncologists, and medical physicists. As part of an effort to advance the science of radiology and improve the quality of radiology services, the College has developed a formal mechanism for establishing and revising standards for the various subspecialty areas that make up the profession. Each standard represents a consensus policy statement on by the College. Effective January 1, 1999, the ACR established new standards for teleradiology and digital image data management.

ACR STANDARD FOR TELERADIOLOGY

This comprehensive standard covers a wide variety of issues related to teleradiology (American College of Radiology 1999b). It stresses that teleradiology must be of sufficient quality to perform the indicated task. When a system is used to perform an official interpretation, there should not be a "clinically significant loss of spatial or contrast resolution from image acquisition through transmission to final image display." From this overriding principle, the document describes in detail the personnel and equipment considered necessary to conduct teleradiology.

Initially, the standard outlines the qualifications of personnel obtaining images at the transmitting site. These individuals must be qualified to perform the specific examination being performed. In all cases, a licensed and/or registered radiologic technologist, nuclear medicine technologist, or sonography technologist is needed. In addition to appropriate technologists, a qualified medical physicist and an "image management specialist" are desirable to have on site or as consultants. The document defines an "image management specialist" as an individual who is "qualified by virtue of education and experience" to provide service to the teleradiology system.

The physician performing the official interpretation of transmitted images must have a basic understanding of the strengths and weaknesses of teleradiology, as well as be "qualified" to interpret the particular diagnostic modality at issue. With regard to what constitutes adequate qualification, the standard refers to other ACR standards for rendering interpretations on the various imaging modalities. Importantly, the teleradiology standard states that this physician should maintain licensure appropriate to the delivery of teleradiology services at both the transmitting and receiving sites. This effectively requires a physician interpreting teleradiology to maintain appropriate licensure in multiple states, if teleradiology is conducted across state lines and the state(s) involved require such licensure. The standard maintains a similar position on staff privileges: If images are transmitted from a hospital, the interpreting physician "should" be credentialed and obtain appropriate privileges at that institution.

Similar to legal requirements faced by physicians interpreting locally produced images, the ACR teleradiology standard holds the physician providing the official interpretation of teleradiology images responsible for the quality of the images being reviewed. Simply put, this position makes it difficult for physicians providing official teleradiology interpretation to escape potential liability for poor-quality images. Physicians providing official interpretations are also cautioned to consult with their professional liability carrier to assure coverage in both sending and receiving sites. A large portion of the teleradiology standard addresses technical and legal issues associated with the equipment used and the images displayed and stored by that equipment. All new equipment acquisition is strongly urged to comply with the Digital Imaging and Communication in Medicine (DICOM) Standard, developed by the ACR and the National Electrical Manufacturers Association. Two matrix categories are established for rending official image interpretation. A small matrix (512×512 resolution with a minimum of 8-bit depth) is deemed sufficient for computed tomography (CT), magnetic resonance imaging (MRI), ultrasound (US), nuclear medicine (NM), digital fluoroscopy, and digital angiography. Computed radiography and digitized radiographs are considered large matrix studies (a minimum of 2.5 lp/mm spatial resolution at a minimum of 10 bit depth).

Image data for teleradiology systems may be obtained by both direct image capture for purely digital images, or secondary image capture for film images that are digitized. Direct image capture is the "most desirable" method of acquisition for primary diagnosis. Regardless of acquisition method, images must have annotation capabilities that allow data such as patient name, identification number, name of transmitting facility, type of examination, anatomic orientation, and method of compression displayed on the image. The standard allows the use of both reversible and irreversible compression, assuming that a qualified supervising physician determines that there is no reduction in "clinically diagnostic image quality." These compression methods should be reviewed periodically by the supervising physician to "ensure appropriate image quality." Data transmission is required to have adequate error-checking capability and there must be no loss of clinically significant data during this transmission.

Display characteristics for the monitors used in officially interpreting teleradiology images are described. These should have a luminance of at least 50 ft-lamberts and be located in areas with suitable room lighting. Image manipulation features should include window and level adjustments, pan and zoom, the capability to rotate or flip images, and the ability to calculate and display accurate linear measurements and pixel values (as appropriate for the modality being interpreted). The images should be accurately associated with the correct patient study and demographic information, as well as note any compression or similar processing. Requirements for displays not being used for official interpretation are noted to be less stringent, though the exact characteristics are not delineated.

Archiving and retrieving image data receives significant attention in the standard. Prior examinations should be retrievable from the archive in a time frame appropriate to the clinical needs of the facility and medical staff. Any system should provide storage capable of complying with all facility, state, and federal regulations regarding medical record retention. Images stored at either the transmitting or receiving site should meet the specific jurisdictional requirements of the transmitting site. Images interpreted off-site need not be stored at the receiving facility. However, if such data is maintained at the receiving facility, the data retention period must meet the jurisdictional requirements of the receiving jurisdiction as well. All policies relating to the storage of image data should be written and equivalent to policies and procedures that exist for hardcopy medical images.

A teleradiology system should have protections to ensure the security of archived data. Specifically, the confidentiality of patient data must be addressed, as well as measures to safeguard the data from intentional or unintentional corruption. These protections should apply to both the network and the software it employs.

Finally, the standard addresses practical, day-to-day issues of teleradiology. Written policies and procedures to ensure a continuity of care consistent with those for hardcopy images is suggested. Mentioned are internal redundant systems, back-up telecommunications links, and a disaster plan.

At least monthly image quality control using a test image is described. Spatial resolution at such testing should be consistent with the specific matrix being employed, that is, small or large.

Currently, there is little indication as to how this revised teleradiology standard may be applied in practice. Given the ACR's reputation and the need for minimum standards in clinical teleradiology practice, many of the details of the standard will probably be adopted by radiologists practicing teleradiology. However, given the rapid advancement of technology, it is virtually certain that some of the standard's technical details will shortly be obsolete. The portions of the document calling for appropriate licensure in both the sending and receiving jurisdictions is likely to be considerably more enduring, as are the provisions applying to the archiving and retrieval of teleradiology data.

ACR STANDARD FOR DIGITAL IMAGE DATA MANAGEMENT

The ACR maintains a separate standard for digital image data management (American College of Radiology 1999a). Its provisions are applicable to any system of image data management, from single modality or single use system to a complete PACS system, as would be used for teleradiology. As such, there is considerable overlap with the ACR Standard for Teleradiology, which focuses on PACS. Like the teleradiology standard, the digital image management standard states that examination that serves as the data source is subject to the specific ACR standard for that modality.

The goals of digital data image management as outlined in the standard include, but are not limited to: (1) initial acquisition or generation of accurately labeled and identified image data; (2) transmission of data to an appropriate storage medium from which it can be retrieved; (3) retrieval of data from available prior imaging studies for comparison; (4) transmission of data to remote sites for consultation, review, or formal interpretation; (5) appropriate compression of image data to facilitate transmission or storage, without loss of clinically significant information; (6) archiving of data to maintain accurate patient medical records in a form that may be retrievable in a timely fashion, meets applicable facility, state, and federal regulations, and maintains patient confidentiality; and (7) administration with appropriate database management procedures.

Most of the document itself is devoted to describing in detail how these goals are to be accomplished. Qualifications and responsibilities for personnel, including physicians, electronic/computer assistant, medical image physicist, and image management specialists are outlined, largely paralleling descriptions in the teleradiology standard. Similarly, compliance with the DICOM standard is "strongly recommended," and image categories for official interpretation are split into those for a small and a large matrix. The definitions for these matrices and the type of imaging modalities in each type of matrix are identical to the teleradiology standard, as are the descriptions of image acquisition and annotation capabilities. Transmission standards likewise mirror those detailed in the teleradiology standard.

Archiving and retrieval sections of the digital image management standard also reiterate those found in the teleradiology standard. Storage capacity must be capable of complying with all facility, state, and federal regulations regarding medical record retention, with images stored at either the transmitting or retrieval site complying with the requirements of the transmitting jurisdiction. Storage is not necessary at the receiving site, but if such storage is undertaken, the retention period of that jurisdiction must be met as well. Security to protect the confidentiality of patient identification and imaging data should be present. All policies relating to the achieving and storage of digital image data should be equivalent to those in existence for hardcopy records and should be in writing. For clinical use, any system must allow timely retrieval of archived images, as well as mechanisms to ensure continuity of care.

AMA POLICIES ON TELEMEDICINE AND TELERADIOLOGY

The American Medical Association (AMA) is the largest medical professional society in the United States, encompassing the spectrum of medical specialties and issues. The growing importance of telemedicine, which includes teleradiology and PACS, has captured the Association's attention at its highest levels. This has lead to the issuance of several reports and implementation of certain policies.

In 1996, the AMA published "The Promotion of Quality Telemedicine," which was jointly issued by the Council on Medical Education and Council on Medical Service (American Medical Association 1996). In this document, the AMA supports the ACR position that physicians providing "authenticated interpretation of images transmitted by teleradiology" should maintain licensure "appropriate to the delivery of radiologic service" at both the transmitting and receiving sites. As noted previously, this position generally requires that a radiologist interpreting telemedicine studies maintain full licensure in both the transmitting and the receiving jurisdictions. However, if the service provided is "curbside consultation," a phrase used to describe an informal second opinion where there is no expectation of compensation, the AMA policy recognizes that a full and unrestricted license is not needed.

AMA policy, however, does not recognize the ACR Teleradiology Standard and related standards as such. Under AMA policy for "practice parameters," as recognized in the AMA Policy for the Promotion of Telemedicine, such parameters serve as "educational tools" and "strategies for patient management that are designed to assist physicians in clinical decision making" (American Medical Association 1999a). This is distinct from the legal concept of a "standard of care," the level of medical care established necessary to defeat allegations of negligence in a malpractice action. Generally, this standard is established by physicians, testifying as experts as to the level of care required. Furthermore, a related policy states that "practice parameters developed by a particular medical specialty or specialties should not preclude the performance of the procedures or treatments addressed in that practice parameter by physicians who are not formally credentialed in that specialty or specialties" (American Medical Association 1999b). Thus, under existing AMA policy, ACR standards on teleradiology and digital image data management serve only an educational purpose and are not acknowledged to establish an actual standard of care.

The AMA has also tracked developments in telemedicine and teleradiology. In 1996, the House of Delegates, the AMA's governing body, adopted a resolution directing the Association to monitor activities of hospitals, specialty societies, and regulatory agencies that affect telemedicine and submit a report (American Medical Association 1996). The result of this resolution was the Status Report of Telemedicine, issued at the 1997 Interim meeting, a substantial portion of which outlined ACR actions in the area (American Medical Association 1997). ACR initiatives such as the DICOM standard, developed in conjunction with the NEMA, were acknowledged. The document also noted that the FDA Center for Devices and Radiological Health had encouraged such collaboration between the clinical community, as represented by the ACR, and manufacturers of diagnostic imaging equipment.

Given the growing importance of telemedicine in general and teleradiology in particular, there is little doubt that the AMA will continue to track developments and generate policy in the area. For the present, it is unlikely that the Association will change its stance requiring full and unrestricted licensure in both transmitting and receiving jurisdictions in the setting of teleradiology, or acknowledge that ACR standards represent the professional standard of care.

GOVERNMENT REGULATIONS

Both the federal and state governments are involved in the regulation of tele-radiology and PACS. This regulatory authority stems from legislation that controls medical devices, healthcare benefits, and the practice of medicine, with the regulations themselves drafted by a variety of administrative agencies. Generally, regulation at the federal level is directed at medical devices and the provision of healthcare benefits. At the state level, the dominant activity is regulation of medical practice.

FEDERAL GOVERNMENT

FOOD AND DRUG ADMINISTRATION   The FDA has its regulatory authority for medical devices grounded in the Food, Drug and Cosmetics Act, as amended by Medical Device Amendments of 1976 and other amendments, which requires that products be safe and effective for their marketed indication(s). The definition of a "medical device" under the Act is extremely broad—broad enough to include devices employed for teleradiology and PACS (Federal Food, Drug and Cosmetic Act 1999). Devices regulated by the Agency are broken down into several distinct groups. Initially, all devices are arbitrarily separated into those legally marketed prior to implementation of the Medical Device Amendments on May 28, 1976, and those marketed after that date. These are known as "pre-amendment" and "post-amendment" devices, respectively.

Pre-amendment devices are further divided into three classes, based on potential patient risk. Devices with the least risk are placed in class I, which is subject only to "general controls." Class I products are not individually regulated. Rather, their safety and effectiveness is assured by general controls, which include manufacturing and labeling controls. General controls are considered important for all medical devices. Accordingly, they also apply to class II and III products.

Class II is the intermediate regulatory category for devices with higher risk to patients than class I but not requiring the highest degree of regulation. Products in this class are subject to "special controls," specific regulations designed to assure their safety and effectiveness. As with class I, these devices are not individually regulated, with each generic product type subject to applicable special controls.

Class III is the most stringent regulatory category. It is reserved for products with either a potentially unreasonable risk of patient injury, or insufficient data to establish actual patient risk. Devices in this class are technically subject to a premarket approval process, requiring demonstration of safety and effectiveness prior to marketing. However, pre-1976 class III products are "grandfathered," and may be legally marketed until such time as the FDA requests such data and the manufacturer either fails to provide it or the data fails to show safety and effectiveness.

Post-amendment devices are generally subject to a premarket notification process, which generally applies to higher risk class II and all class III products. This requires that a manufacturer provide the FDA notice of their intention to market a product. If the Agency determines that the product is "substantially equivalent" to a pre-amendment device (or a post-amendment device that has been reclassified to class I or II), that device may be legally marketed subject to the regulations currently applicable to its "predicate" device. Should there be no pre-1976 equivalent, the device is automatically placed in class III, subject to the premarket approval process. Lower risk products may be reclassified to class I or II, although this generally requires evidence that the device's risk is appropriate to the new classification.

Teleradiology and PACS system were not in existence in the pre-1976 world of medical devices. Though these post-amendment devices could have been automatically placed in class III, the FDA treated teleradiology and PACS equipment as accessories to the imaging devices that they serviced, avoiding the premarket approval process. However, this made marketing approval for the devices somewhat complicated, as the products were not themselves classified.

The FDA moved to end this system in 1996, issuing a policy statement on "Telemedicine Related Activities" (1996). While reinforcing the Agency's authority to regulate teleradiology and PACS devices, the statement proposed formally classifying the products. Image storage devices and medical image devices were to be placed in class I, and exempted from the premarket notification requirement unless irreversible compression was used. Medical image digitizers, medical image hardcopy devices, and PACS systems were to be class II products. General purpose products used in a medical setting were not to be regulated, unless labeled for a medical use. The latter category could include such items as word processing software employed in a PACS system.

The Agency issued its final rule effecting these changes on April 29, 1998 (63 *Federal Register* 1998). As proposed in Teleradiology and Related Activities, these regulations placed medical image storage devices in class I, exempt from the premarket notification requirement unless irreversible compression is used. Medical image digitizers, medical image hardcopy devices, and PACS were made class II devices. A number of "voluntary standards" are to serve as special controls for these devices: (1) DICOM; (2) Joint Photographic Experts Group (JPEG), which specifies methods for reversible and irreversible compression of digital medical images; and (3) the Society of Motion Picture and Television Engineers test pattern, used to test monitors and printers for acceptance and quality control purposes.

HEALTH CARE FINANCING ADMINISTRATION   The Health Care Financing Administration (HCFA) oversees the federal Medicare program, disbursing vast sums of money to health care providers and institutions nationwide. Given the scope of Medicare, HCFA regulations applicable to Medicare fund recipients have a broad impact on the provision of U.S. healthcare. HCFA itself is governed by the Privacy Act of 1974, a federal statue that protects the confidentiality of individually identifiable data. In practice, the Act requires that HCFA keep the records of its Medicare patients confidential. HCFA is also subject to certain provisions of the Health Insurance Portability and Accountability Act of 1996, in which Congress mandated certain security and electronic signature requirements.

Recently, HCFA has become concerned that certain electronic data transmissions have the potential to violate patient confidentiality and hence the Privacy Act 1974. Its response was the HCFA Internet Security Policy, issued in November 1998 (Health Care Financing Administration 1998a). This document applies to what HCFA describes as "HCFA Privacy Act-protected and/or sensitive HCFA information," which includes: (1) all individually identifiable data held in systems of records; (2) payment information that is used to authorize or make cash payments to individuals or organizations; (3) proprietary information that has value in and of itself and that must be protected from unauthorized disclosure; and (4) computerized correspondence and documents that are considered highly sensitive and/or critical to an organization and that must be protect from unauthorized alteration and/or premature disclosure.

The HCFA Internet Security Policy allows covered data to be transmitted via the Internet, as long as "an acceptable method of encryption" is utilized to provide confidentiality and integrity of the data. Furthermore, authentication or identification procedures must be employed to assure that both the sender and the recipient of the data are known to each other and are authorized to receive and decrypt such information. The policy covers all systems or processes that use the Internet or interface with the Internet to transmit sensitive data. However, it does not apply to local data-at-rest or local host or network protections, although it is explicit that such local data must still be protected by "all necessary measures."

The HCFA Internet Security Policy describes in considerable detail the technical specifications of acceptable practices. Minimally acceptable encryption methods as of November 1998 include algorithms such as Triple 56-bit DES (defined as 112-bit equivalent) for symmetric encryption, 1024-bit algorithms for asymmetric systems, and 160 bits for Elliptical Curve systems. The Agency explicitly reserves the right to increase these minimum levels when "deemed necessary" by advances in techniques and capabilities associated with the processes used by attackers to break encryption.

Acceptable authentication approaches, accomplished over the Internet via an "in-band" process, include: (1) formal certificate authority-based use of digital certificates; (2) locally managed digital certificates, provided that all parties to the communication are covered by the certificates; (3) self-authentication, as in internal control of symmetric "private keys"; and (4) tokens or "smart cards." Acceptable identification approaches, undertaken outside of the Internet via an "out-of-band" process, include: (1) telephonic identification of users and/or password exchange; (2) exchange of passwords and identities by U.S. Certified Mail; (3) exchange of passwords and identities by bonded messenger; (4) direct personal contact exchange of passwords and identities; and (5) tokens or smart cards.

Entities subject to the HCFA Internet Security Policy must modify their security plan to detail the methodologies and protective measures used if they employ the Internet for transmission of covered data and to adequately test these implemented measures. HCFA reserves the right to audit these organizations and their security policies. Finally, any organization wishing to transmit covered data via the Internet must inform HCFA of its intent to do so.

HCFA is in the midst of promulgating formal regulations addressing security of electronic individual healthcare information, as well as health plan use of electronic signatures (Health Care Financing Administration 1998b).

STATE GOVERNMENT

LICENSURE At its most basic level, teleradiology is the practice of medicine. The right of the individual states to license such practice has been settled law in the U.S. since the turn of the century, when the U.S. Supreme Court upheld a West Virginia statute requiring that physicians practicing in that state obtain a license based on criteria established by the state (*Dent v West Virginia*). Today, states enforce their licensure prerogative through medical practice statutes, which typically define what constitutes the "practice of medicine" and therefore who is subject to medical licensure. The definition of the practice of medicine is usually broad, as with North Carolina's statute:

" . . . any person shall be regarded as practicing medicine or surgery . . . who shall diagnose or attempt to diagnose, treat or attempt to treat, operate or attempt to operate on, or prescribe for or administer to, or profess to treat any human ailment, physical or mental, or any physical injury to or deformity of another person . . . " (North Carolina General Statutes 1998)

Although teleradiology is not specifically mentioned in this and other statutes, there is little doubt that the broad definition of medical practice encompasses the in-state teleradiology practitioner. The impact on out-of-state physicians who consult about patients located within the jurisdiction is less clear. To eliminate this confusion, many states have amended their medical practice statutes to clarify their applicability to out-of-state teleradiology practitioners (Goldberg and Gordon 1998). In states where statutes have not been altered, the impact on out-of-state practitioners remains uncertain.

Many states have various exceptions to their licensure requirement. For example, out-of-state physicians rendering emergency treatment are often exempt. "Occasional" consultants may be exempt, but the definition of what level of activity qualifies differs between states. Several states have "border states exceptions," which exempt licensed physicians in immediately neighboring states from the state's licensure requirement. Given the nature of teleradiology practice, with its typically nonemergent, recurrent nature and broad reach, it is likely that the applicability of all of these exemptions will be limited.

With current medical practice statutes and their exemptions, licensure requirements for out-of-state teleradiology practitioners fall into one of three general categories: (1) full licensure is either expressly required by statute or presumed because teleradiology and/or telemedicine is not specifically mentioned in the applicable medical practice act and no exemption applies; (2) a "special purpose" license for out-of-state teleradiology practitioners is available; and (3) full licensure is not required, though something short of full licensure may be necessary. The last two categories are infrequently encountered.

Given the potential consequences of violating medical practice statutes, it is advisable to exercise caution in all questionable practice situations. Loss of licensure in a practitioner's home state, exclusion from federal Medicare and Medicaid programs, and/or loss of malpractice insurance may all be indirect consequences of practicing without an appropriate license (California Business and Professions Code 1998a; 42 U.S.C.A. 1998; NORCAL Mutual Insurance Co.). Interestingly, violation of the medical practice statute itself is typically only a misdemeanor (California Business and Professions Code 1998b).

Licensure requirements, current as of April 1999, for the 50 states appear in Table 14.1. Also included are pertinent, specific state requirements. Given the myriad of state licensure requirements, some have advocated a more uniform system of licensure for telemedicine/teleradiology. In 1996, the Federation of State Medical Boards suggested that the states adopt limited telemedicine licenses (Federation of State Medical Boards of the United States, Inc. 1995). However, leading national medical organizations, such as the American College of Radiology and the American Medical Association, have adopted policies advocating full licensure in each state where a physician practices teleradiology. The states themselves heavily favor full licensure for physicians treating patients within their borders and appear extremely reluctant to surrender any authority to regulate such medical care. In this current climate, it is unlikely that any type of national licensure for teleradiology practice will emerge in the foreseeable future.

OTHER STATE ISSUES   In addition to licensure, many states have enacted legislation that affects teleradiology. Generally, these laws and regulations address teleradiology/telemedicine initiatives within the state, or attempt to coordinate such activities to achieve a public health goal. For example, some states are actively promoting telemedicine to provide care to their rural populations. A complete description of these nonlicensure activities is beyond the scope of this discussion.

RELATED LEGAL CONSIDERATIONS

The practice of teleradiology and PACS storage of image data raise a number of legal concerns, mostly related to state law doctrines. These include

TABLE 14.1
Licensure Requirements (1999)

State	Code	Specific Requirements
Alabama	3	Grants a three-year special purpose license to nonresident telemedicine practitioners. Excludes informal or uncompensated consultations. Subjects licensee to Alabama medical board jurisdiction and requires licensee's home state to issue reciprocal telemedicine licenses to Alabama physicians.
Alaska	1	
Arizona	2	"Single or infrequent" consultations are exempted.
Arkansas	2	Episodic consultations with Arkansas physicians, provision of services unavailable in Arkansas, or physical travel to the state to provide care are exempted.
California	3	No license required so long as the telemedicine consultant does not have ultimate authority over the patient; requires specific informed consent from the patient to use telemedicine consultation; exempts telephone conversations and e-mail messages between patient and practitioner.
Colorado	2	"Occasional" consultations exempted.
Connecticut	2	"Occasional" consultations exempted.
Delaware	1	
District of Columbia	1	
Florida	2	Full licensure for physicians providing official authenticated interpretations through an ongoing regular arrangement.
Georgia	2	
Hawaii	3	Telepractitioners exempted from licensure if local physician maintains primary control over the patient's care.
Idaho	2	
Illinois	2	Out-of-state physicians practicing telemedicine subject themselves to the jurisdiction of Illinois courts.
Indiana	2	Full licensure for telemedicine on a regular routine or nonepisodic basis.
Iowa	1	
Kansas	2	Exemption for occasional consultation; border states exemption.
Kentucky	1	
Louisiana	1	No consultation exception.
Maine	1	No consultation exception.
Maryland	1	
Massachusetts	1	Opinion of medical board attorney that full licensure needed.

Michigan	1	
Minnesota	1	
Mississippi	2	Exemption if local physician requests nonresident physician's services. The resident physician must have a prior relationship with the patient being treated via telemedicine.
Missouri	2	Exemption when consulting with local physician.
Montana	3	A bill pending in the legislature would require a telemedicine certificate issued by the medical board; passed House, pending in Senate as of 2/22/99.
Nebraska	2	
Nevada	2	
New Hampshire	1	Bill pending in legislature to explicitly require full licensure for physicians who provide teleradiology services on a regular contractual or frequent basis.
New Jersey	1	
New Mexico	1	
New York	1	Border states exception.
North Carolina	2	Exemption for infrequent consultations. Residents may bring malpractice claims against telemedicine practitioners in North Carolina courts.
North Dakota	1	Bill pending in legislature to require full licensure.
Ohio	1	
Oklahoma	2	Brief consultation exception; telemedicine practitioners submit to the jurisdiction of Oklahoma courts.
Oregon	1	Bill pending in legislature to require a special telemedicine license that is not a limited license but still does not allow the out-of-state physician to practice in the state, except across state lines.
Pennsylvania	1	
Rhode Island	1	
South Carolina	1	
South Dakota	2	Consultation exception limited to maximum 24-hour period in any one year.
Tennessee	2	On 5/15/96 the medical board was authorized by the legislature to issue special telemedicine licenses; as of 2/25/99 there is a bill pending in the legislature that would make transmission of patient medical information via telemedicine technology to a person in another state who is not licensed in Tennessee grounds for license suspension or revocation.
Texas	3	The state board of medical examiners is authorized to issue special purpose licenses for telemedicine; otherwise, full licensure required.
Utah	2	Consultation exception repealed.

(Continued on next page)

TABLE 14.1
Licensure Requirements (1999) (*continued*)

Vermont	1	Bill pending to authorize special purpose license.
Virginia	1	
Washington	1	Bill pending that would require telemedicine practitioner to be sponsored by a local physician.
West Virginia	2	Consultation exception provides that consultant can not consult for more than three months in his lifetime.
Wisconsin	1	
Wyoming	1	

KEY: 1: States that have not specifically addressed the telemedicine licensure issue, so that full licensure is presumed.
2: States that specifically include telemedicine in their definition of medical practice and expressly require full licensure.
3: States requiring something other than full licensure, such as a special purpose license or no license in the state.

medical malpractice and record keeping issues. To date, there are no known cases known to the authors or other commentators directly addressing teleradiology and PACS (Caryl 1998). Accordingly, most analysis in this area is by analogy to conceptually similar fact situations.

MEDICAL MALPRACTICE IN TELERADIOLOGY

ESTABLISHING A CLAIM   Teleradiology is medical practice, and as such, exposes a physician to liability under state tort law, commonly known as medical malpractice. Successful malpractice actions require four elements: (1) a duty to the patient; (2) a negligent breach or violation of that duty; (3) patient injury as a result of that negligence; and (4) actual damages from the injury. Assuming that a patient has suffered injury that has resulted in damages, as is the case in most malpractice actions, the question becomes whether the teleradiology practitioner owes a duty to the patient whose images he or she interprets and what constitutes negligence in that interpretation.

There is no definitive case law addressing the existence of duty owed to a patient by a teleradiology practitioner. However, most commentators believe that a doctor-patient relationship exists between a radiologist interpreting teleradiology images and the patient whose images he or she reviews, a relationship that establishes a duty to that patient (Caryl 1998; Cuzmanes and Orlando 1997). A court decision supporting this proposition is *Hand v Tavera* (1993), in which a physician under a managed care contract who refused to hospitalize a patient was held to have formed a doctor-patient relationship, despite that fact he had never met or spoken with that patient. The court reasoned that the relationship was established as the patient had paid for the physician's services. Another decision is *McKinney v Schlatter* (1997), which found that a telephone consultation is sufficient to establish a doctor-patient relationship, when a physician relied on a cardiologist's advice that a clinical problem was not cardiac in nature. Given that a teleradiology practitioner is paid for his or her interpretation, and that interpretation is ordinarily relied on to guide clinical decision making, these cases indicate that typical teleradiology consultations will be sufficient to establish a duty to the patient.

It is less clear that a doctor-patient relationship is established when the consultation is informal, no compensation is received, and no official interpretation is rendered. Specifically, if the teleradiology practitioner is engaged in a "curbside consult," there is the possibility that no relationship will be found (Berger and Cepelewicz 1996). However, if the radiologist receives or expects any compensation from the consult, it is doubtful that any "curbside consult" exception would apply.

A second key requirement of a successful malpractice action is negligent breach of a physician's duty to the patient. Negligence exists when a physician has violated the medical standard of care, a legal concept whose exact definition varies between jurisdictions. Generally, this standard is established by physicians, testifying as experts, as to what constitutes acceptable medical practice in the fact situation before the court. Although these standards were originally based on practice patterns in the local community where injury occurred, there has been a growing trend in medical malpractice to a national standard of care, applicable across jurisdictions. Teleradiology, with its wide geographic sweep and cross-jurisdictional nature, will almost certainly involve a national standard of care. The exact form this standard takes will depend on case law developed as malpractice cases involving teleradiology inevitably come before the courts.

CHOICE OF LAW Medical malpractice is a legal action based in state law—law that may differ greatly between jurisdictions. These differences become problematic when the teleradiology practitioner interprets images of a patient who resides in and was imaged in another state. Here, the question becomes which law, that of the transmitting or the receiving state, to apply.

Although teleradiology and PACS are new technologies, the choice of which state law to apply when a plaintiff and defendant are residents of different jurisdictions is not new for the courts. Under well-established law, a state may exercise jurisdiction on an out-of-state individual or corporation provided that there are "minimum contacts" between the state and the individual or corporation (*International Shoe v Washington* 1945). Three criteria must be met: (1) the defendant must have purposefully availed him- or herself of acting in the state; (2) the cause of action must have arisen in the state; and (3) the defendant's acts must have a substantial enough connection to make exercise of jurisdiction reasonable (*Compuserve, Inc. v Patterson* 1996). In the setting of commercial activity, it is widely acknowledged that committing an act of negligence in a state or doing business in that jurisdiction satisfies these requirements. Commentators examining teleradiology believe that this doctrine will be used to subject practitioners to the laws of the transmitting jurisdiction, although in the absence of applicable court decisions, the question remains unresolved (Caryl 1998). Some states have acted to remove this uncertainty by enacting legislation that specifically subjects out-of-state telemedicine practitioners to the state's jurisdiction.

The practical implications of a teleradiology practitioner being subject to the laws of the transmitting jurisdiction may be profound. A radiologist could find him- or herself facing a local judge or jury potentially hostile to an out-of-state defendant. Perhaps even more important, applicability of another state's jurisdiction may destroy protections a physician enjoys in his or her home state, such as award limits on the amount of allowable damages.

INSURANCE ISSUES   Interstate teleradiology practice raises professional liability insurance coverage issues related to the interpretation of images generated outside of the practitioner's home state. Coverage of out-of-state teleradiology activities should not be presumed. Not all insurance carriers are licensed in every state and underwriting criteria between jurisdictions may vary. Accordingly, many policies specifically exclude coverage for out-of-state incidents, unless a rider has been added to specifically provide such coverage. This means that the unwary teleradiology practitioner subject to an out-of-state malpractice action may find his professional liability carrier reserving coverage rights or completely denying coverage.

RECORD KEEPING

Data generated from teleradiology and PACS activities are medical records. As such, there are a myriad of considerations regarding data storage, including where the data must be maintained, its form, and the period of retention. Confidentiality of data is another consideration. Laws, regulations, and institutions' policies for film and paper records may serve as a guide, though the vary nature of electronic data will necessarily demand special considerations.

Initially, when electronic data is acquired at one state and stored at another, it is unclear whether this data must be maintained at the transmitting site, the receiving site, or both sites. As discussed previously, the ACR Standard for Teleradiology only requires that data be maintained at the transmitting site. Certainly, any applicable law, regulation, or institutional policy with regard to where data must be maintained should be observed.

The form of stored image data is another consideration. Given the present cost of electronic storage and the amount of that storage necessary to archive medical images, many centers compress data to save resources. If compression is reversible, there is no intrinsic problem. However, when irreversible, "lossy" compression is employed, there is a question of a medical record being altered and clinically relevant data being lost. In the somewhat analogous setting of hardcopy medical records, any alteration may be extremely problematic legally, as it calls into question the validity of the entire record (Andrews 1992). It remains to be seen whether storage with lossy compression practice will become an issue for the courts.

The retention period of medical records is subject to federal, state, and institutional laws and policies. Laws and policies for the jurisdiction where electronic data is being stored should be followed. In addition, the "ACR Standard for Teleradiology" suggests that teleradiology data being stored at the receiving facility meet the storage standards at the transmitting facility. This policy is prudent, given the probable applicability of the transmitting state's laws to the teleradiology practitioner.

A final consideration with any stored medical record is confidentiality. Various authorities, the physician/patient privilege, ethical considerations, the constitutional right to privacy, and some state statutory law demand that this confidentiality be maintained (Andrews 1992). Although electronic storage may be a more convenient and accessible format for storing and accessing medical records, this form of record keeping may be more vulnerable to security breaches.

As described in the "ACR Teleradiology Standard" and the Standard for Digital Image Data Management, security is needed for electronically stored medical records. The ACR standards notwithstanding, there is virtual certainty that the courts would apply the same privacy standards to electronic records that have been applied to traditional medical records (*Alberts v Devine* 1985). This imposes a duty on the physicians and institutions using teleradiology and PACS to develop policies that assure reasonable patient confidentiality, or face potential liability for breaches of confidentiality.

CONCLUSION

Teleradiology and PACS technology and application have expanded greatly in the last decade, in many ways leaving behind the laws and policies intended to regulate and control the field. Even where policies have been developed, such as the ACR Standard for Teleradiology and the Standard for Digital Image Data Management, it is unclear the impact these policies will have on the practice of teleradiology and the use of PACS. Many of the legal and policies questions being asked by radiologists and others today will not be answered for years, as legislatures, courts, and professional societies develop approaches to the novel problems posed by the technology. Until that time, physicians using teleradiology and PACS technology should use caution and common sense when confronted with unsettled legal or regulatory questions.

▶ REFERENCES

42 *USCA* Section 1320a-7 (1998).

Alberts v Devine, 479 N.E.2d 113 (Mass. 1985), *cert. denied*, 474 U.S. 1013 (1985).

American College of Radiology: *ACR Standard for Digital Image Data Management*. Effective January 1, 1999. Reston, VA (1999a).

American College of Radiology: *ACR Standard for Teleradiology*. Revised 1998; effective January 1, 1999. Reston, VA (1999b).

American Medical Association: House of Delegates Resolution 117 (I-96). Interim Meeting. 1996.

American Medical Association: *Status Report on Telemedicine*. Council on Medical Service Report 8-I-97. Chicago 1997.

American Medical Association: *The Promotion of Quality Telemedicine*. Joint Report of the Council on Medical Education and Council on Medical Service, 1996. In: American Medical Association: *Continuing Medical Education Resource Guide*. Chicago, 1996.

American Medical Association: *The Promotion of Telemedicine.* Quoting AMA Policies 410.973 and 410.987. American Medical Association. Chicago 1999a.

American Medical Association: Policy 410:987[3]. American Medical Association. Chicago 1999a.

Andrews, BW. *Medical records liability.* 6 Health Lawyer 11 (Summer 1992).

Berger S, Cepelewicz BB. *Medical legal issues in teleradiology.* AJR 166:505–510, 1996.

California Business and Professions Code. Section 2305 (1998a).

California Business and Professions Code. Sections 2314, 2315 (1998b).

Caryl CJ. *Malpractice and other legal issues preventing the development of telemedicine.* 12 Journal of Law and Health 173 (1998).

Classification for Five Medical Image Management Devices: Final Rule. 63 *Federal Register* 43242 (April 29, 1998).

Compuserve, Inc. v Patterson, 89 F.3d 1257 (6th Cir. 1996).

Cuzmanes PT, Orlando CP. *Automation of medical records: The electronic superhighway and its ramifications for health care providers.* 6 Journal of Pharmacy and Law 19 (1997).

Dent v. West Virginia. 129 U.S. 114 (1889).

Federal Food, Drug and Cosmetic Act, Sec. 201. Codified at 21 USCA 321 (1999).

Federation of State Medical Boards of the United States, Inc.: *A Model Act to Regulate the Practice of Telemedicine or Medicine by Other Means Across State Lines, Executive Summary.* Euless, TX (October 31, 1995).

Goldberg AS, Gordon JF. *Telemedicine: Emerging Legal Issues.* American Health Lawyers Association. Washington, DC 1998.

Hand v Tavera, 864 S.W.2d 678 (Ct. App. Tex. 1993).

Health Care Financing Administration. *Internet Security Policy.* Washington, DC (November 24, 1998a).

Health Care Financing Administration. *Proposed Rule: Security and Electronic Signature Standards.* 63 *Federal Register* 43242 (August 12, 1998b).

International Shoe v Washington, 326 U.S. 310 (1945).

McKinney v Schlatter, 1997 WL 67702 (Ohio App. 12 Dist. 1997).

NORCAL Mutual Insurance Co. *Professional Liability Insurance Policy. Part III Exclusions, A-7.* San Francisco 1997.

North Carolina General Statutes. Section 90-18 (1998).

Telemedicine Related Activities. Center for Devices and Radiological Health, U.S. Food and Drug Administration. Rockville, MD (July 11, 1996).

CHAPTER 15

RESEARCH AND EDUCATION

DAVID AVRIN

In our lifetime, education and research have been synonymous with books and print publications. Five centuries have passed since Gutenberg invented the printing press, but not even a decade since publication on the World Wide Web and widespread publication of educational material on CD-ROM. I recently received my subscription copy of Windows magazine, which contained a mailer for new subscriptions, but also an apparently hastily written note from the publisher in the contents section to the effect that this was the last print copy I would receive, that all future effort will be devoted to the Web version of their publication, and that I would be compensated in some way. Now, that is the sign of a revolution.

Several years ago, I was at a meeting with Steve Horii, radiology's fearless DICOM leader and warrior, who talked about a "place" on the Internet called the "World Wide Web." Shortly after, an Italian neuroradiologist friend of mine was visiting, and scoured computer stores and bookshops for HTML (hypertext markup language) information and tools. Four months later, I could use a browser to view his case-of-the month Web site in Italy from my home in California, with reasonable speed and excellent image quality. How prophetic this was of the changes that were about to occur, not only in commerce and entertainment, but in the building blocks of education: where learning will occur in a virtual rather than physically bound environment; where potentially every significant document and instructive case (images and associated information) can be cross-referenced and viewed no matter where in the world the case and the user physically reside.

Education and research in radiology are largely image-based. The mission of the academic radiology department is often described as being supported by a three-legged stool, the legs of which are: clinical study, education, and research. In this book, the clinical impact of digital technology has been fully explored. This chapter examines the ways in which the digital department is enabling technology that can support the teaching and research missions of an academic department. We review and describe some of the methods used to create a continuum of image and data integration from the clinical environment to the research and educational efforts.

BACKGROUND

Seshadri and Arenson assessed the potential impact of PACS on research and education in 1992. Jaffe reviewed the impact of new information technologies on education in radiology in 1996. He made the observation that computers "permit image organizing, collection and storage." He also commented that current technology renders production of educational materials relatively easy, "leaving distribution as the only publishing hurdle." His article compared print and electronic media, and also reviewed some of the early capabilities of the Internet and World Wide Web (WWW), including Mosaic and early browser developments, as well as mentioning HTML, universal resource locaters (URLs) and Java (java.sun.com). "Most importantly (with computers) electronic indexing, search, and hyperlinking all become dynamically possible." Needless to say, the Web solves the distribution problem. I don't think that many of us could foresee the truly incredible acceleration of technology in short years that has brought us to where we are with almost universal access to the Internet, the beginning of a new era of widespread high speed telecommunications (cable modem or broadband and digital subscriber lines (DSL)), hard disk storage costs of less than a penny per megabyte, DVD with capacity of upwards of 10 GB, inexpensive personal computers, software development and multimedia authoring tools, and new standards such as extensible markup language (XML) (Bosak and Bray 1999) that have great potential for educational use of documents and images in the broadest sense.

In radiology education, compared with many other medical disciplines, it is particularly true that "a picture is worth a thousand words." Indeed, images are the *lingua franca* of radiology education and research, and therefore methods to facilitate their handling in cyberspace, rather than through the traditional photographic process and print media publishing methods, are of utmost importance.

The goal for those of us working in this arena is seamless integration and interoperability between the clinical and academic applications to simplify the creation of computer-based diagnostic imaging educational and research resources. Interoperability is the capability of two or more physically distinct computers to communicate such that data can be transferred between two separate processes running on these machines in a controllable and useful way. Furthermore, the processes must work in harmony, and often by command from the second device.

I heard a cyber philosopher (Evans 1999) describe the digital revolution as a product of the combination of *technology, content, and distribution*. I think this applies equally well to healthcare, including education and research, as it does to business. We will focus on the issues specific to education and research in comparison to the clinical mission.

1. *Technology*. My colleagues and I believe in COTS (components off the shelf) network devices and protocols, ubiquitous computers running on a few platform operating system configurations, nonproprietary or open standards, commercially available application software (desktop publishing, presentation, authoring, and Web tools), supplemented by custom radiology applications to be described later in this chapter.

2. *Content*. Image data, patient data (clinical information etc.) follow-up (pathology results), accessory educational information (teaching module), basically the "stuff" or substance of radiology education, heavily weighted towards image content.

3. *Distribution*. Getting the content to the person with the need to know. In the past, print and conventional (snail) mail. Now CD-ROM, CAI (computer aided interactive instruction), intranet and Internet via Web technology.

THE TWO CHALLENGES

There are two main components of the research and education challenge to PACS: migrating content and authoring tools. At University of California,

San Francisco (UCSF), we have focused our efforts on seamless migration with database support, because we believe that this provides a common pathway or source of imaging data for both research and education in radiology. On the other hand, the group at the Advanced Imaging Laboratory at Massachusetts General Hospital (MGH) (Mehta and Dreyer 1999) have focused on the authoring problem with the RAPS (Radiology Annotation and Publishing System) project. They determined, rightly so, that commercial authoring tools require so much expertise that they are themselves the main obstacle to creating educational materials, and therefore created a DICOM-compliant input authoring tool specific to radiology.

Although some miniPACS (e.g., for ultrasound) have a built-in capability to mark and annotate interesting cases (a *virtual* interesting case file), we do not believe that this approach is scalable for a department-wide PACS at the present time. Two principle difficulties are that large-scale systems must utilize hierarchical storage solutions that make older cases less accessible, or short-term archives get populated with cases of research or educational interest rather than clinically current studies, even though the number of cases of high interest is small by total percentage. Second, contention between the clinical and academic environments for system resources and timely response is unacceptable for both activities. Therefore we adopted the approach of migrating the cases of high interest, with their associated information, to a separate image-capable database, as shown in Figure 15.1.

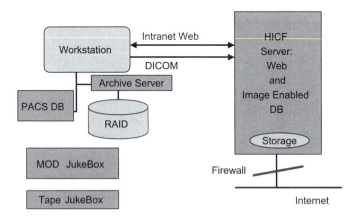

FIGURE 15.1

Recommended high interest case file (HICF) architecture for large systems.

In this era of commercially available PACS, even with DICOM, the biggest obstacle to overcome is moving digital image data and related information from the commercial system to the academic system. Commercial PACS archives, databases, and workstations, even on standard platforms and networks, have the mysterious and impenetrable "black box" appearance to those outside, i.e., who have no access to proprietary information and source code.

As an example, consider first a system with a Unix workstation, displaying images in DICOM format. Choose an image (CT for example), with which you want to do something educational, or add to a research project database. In DICOM3, each image is in a separate file. The file contains two parts. The first part (the header) contains information about the study, the patient, and how the image data is stored. The second part contains the image data, row by row, pixel by pixel.

The first task is to *export* the selected images to a separate repository. The image format in that repository can be DICOM, but we chose to also *convert* the images at this point into a format directly acceptable to desktop publishing (DTP) applications, the most common being known as GIF (graphics interchange/graphics programs), JPEG (Joint Photographic Experts Group), TIFF (tagged image file format—Microsoft) and PICT (Macintosh). All of these standards represent grayscale images with only 8 bits per pixel, or 256 shades of gray. They all do compression of varying degree and quality. JPEG has been compatible with all browsers since 1995, and has a lossless (bit-preserving) version, as does PICT and TIFF. The format conversion therefore requires mapping of larger range of density into a narrower range, as shown in Figure 15.2. For images other than CR and mammography, spatial resolution is usually not an issue.

The infrastructure must also be able to move the image data over a network on command to the desktop publishing application, or put it on removable media that can be read by the desktop system. This problem is only slightly less daunting even when using a workstation running under the Windows NT operating system on a PC type computer.

Some commercial and shareware packages are available for format conversion from DICOM (e.g., LeadTools, www.leadtools.com).

There is a generalized need for a DICOM AE (application entity) that acts as a storage SCP (Service Class Provider), and performs a DICOM to DTP (desktop publishing) format conversion. The output of this process should be managed by a database, in a semi-automated rather than manual way. Otherwise the repository quickly becomes an unqueriable and random collection of images and studies sent to it by many individuals. At a minimum, the identification of the inserter should be cataloged, if only for maintenance purposes.

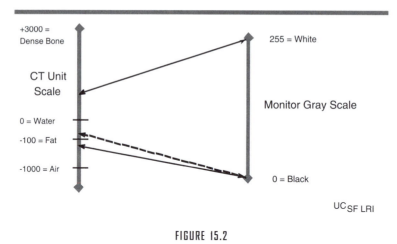

FIGURE 15.2

CT window/level mapping for Web and desktop publishing.

In summary, not only is access to PACS data required, but the access must be useful and seamless. Systems must communicate, must be interoperable, must follow protocol standards for communication and format, and must convert image data format. Associated study and patient information must be able to be transferred with the image data, and be capable of being stored, catalogued, and queried. The educational and research needs share many common requirements.

TECHNICAL ISSUES

IMAGE FORMAT, WINDOW/LEVEL, AND COMPRESSION ISSUES

Clinical image data is usually stored in a PACS in DICOM format, usually 12 bits deep (4096 step density scale). Most DTP (desktop publishing applications) use 8 bit (256 step grayscale) JPEG, TIFF, PICT or GIF format. Therefore, appropriate conversion from DICOM to one of these formats is necessary, with appropriate handling of window and level. Furthermore, computed radiography is usually presented with nonlinear lookup table transformations, and these must be emulated for a faithful rendition of the image in the DTP format.

In fact, the human eye and brain, in conjunction with a computer monitor, cannot perceive more than 256 shades of gray[8]. The problem is that CT and MR images have a tremendous range of density discrimination, and the range of interest depends on the characteristics of the anatomical region and clinical question under consideration. For example, examination of the lung by CT requires a very wide and low range of attenuation, whereas the liver or brain requires a narrow and higher range. Whatever range is selected, though, it must be mapped to 256 shades of gray, as shown in Figure 15.2.

For creation of educational materials, or reference images for research, there is a significant advantage to using the extensive desktop publishing tools available commercially, and the vast majority of these treat images as 8 bits (256 shades of gray).

Wavelet compression has tremendous potential, and is described by Paul Chang and his associates (1998) as an "alternative data representation with progressive resolution." An attraction of this "format" is that it can deliver image data appropriate to the resolution needs and abilities of the viewer. It is not a DTP format, but can be converted to one of the DTP formats described above.

SECURITY ISSUES

Teaching file or case file servers that connect to the clinical PACS secure intranet and also to the departmental network (and therefore to the Internet) are a potential security breech that needs special attention. Appropriate firewall, encryption, and username/password techniques should be utilized.

UCSF APPROACH AND REQUIREMENTS: THE UCSF/AGFA HICF/TF PROJECT

Early on, we developed a consensus within our radiology department regarding the requirements for our academic PACS interface and infrastructure known as the HICF (High Interest Case File) (Avrin et al. 1996). These requirements included:

1. uniform department-wide solution.
2. integration with diagnostic workstations for automated case insertion, since the ideal time for case insertion is at the time of inter-

pretation (no 3×5 card in the pocket with names and medical record numbers).

3. minimal conflict with the clinical environment, and therefore a separate, not virtual, high interest case file database.

4. support for desktop publishing applications (standards).

5. cross platform (heterogeneous).

6. access to PACS/HICF from the desktop, initially by client-server software such as the Radiology Workshop (Ramaswamy et al. 1994), and now by the Web (intranet/Internet).

We chose to develop a separate HICF database to which image and related data were migrated, rather than a "virtual" approach. The virtual approach essentially consists of flagging or saving pointers to cases and images of academic interest in the clinical PACS. The two main reasons that we did not pursue this approach are to avoid contention with the clinical environment for network and archive resources (clinical performance), as discussed previously, and security. In the past, limited desktop access to the clinical PACS was provided for query and retrieve via a client-server software suite called the Radiology Workshop, well described elsewhere. This suite had no associated database or persistence, but could download images to DTP applications. Technical advances including network speed, archive size and retrieval speed may make the virtual approach feasible in the future. It is currently implemented in many miniPACS, for example the Accuson Aegis for ultrasound, where the number of concurrent clinical and academic users is small.

Our long-term goal, which has now been realized, has always been to populate a separate database from the clinical PACS diagnostic workstations. This is a somewhat difficult problem even in a "home-grown" system where the internal software structure and workstation source code software are understood and available to the database developer. It is a tough interoperability, interface, and conversion problem. When commercial workstations are in primary use, they are essentially "black boxes," the inner software workings of which are usually confidential and unavailable. Most commercial vendors are not interested in this problem.

Fortunately, we had a vendor that understood the value of this application, particularly in an academic department. A "minimally intrusive" solution was worked out that utilized existing capabilities of the workstation: summary series and DICOM series send, and intranet Web techniques to access and populate a Web-enabled image-enabled database. Other than installing a Web browser button, only minimal modification of the commercial production workstation software was required.

TECHNICAL DETAILS OF THE UCSF HICF PROJECT

Following is an explanation of the implementation of the HICF project as an example of some of the concepts presented in this chapter (Tellis et al. 1998). This project consists primarily of the following server applications: the HICF 4th Dimension (www.acius.com), object-oriented database Web- and image-enabled application; and a DICOM receive AE (application entity) SCP (Service Class Provider) for receipt of image data, both running under Windows NT 4.0. At the Impax Display Station (Agfa Corp.), Netscape Navigator Web browser provides access to a database input form of the Web-enabled 4D database. In addition, some minor modification of the workstation software was provided by the vendor to automatically populate various fields of the database record, such as medical record number, type, date, and time of exam. The HICF file creation form also allows manual entry of clinical discussion and radiologic findings, as well as ACR code pairs.

The integration is demonstrated in Figure 15.3. A study is displayed

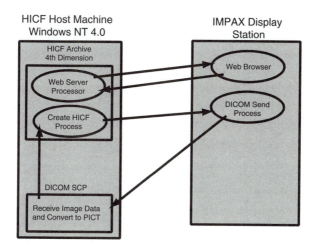

Key:

A- Send create HICF form to display station
B- Submit form back to web server
C- Send reference ID to display station
D- Send images in summary series to DICOM SCP
E- Images imported into HICF

FIGURE 15.3

UCSF/Agfa HICF project design.

on the clinical workstation. Images are windowed and leveled for optimal appearance and then selected and saved into a conventional summary series. The browser button is activated, and the browser accesses the high interest case file (HICF) server. The browser opens a page on the workstation containing the input form for a new record of the HICF database, with demographic and exam fields automatically populated from the current study on the diagnostic workstation, as shown in Figure 15.4. At this point the user enters a variable amount of information, the minimum requirement being a single ACR code pair for anatomy and pathology. Dropdown, categorized alphabetic lists are provided through the browser. Optional fields include key words, findings, differential diagnosis ACR codes, clinical information, and radiographic findings (these final two being free text). The user is automatically known by login and recorded by the database. A verification dialog follows, checking for at least one ACR code pair, and upon acknowledgement by the user of accuracy, the new record is posted, the images are DICOM-sent by the workstation to the server,

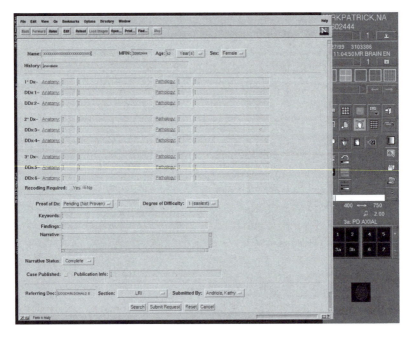

FIGURE 15.4

Web integration for HICF input at the diagnostic workstation.

with the selected window/level in the header. Upon reception by the DICOM receiver AE, the images are converted to JPEG DTP 8-bit format by applying the window/level and inserted into the new record automatically.

The new images and associated information are immediately accessible from the client side via intranet/Internet using standard browsers, and the images are pastable into DTP applications like PowerPoint or more sophisticated authoring tools. This functions well on Macintosh as well as PC platforms, and cases can also be queried, selected, and recalled for educational and comparative viewing from the clinical commercial workstations via the same browser that is used for insertion. The HICF is accessible with powerful database search criteria, as shown in Figures 15.5 to 15.8. The database viewing client also contains a tool to create a conference list and set of images, with hidden diagnoses, for quick conference preparation, with projection via an LCD projector.

AUTHORING TOOLS AND CAI (COMPUTER-AIDED INTERACTIVE INSTRUCTION)

A number of interactive multimedia authoring tools now exist. One of the ones we used early on was Authorware (www.macromedia.com). It provided a good environment for multimedia development, and had branching logic for question and answer. It was used successfully to implement the first several CD-ROMs in the UCSF Department of Radiology courseware for independent learning and review that is currently being developed for publication and CME credit (Webb, 2001).

"Smart" CAI can alter the path and difficulty of questioning in response to the performance of the learner. Most of these applications also include the ability to score the user.

MGH RAPS PROJECT

Mehta and Dreyer (1999) have described the difficulty of creating digital educational material, requiring detailed understanding of one of several multimedia authoring tools such as Macromedia Director or Authorware, Hypercard, Supercard, or Visual Basic. This creates a significant obstacle to the creation of teaching files, with the consequence that "few are cre-

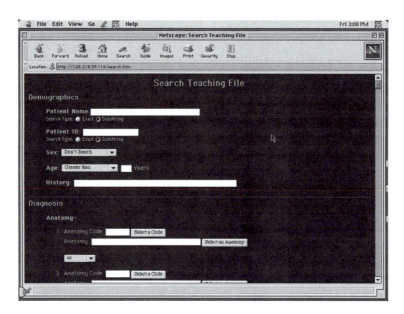

FIGURE 15.5

Comprehensive search capabilities of HICF.

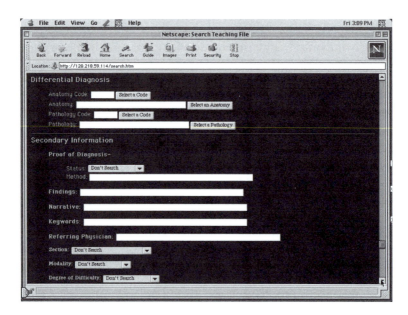

FIGURE 15.6

Search HICF for differential diagnosis.

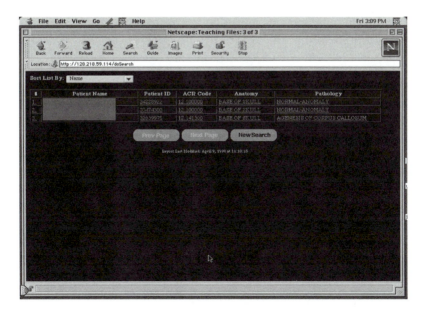

FIGURE 15.7

Results of search.

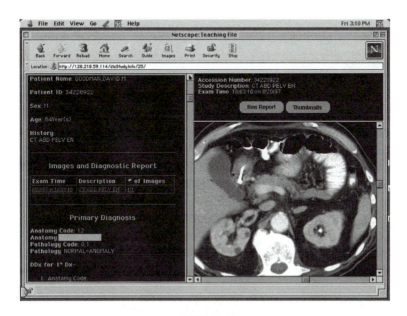

FIGURE 15.8

Display of selected case with images through Web browser.

ated and thousands lost" despite the best intentions. Alternatives, such as hiring a content programmer, are prohibitively expensive for most institutions and separate the medical/radiology "author" from the actual authoring process.

Therefore they created a package called RAPS (Radiology Authoring Program System), which summarized in Figure 15.9, for easy creation and robust distribution of content via CD-ROM or Web, using LeadTools as the format conversion engine. Image data is DICOM-transferred to a temporary repository, from which RAPS can retrieve it for selection, cropping, sizing, window/level, and overlay annotation with graphics and text. It also organizes the case material according to traditional radiology indices.

CONFERENCING

We are close to realizing our goal of conducting some of our major weekly rounds, such as neuroradiology, on a workstation with an LCD projection system. Our plan is to create summary series of the cases and images to be presented and send them to a designated conference workstation. A conference worklist can then be created and the relevant cases sequentially presented. Some institutions have already placed large monitors over workstations for working rounds with housestaff.

More ambitious undertakings include multi-site image-enabled video conferencing with the markup and realtime pointing capabilities described above.

CONSULTATION

Workstations have been demonstrated that can associate with other workstations with shared mouse-driven markup and annotation in user keyed colors, while displaying the same image for consultation. This technology can be Web-enabled for consultation with referring physicians as well as other radiologists. It is a very powerful technique.

OTHER APPROACHES

European (Caramella et al. 1999) and American (Freckleton et al. 1997) shared teaching file projects have been developed. Internet access to in-

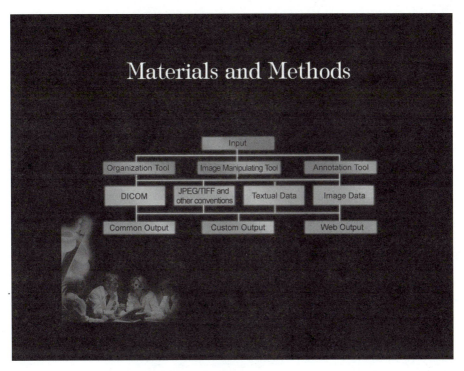

FIGURE 15.9

Summary of MGH RAPS project.

teresting cases has been demonstrated for several years, and facilitated by the Web and browsers. There are some very exciting activities, exemplified by Eurorad, shown in Figures 15.10 to 15.12, consisting of multi-site shared resources with a centralized database. This is an excellent example of how the Web transforms the traditional fixed-site medical school-based center of learning to a virtual and collaborative resource.

ICON was a teaching file concept developed to show interactively cases of similar radiographic findings or cases with the same differential diagnoses. This concept that should be revisited for on-line assistance at a diagnostic workstation, as well as within a pure educational environment (Mutalik et al. 1990).

In summary, all of these tools are coming together for creation of interactive digital educational media with content distributed via the Web or CD-ROM and a digital research resource for diagnostic imaging.

NEW DIRECTIONS

FREE TEXT REPORT SEARCH ENGINE WITH IMAGE LINKAGE

This research application can conduct sophisticated real-time searches of huge volumes of diagnostic reports on the basis of patient characteristics, modality, anatomy, and imaging findings in free text, without keywords. Used in combination with the Radiology Workshop previously developed by Ramaswamy et al. (1996) or with linkage to a clinical Web server with retrieval ability, the associated images matching the retrieved reports can be reviewed.

Ramaswamy makes the point that when "pursuing a variety of teaching and research activities, it is important to be able to find cases that demonstrate certain imaging findings." One of the shortcomings of the ACR coding system, pointed out by Arenson, is that it needs a "third axis"

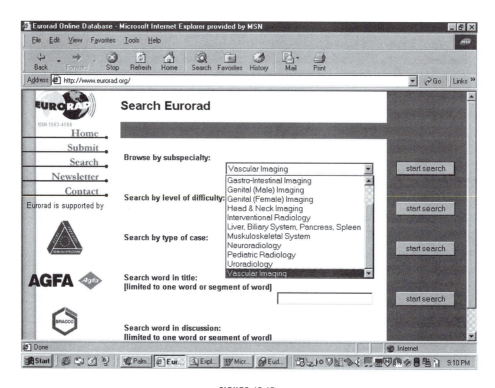

FIGURE 15.10

Eurorad search page via WWW browser.

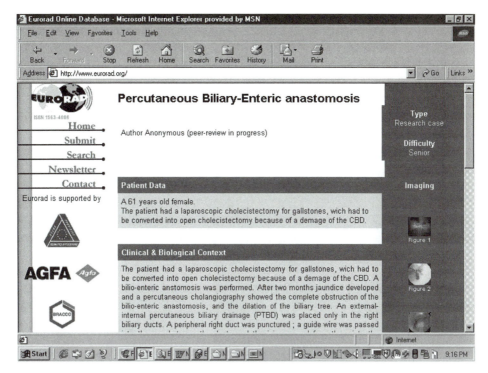

FIGURE 15.11

Eurorad selected case.

of radiological findings, in addition to the traditional axes of anatomy and disease entity or process. MoSearch enables rapid searching of a large volume of reports for findings, and as Ramaswamy, Seshadri, and Arenson observe: "This capability is particularly powerful when combined with access to the actual imaging data stored in a PACS" (Ramaswamy et al. 1996).

THE FUTURE: THE WEB, XML, AND DVD

With faster access to the Web beyond the campus via cable modems and ADSL, and the proliferation of authoring tools, the potential is truly exciting. Although the exact face of the future can only be surmised, it is clear that the Web has probably been a landmark event in education and publication development—a unique enabling technology.

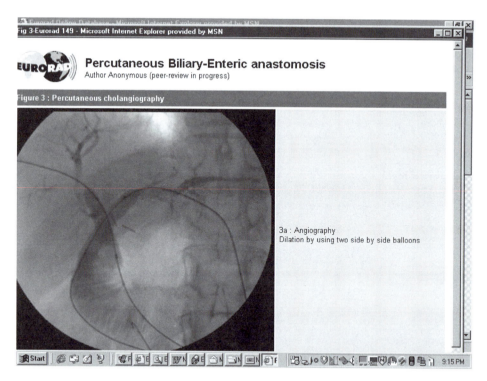

FIGURE 15.12

Eurorad selected case image viewed via browser.

While CD-ROM has a capacity of about 670 MB (thousands of CT images, tens of thousands of MR images), the new DVD media can store more than 10 GB, at least 12 times the capacity, at similar cost.

XML will be replacing HTML, with the advantage that content can be self describing to a receiving database or client (Bosak 1999), not merely describe its visual presentation. This will be useful for the infrastructure described here, as well as combining content including images from the medical enterprise beyond radiology.

CONCLUSION

We have tried to demonstrate how and why PACS is enabling technology for research and education in radiology. The fusion of unique content, in the form of a high interest case file database, with digital technology can create powerful opportunities for learner-directed training and education, based on a range of media and interactivity from the Web to DVD. Convenient migration of images and related information to a separate database is a powerful tool for conducting image-based radiology research.

▶ REFERENCES

Arenson RL. *The digital imaging workstation.* Radiology 176:303–315, 1990.

Avrin DE et al. *Integration of a digital teaching file at the diagnostic workstation.* SCAR 1996:56–61.

Bosak J, Bray T. *XML and second-generation Web.* Scientific American May, 89–93, 1999.

Caramella D et al. *European Radiology Online Database.* RSNA inforad 1999. (www.eurorad.org)

Chang PJ et al. *Dynamic transfer syntax: A flexible representation and interactive image data delivery protocol for enterprise-wide image distribution and integration.* RSNA 209:677, 1998.

Evans JD. *How digital technology will revolutionize medical science and care.* University of California, San Francisco presentation. June 27, 1999.

Freckleton MW et al. *Creating a Multi-Institutional Internet-based Teaching File with a Common Database Schema and Distributed Query.* RSNA 83rd Scientific Assembly, November 1997. 205:730, 1997.

Jaffe CC, Lynch PJ. *Educational challenges.* Radiology Clinics of North America 34:629, 1996.

Mehta A, Dreyer K. Joseph E. Whitley Award. Association of University Radiologists, San Diego, CA. March, 1999.

Mutalik P, Fisher P, Swett H. *Radiologic knowledge representation and axis display in the IMAGE/ICON system.* 1990:185–190.

Ramaswamy MR, Patterson DS, Yin L, Goodacre BW. *MoSearch: A radiologist-friendly Tool for Finding-based Diagnostic Report and Image Retrieval.* RadioGraphics 1996; 16-923–933.

Ramaswamy MR et al. *Accessing picture archiving and communication system text and image information through personal computers.* AJR 163:1229–1243, 1994.

Seshadri SB, Arenson RL. *The impact of PACS on research and education.* 30:263–266, 1992.

Tellis TW et al. *Web technology in the integration of a digital teaching file at the diagnostic workstation.* Journal of Digital Imaging 11(suppl 1):117–119, 1998.

Webb R. *High Resolution Lung CT.* The University of California San Francisco, Interactive Radiology Series. (CD-ROM) Lippincott, Williams & Wilkins, Hagerstown, MD, 2001.

CHAPTER 16

MEDICAL UTILIZATION AND MANAGEMENT

ROBERT T. BRAMSON

"Nothing so needs changing like other people's habits. . . . "
Mark Twain

In 1996 healthcare expenditures in the United States exceeded one trillion dollars. By the year 2003 it is estimated they will exceed two trillion dollars. According to figures from the American College of Radiology (ACR), diagnostic radiology accounts for at least 4% of annual healthcare expenditures. In some cases radiologists have demonstrated that using more radiology may save money from other parts of the healthcare system, for example by avoiding surgery when the diagnosis of appendicitis is in doubt. However, some studies suggest there may be as much as 20% too much radiology in the medical system. If this is so, there is no valid information about which 20% of the forty plus billion dollars spent annually on radiology should be eliminated, and little information about when we should use more radiology.

As increasing numbers of Americans age, the demand for medical care increases. Older people require more medical resources to remain healthy.

OVERVIEW

Background

1. Medicine is the largest service industry in the United States and is growing.
2. Demand for medical care is growing.
3. Older people consume more resources (Medicare 2.8–3.0 times non-Medicare age).
4. Baby boomers are aging.
5. Radiology is increasing in importance in evaluation of patients.
6. Perception is that radiology/lab/pharmacy usage is not optimum.
7. Studies show 20%–30% unnecessary radiology.
8. Studies show more radiology may save dollars from other parts of the system.
9. Proper use of radiology/lab/pharmacy could lead to decreased cost and increased quality.
10. Medical knowledge on proper role of radiology is inexact.
11. Data currently collected has no value to change behavior.

Goal

Improve quality, decrease cost.
Need data to determine guidelines.

Data collection

Information currently collected.
Data needed to affect change.
How to collect data.
Elicit cooperation from providers.
Expensive investment of time and money.

Goal

Change behavior with data (intellectual knowledge management).
Goal accomplishment worth capital investment.
Digital revolution allows collection of quality data.

The average use of radiology services for people of Medicare age is 2.8–3.0 times the use of services of the population below age 65.

Since the advent of Medicare in the late 1960s, the use of radiology has increased dramatically. Radiology has developed a multitude of new innovations, largely since 1970. These include CT, MRI, and high-resolution ultrasound. These new innovations are expensive. Some observers have argued that the expense of the new technology is at least partially to blame for the rising cost of medicine. More and more physicians order high technology studies on their patients. They have discovered that high technology radiology studies provide important information about their patients. Each year radiology assumes a bigger role in the diagnostic evaluation of patients.

Since 1992 the number of radiology studies performed on patients has remained fairly constant. In contrast, the number of radiology relative value units (RVUs) used in the United States has dramatically increased (Figure 16.1). In other words American physicians now order fewer of the lower technology studies, and more of the expensive high technology radiology studies on their patients than they did just a decade ago. None of these trends show any signs of changing, and that suggests that the study of utilization will become increasingly important.

As previously mentioned, there are some indications that 20% or more of the radiology done in the United States is redundant and unnecessary. A multitude of explanations have been advanced to explain this excessive radiology. Regardless of whether the alleged overutilization of radiology is

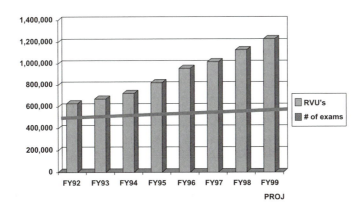

FIGURE 16.1

Upswing of RVUs with flat usage by examination.

RELATIVE VALUE UNITS

Relative value units (RVUs) were developed by Health Care Financing Administration (HCFA) for Medicare payments. The concept was that it required more work (technical expertise, educational training, and more expensive technology) to interpret an MRI of the knee compared to the performance and interpretation of an x-ray of the knee. Relative value units were developed to allow compensation for these more complex studies as opposed to the simpler studies. The theory followed the logic that a knee x-ray might be given a value of 1, and the knee MRI would be given a value of 12.

Third-party payers would then assign a fixed amount of money per relative value unit, for example $1 per relative value unit. In this example, the MRI of the knee would be paid at 12 times the rate of the plain film of the knee.

The theory of RVUs and the reality quickly diverged because of a failure to agree on the arbitrary weighting of the complexity of the various studies. Nevertheless, the general concept is that the more RVUs per study the more complex and expensive the study will be.

Since 1992, RVUs have increased drastically at the Massachusetts General and Brigham & Women's Hospital while the number of studies has remained fairly constant, as seen in Figure 16.1. In conversations with other academic institutions across the United States, this trend is consistent. The implication is that physicians are ordering the more complex studies on their patients instead of the less expensive and simpler studies. One could speculate this means that referring physicians are gaining more valuable information by ordering complex studies than they do by ordering some of the simpler studies.

secondary to defensive medicine or is a style of practice that has been learned by the current generation of physicians, the fact remains—American medicine spends more on healthcare than some people think is necessary. This leads to the desire to eliminate unnecessary radiology in the system, and a desire to exploit radiology when it can save money from other parts of the system.

Many observers argue for a healthcare system that has the highest quality of medicine at the lowest possible cost. Most would agree that these two objectives form the ultimate goal of good utilization and medical management. Although this discussion will focus on radiology, the same principles apply to other services ordered by physicians, such as laboratory and pharmacy usage.

When one starts to define optimum care for a patient, one must know how an intervention will affect the patient. Many physicians feel they learned this either in medical school or their subsequent residency training and continuing medical education. In reality, radiologists frequently find that referring physicians are often quite dogmatic about what they order on their patients, and sometimes don't understand the limitations of diagnostic radiology. Some of this ignorance about radiology occurs because research into the value of performing diagnostic studies has not been done very well in the last quarter century. Therefore, physicians determine the effect of a radiology intervention based on common use among their peer group or an outdated or sometimes even faulty information. Radiology research has focused on describing new innovations and demonstrating how valuable these innovations are for diagnosing diseases. Little work has been done on the actual impact on the patient of using one imaging modality vs. another, or on how the care of a patient is affected by a radiology intervention. The volume and quality of outcomes research as it pertains to radiology has been minimal, and this type of research must be emphasized in the 21st century.

When physician practice patterns are studied for how physicians order radiology, it is apparent that there is often little agreement among doctors on how to approach a problem. There is often a striking inconsistency in the number and types of interventions ordered by physicians for patients.

Examining radiology use from different areas of the country demonstrates little agreement about which radiology studies should be ordered in individual clinical situations. The differences in physician ordering patterns are not just geographic differences, or differences between academic centers and community practices, but within groups of physicians practicing together (Figure 16.2).

Actuary firms sell data that demonstrate that the cost for radiology can run from approximately $13/member/month in the Northeast to as low as $4/member/month on the West Coast. If one evaluates the numbers of exams rather than the dollars, there are approximately 850 exams/1000 covered lives in the Northeast and 330 exams/1000 covered lives in the West. These numbers come from examples for commercial populations below age 65. Above age 65, as previously mentioned, the number needs to be multiplied by a factor between two and three.

OUTCOMES RESEARCH

Thornbury in his 1994 Caldwell lecture describes a research system on how a radiology intervention changes what happens to patients. He categorizes research into 1 of 6 levels that affect patient outcomes. A level 6 study will yield results that will have the greatest impact on both patients and society. Every researcher strives to perform a level 6 study and have it published in a journal like the New England Journal of Medicine. Thornbury's papers, many of which were done with Dennis Fryback, rank as required reading for anyone contemplating utilization management. A synopsis of the levels follows (with my apologies to Dr. Thornbury for oversimplification of his work):

- Level 1: Technical efficacy. Research done at this level usually evaluates physical parameters, such as resolution of line pairs, grayscale images, and digital resolution.
- Level 2: Diagnostic-accuracy efficacy: Studies at this level measure the diagnostic accuracy of a test. ROC analysis is an example at this level.
- Level 3: Diagnostic-thinking efficacy: How the imaging information may change the ordering physician's diagnostic certainty.
- Level 4: Therapeutic efficacy: "An imaging examination can influence diagnostic thinking and still not affect choice of treatment." At this level, patients may interact with physicians in evaluating results and making decisions about their treatment.
- Level 5: Patient-outcome efficacy: Studies at this level improve both life expectancy and the quality of life. Some studies at this level may weigh the cost of a study against the benefits.
- Level 6: Societal efficacy: Studies at this level address costs to society. An imaging examination may be an efficient use of resources to provide benefits to society. (Source: Thornbury J. *Clinical efficacy of diagnostic imaging: love it or leave it.* AJR 162:1–8, 1994.)

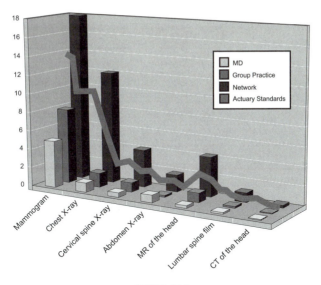

FIGURE 16.2

Graph showing the difference in ordering patterns among individual physicians and the other members of the same medical group (group practices) and the other physicians in the same geographic area (network) versus what an actuary firm recommends.

Utilization management requires several pieces of information. First, there must be some understanding of what studies are ordered in a medical practice. Second, there needs to be an understanding of why the study is ordered. And finally, there needs to be some agreement about the best use of radiology to evaluate a patient. Unfortunately, it is only the first of these three requirements for which good data currently exists.

Most insurance companies have data that can list the numbers of studies per patients in an insurance plan or the amount of money, usually listed as dollars/member/month, spent for radiology (Figure 16.3). A few insurance plans can present this as a crude profile that assigns the radiology studies to a primary care physician responsible for the care of the patient. Most insurance companies are not able to track the ordering habits of the specialists to whom the primary care physicians referred their patients. When aggregate data of this type is presented to primary care physicians who order studies, the physicians usually find little value in the information. They have no idea what studies the specialist ordered on the patient. They certainly have no control over what the specialist orders.

Dr.	Number of studies/1000	$ (PM)^2
1	850	12.02
2	783	11.53
3	462	12.95
4	527	10.52
5	838	12.00

FIGURE 16.3

Usually insurance companies list data like this by physicians. It does not tell the physician much. PM^2 = per member per month

To change physician behavior will require much improvement in the data collected. The usual response of a physician confronted with data that would suggest that he orders too many studies is that his patients are sicker than patients of other doctors. This is rarely true, but points out the necessity for some adjustment for disease severity. Data also must be adjusted for the age of the patient as well as the gender. As mentioned, older patients require different types and amounts of radiology compared to younger patients (Figure 16.4).

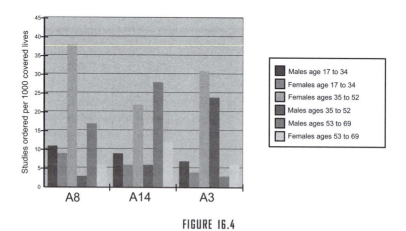

FIGURE 16.4

Graph showing how three different physicians in the same group practice use ultrasound depending on the age of the patient.

To obtain really significant behavior change requires an understanding about why a particular physician requests a study on his/her patient. Whether a study was positive or negative is also important, as well as whether the information gave some unexpected result.

Finally, proper utilization management needs to compare radiology usage to some standards that are accepted in the community as representing high quality. Quality is defined inversely as the deviation from an expected result. This means that, if a patient has a particular disease, there is some expectation from both the physician and the patient that the patient will get better, will die, or will be left with some residual defect from the disease. That is the expected outcome. Granted, the patient may frequently have a different expectation from the best judgment of the medical experts. But deviation of the actual outcome from the expected outcome represents a lower quality then expected. It may mean the expected outcome was not realistic. In that case, future expected outcomes need to be adjusted either to a better or worse expectation. The goal is to have as little deviation from the expectation as possible. Medical science continually tries to make the expectations both as clear as possible and as good as possible. The ultimate hope is that every patient will always get better from every disease and be left with no residual defect.

Analysis of the available information suggests that most standards of utilization are geographically local. Even within local communities, however, there may be disagreement about which studies to order and with what frequency (see Figure 16.2). In some cases physicians practicing together in

QUALITY

The medical literature is replete with articles on the quality of medical care. Physicians frequently invoke the concept of quality, but know little about measuring it. To many physicians, quality is much like the old story about good art: " . . . I know it when I see it."

In the 21st century, that isn't good enough. Physicians must understand how to measure quality and compare the quality among different providers. Nonphysician organizations are increasingly finding ways to measure quality and supply this information to consumers. In general, any deviation from an expected outcome is a deviation in quality. It can be measured.

a group disagree on how to evaluate a patient. The science of medicine has not yet evolved to the state that allows certainty on how one should care for every patient. Nevertheless, one needs a standard of radiology utilization, however crude, to compare to a practice. As more data is accumulated, the standard can be altered, discarded, or marked as acceptable. A standard presents an early target with which to compare the utilization within a group of physicians. Ultimately, standards will result from decades of outcomes research. Until that work is completed, we need to use crude targets as standards.

COLLECTING DATA

There is a need to collect specific data as to what physicians order. The demographics of the patient population on whom the studies are ordered are important. The positive or negative rate of the studies requested also needs to be recorded. Most important in really changing physician behavior is that the physicians being evaluated must agree on a guideline that focuses on how to evaluate a patient with a particular disease. This latter objective is both the most important and the most difficult to achieve. To accomplish this objective requires specific data. Collection of that data requires cooperation among providers and a real desire to achieve the information necessary to establish good guideline.

There are several ways to build guidelines. One can simply collect data, guess where deviation from expected usage occurs by looking at crude standards, and make gradual changes. Another more elegant way would be develop a grand plan by attacking diseases that commonly affect the population. Then pathways that incorporate radiology, lab use, pharmacy, hospitalizations, and so forth could be developed and followed. Common diseases like atherosclerotic heart disease, breast cancer, and degenerative hip disease all form likely candidates for this latter type of guideline development.

Thrall emphasized this point and cogently argued that the ultimate goal was to obtain a clear understanding of when interventions happen and how they affect the management of a specific disease. For example, Thrall discusses women at risk for breast cancer. Today we expect women to get a screening mammogram between the ages of 35 to 40. Women then follow guidelines that give them mammograms on a regular basis. At some point a breast lump may be discovered and it may be necessary to do a diagnostic mammogram. This might require needle localization and biopsy. Depending on the result, the woman may have surgery and follow a guideline that uses a bone scan every year and other studies that evaluate the spread of the disease. Later, it may be necessary to do certain interventions because of expected complications of therapy. Ultimately, the patient, family, and physicians need guidelines on what is needed to make the last few years of life for a woman with breast cancer comfortable and of a high quality. At the present time, the last few months of a woman's life with breast cancer often comprise frenetic efforts to diagnose complications with minimal concern at to what is actually happening to the woman and her disease process. Done properly, guidelines will allow a rational approach to alleviate the problems of the disease and intervene at appropriate times with some consistency of outcome. In this hypothetical scenario an organization could look at the female population that they serve, predict the incidence of breast cancer, and calculate what resources and interventions will be needed and at what time. The organization then has a clear understanding of the management of breast cancer and ensures that all women get the best quality care at the lowest cost. The problem, of course, is developing acceptable guidelines and keeping them current with the advancing knowledge about the diseases that affect the American public. That, however, is both the challenge and the opportunity inherent in medical utilization management. The digital revolution allows collection of the data necessary to develop these guidelines of high quality medicine with consistent outcomes and optimum cost efficiency. Occasionally, even today, this data is available and there is little disagreement about its validity. In many instances that is not true and that forms our challenge for the future.

The Massachusetts General Hospital (MGH) radiology department developed a system to profile the radiology studies ordered by both primary care physicians (PCPs) and specialists. They collected data that included the patient's demographics by age and gender. Furthermore, the data tracks the reason the physician ordered the study. Additional features that are currently being introduced into the system is whether the study was positive or negative.

The MGH system tracks both PCPs and specialists and can link the studies requested by specialists back to the primary care physician who referred the patient to the specialist. The system profiles separately all types of physicians. This allows a primary care physician to see the ordering patterns of the specialist to whom he refers, and to view aggregate data by various specialists' groups. In theory this type of information could let a PCP select specialists to whom he refers his patients by their radiology ordering habits.

Each organization needs to agree on the goals of their utilization management project prior to data collection. For example, a group of physicians at MGH sat down and brainstormed over a period of several days about what was needed to change the ordering patterns of physicians. That was a worthwhile exercise in its own right as it clarified the group's objectives and told them what changes were needed in their information systems to collect the required data. The resulting plan was then presented to the ordering physicians, who made suggestions as well. Other organizations may desire to collect different information than MGH, but the need to feed the information back to the referring physicians can not be emphasized too strongly. For ordering physicians to cooperate in a profiling system, they must feel they are part of the development process and agree that what has been decided is acceptable. Any organization always has physicians who express anxiety about how the information of a profiling system is going to be used. A cooperative development system with a lot of physician input has a better chance of success than a confrontational system imposed on physicians. Physicians want to develop both the goals of a utilization management project and the process.

Insurance companies and other payers should consider the increased value in developing a profiling system in close cooperation with the physicians involved. Physicians tend to be an autonomous group. In addition they often see practical problems in a lot of different proposals sent to them by nonphysicians.

Most physicians are familiar with confrontational methods employed by insurance companies to lower utilization of medical services. These usually take the form of rules and regulations that are simply issued by the insurance companies, who promulgate new policies about the care of patients. Such policies often require telephone approval of certain expensive studies prior to the physician's ordering the studies. Sometimes the request for the study is denied, but often it is simply a hassle factor that drives down the utilization. In most physician's opinion, the experience of insurance companies regulating how to practice medicine has usually been bad: bad for patients, bad for insurance companies, and bad for providers. In fact, currently at many levels of government there are initiatives to pass legislation concerning who sets the rules for practicing medicine.

A cooperative system of utilization management is in everyone's best interest. Patients talk to their physicians, not usually to insurance company administrators. If physicians are unhappy about a system, they convey that unhappiness to the patients. Unhappy patients in turn often find another insurance plan to join at the earliest opportunity. Patients are much more likely to search for a new insurance plan than they are to search for a new physician.

Once some degree of cooperation with ordering physicians is obtained,

PHYSICIAN COMFORT WITH PROCESS CHANGES

Physicians are notoriously poor at understanding the development of a process. Physicians receive little education about management techniques. A physician encounters a patient and takes care of the patient's problem during that encounter. The patient presumably is happy, the physician is happy, and at least for a while that transaction has accomplished the initial task and the physician moves on to the next task.

Managers are used to setting up processes. That process might establish the steps whereby the physician would see a number of patients per day, the various physician-patients encounters that would occur, the operating rooms that would be available for surgery on a particular schedule, how and what types of drugs from a pharmacy would be available, how those drugs would be delivered to the patient, how other ancillary care would be delivered to the patient, when bills would be sent out, when the patient would be discharged, and when the schedule for the follow-up visit would be made. This entire process falls into the realm of managers. Physicians are not good at working through the process. They want the immediate satisfaction and immediate results of their one-on-one encounter. Therefore, physicians have a difficult time thinking about how a process works and little experience in actually setting up processes.

Managers, on the other hand, are trained in developing the process so that it works at a level of maximum efficiency. This process development coordinates the allocation and deployment of resources within an organization. The satisfaction comes to the manager from designing and running an efficient process in the organization. There is no immediate feedback on an individual basis to the manager, and perhaps that is why physicians are sometimes not interested in developing a process.

then an organization should collect the data that they require. It is here that the digital revolution allows not only collection of data but manipulation of the data to yield the information requested. In the MGH database, the data can be evaluated in almost any form desired. It is frequently only by interaction and study of the data that insight is acquired into trends or areas that might require more fruitful exploration.

CLASSIC DATA MAY NOT BE SUITABLE FOR CHANGING PHYSICIAN BEHAVIOR

Insurance companies today usually collect claims-based data. The information is provided to them to request payment on an insured patient. Most companies, but not all, can generate information about what study was ordered on a particular patient. Many companies can track the information back to the primary care physician taking responsibility for the patient. Very few can track the study ordered back to the doctor who actually requested the study. Sometimes the insurance company determines why the study was ordered by the ICD9 code. There are, however, in excess of 14,000 ICD9 codes. Some of these codes are confusing. In fact, at least eight ICD9 codes address complaints of low back pain. Which ICD9 code a provider should list to trigger payment for a claim often becomes a guessing game between the provider and the payer. Payers frequently do not give any help to providers who inquire about which code should be used to trigger payments. Often the ICD9 code listed on a claims form may have little relationship as to why a particular study was ordered. The code may represent the code that was attached to the patient at discharge from the hospital or clinic. The code could simply be the code of the patient's underlying disease. In summary, it is not easy to obtain any understanding why a particular study was ordered with most claims-based data. Almost never will the result of the study be listed by the claims data.

I believe, therefore, that insurance companies need to reevaluate the data they collect. Most insurance company data is aggregated into some variation of either the number of studies done per 1000 patients in the plan, or the amount of money spent on radiology per patient. These numbers are grouped so that they appear as something like $11.22/member/month (PMPM) or 852 studies/1000 covered lives. Frequently the insurance company breaks the data into types of studies so they can identify that $3.44 PMPM was spent on ultrasound, and $2.50 PMPM was spent on CT studies. Because this data is tracked back to the primary care physician, these numbers might yield a report card for the physician that looks like something in Figure 16.5.

What the physician in Figure 16.5 sees is a report that lists all the studies done on his patients by both him and the specialists to whom he refers his patients. If that number is above some arbitrary standard, he may be admonished by the medical director of the health plan. This probably simply irritates him and makes him prone to throw the report in the wastebasket—and rightfully so. The medical director has

Dr.	CT Studies/1000 (PM)^2	U/S Studies/1000 (PM)^2	Plain Film/1000 (PM)^2
A	42 (5.25)	21 (1.26)	140 (2.8)
B	17 (2.13)	18 (1.08)	100 (2)
C	100 (12.5)	85 (5.1)	54 (1.08)
D	162 (20.25)	15 (0.9)	89 (1.78)
E	51 (6.38)	28 (1.68)	115 (2.3)

FIGURE 16.5

Example of the type of data sometimes given by insurance companies to physicians in the form of a report card. This report card indicates how physicians' use of high technology studies compare to their peers. Usually the number of studies per thousand patients is listed as well as the cost per member per month of these radiology studies.

no idea as to why the physician's ordering profile is abnormal, and certainly has no way to help the physician understand how to change his behavior.

Historical claims-based data is of little value to reach the goal of highest quality at the lowest cost. The information needed to affect change has been discussed earlier, but amounts to some variation of the following: patient demographics by age and gender, ordering physician, specialty of ordering physician, type of study ordered, reason the study was ordered, and the result of the study.

Comparing the radiology usage for a physician or group of physicians requires some standard and is the reason for guideline development. Profile the group that you are evaluating and try to determine where problems are located.

Figure 16.6 shows a bar graph of the five most expensive (by aggregate dollars) of radiology studies done in a healthcare plan in New England. These are compared to an arbitrary standard from a health actuary firm for the numbers of studies that should have been ordered in that population for these types of problems. Several variations from the expected are identified. The bar marked with the asterisk is the number of studies done (aggregate dollars spent) on patients who present with low back pain. Notice in this example that it is significantly higher than the standard to which it is compared. In this example the standard was based on an actuary firm's aggregate data. It demonstrates no real truth in the philosophical sense, but it provides a crude starting point to focus on where to start the effort.

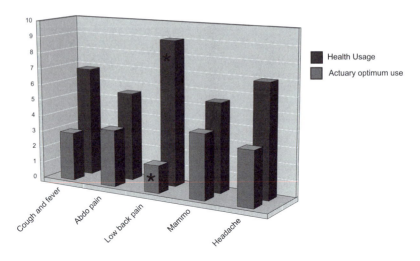

FIGURE 16.6

A bar graph of the actual use of radiology studies in a New England health plan for five different clinical categories versus what the health plan's actuary felt should have been used for these types of symptoms and patient complaints.

DEVELOPING A CONSENSUS ON GUIDELINES

A variety of techniques adapted from nonmedical sources can be used to develop guidelines. The easiest way for an organization to use guidelines is to adopt a guideline that someone else has developed. Multiple guidelines prepared by a variety of organizations exist on things like back pain and a host of other afflictions. Some of these guidelines are quite elaborate and are available to the public at large because they were developed with government funds. Other guidelines are proprietary but are often available just by asking. One should study these to decide if they are useful and if the physicians in your organization will agree to follow them.

Many times, however, there are no acceptable guidelines or none germane to the particular problem of an organization, in which case the organization must develop its own. Several techniques are used. The general concept is to reach consensus among the parties affected by these guidelines.

With data such as given in Figure 16.6 a group could decide to develop a guideline on how a physician should use radiology in patients who present with low back pain. Either an existing guideline could be used, the organization could develop their own guideline with experts from inside or outside of their organization, or they could simply agree to follow certain standards. Consensus must be reached so that this will be a cooperative effort.

Once a guideline is adopted, then the data system should track every study ordered on patients with low back pain. The data should create profiles on the ordering patterns of the physicians. All physicians need to have the information fed back to them on a regular basis. Outliers, physicians who order too few or too many studies, need their use patterns analyzed more carefully and fed back to them and their chief medical officers. The medical administrator may need to schedule educational sessions on how to evaluate patients with low back pain.

An insurance company can also put other incentives in place to force physicians to follow guidelines, but the group initiative must be cooperative to achieve the goal of optimum quality. In theory, if a physician refuses to cooperate, then an insurance plan has a host of remedies available to them. If they chose to terminate a physician, they can base that decision on the failure of the physician to follow guidelines based on an agreed standard of high quality medical care.

Results coding can help in both developing and refining guidelines. A radiology profile company located in Chicago devised the concept of "negativity" of a study. They would record whether a study was positive or negative and then attached a percentage of negativity to the physician's profile. Any data using results coding must be considered in the total context of the patient care. Dr. Jones may have a negativity rate of 25% on chest CTs ordered for cancer of the lung, which in some groups might be a relatively high yield for CTs of the chest. More importantly, it might be that some studies were unnecessary because the information about cancer of the lung may already have been known from chest X-rays. One could argue a study was done to stage the operability of the tumor. Again, all data must be placed in context. A chest X-ray or bone scan may already have demonstrated that metastatic spread of the tumor had occurred prior to the chest CT.

Results coding may be useful when one gathers data and discovers that 90% of the chest X-rays are negative by one physician and 50% are negative by another. That should alert people to the fact that a different practice pattern exists that requires some investigation into the indications or types of patients seen by those two physicians. It doesn't mean either is wrong. It just is a signal that more inquiry is needed to discern the differences. Blindly following negativity rates is no more useful than comparing numbers of studies done per thousand population. All data needs to be evaluated and analyzed by experts to identify trends and differences in practice behavior. In short, results coding is very powerful and can be an excellent

MODIFIED DELPHI APPROACH

In 1995 the American College of Radiology released work on the appropriateness criteria for imaging studies. They are of little value for what we are discussing here, but the methods they used are worth examining. They use a modified Delphi approach to reach consensus among recognized experts in the field. A clinical problem was selected. Peer-reviewed articles on the clinical problem were collected. A team leader then developed an evidence table for the topic under investigation. A panel of experts received a series of surveys on the topic. These experts had to reach 80% agreement on the surveys to reach consensus. This technique is discussed in greater detail in the *ACR Appropriateness Criteria for Imaging and Treatment Decisions*, Volume 2, 1996, page 3.

Some variation of this technique is an excellent way for an organization to reach consensus on clinical pathways.

Delphi Approach: Same concept as the modified Delpha approach; it is just necessary to reach complete agreement. This is probably impractical in most organizations.

Forced choice matched pairs: This technique compares a series of items in a list in which participants choose between one of two paired items. These items are then revisited from every possible permutation and combination. What emerges from this exercise is a degree of confidence that a group has priorities on which of these items is most important. This technique is powerful and can result in agreement on what a group of people think about something. I have no knowledge that this technique has been used in developing guidelines for medicine, but the concept is excellent, and in theory, this would lead to appropriate guidelines.

Almost all of these techniques require expert consultants skilled at developing consensus. An organization would be well advised to spend some money up front, find the right consultant, and then proceed with guideline development.

tool. It simply must be used in conjunction with other information and data. Remember that the ultimate goal is to develop quality guidelines on how to practice better, more effective medicine.

Good utilization management demands intensive cooperation among all players. It requires investment of capital to develop the database, and then it requires dedicated people to analyze the data and make the information meaningful. The very best utilization management programs have not yet been developed. They will require close cooperation between providers and payers, a lot of time, and a lot of dedicated work.

The ultimate guidelines will save lots of money. To put this in perspective requires some calculations. In Boston the global outpatient and pro-

COST SAVINGS FROM CT-FOCUSED APPENDICITIS

In 1998 Rao and associates published an article in the New England Journal of Medicine about how the use of CT in diagnosing people with appendicitis could save money from unnecessary surgery. For decades the rate of removal of a normal appendix in the setting of acute appendicitis was 20% in a hospital population. In fact, some organizations have used that number as a measure of quality. If the surgeons in your hospital took out more than 20% normal appendixes, they were operating too frequently on patients with suspected appendicitis. If they took out fewer then 20% normal appendixes, then they weren't aggressive enough, and the fear was that the morbidity and mortality from missed or ruptured appendixes was too high.

Rao and his colleagues did a study to see if they could safely drive the percentage of normal appendixes removed to a much lower number, say 2% to 3%. They found that if they did a focused CT study in the clinical setting of acute appendicitis, they did not miss any patients who had an inflamed appendix and could identify those patients who did not have appendicitis. From a strictly cost savings measure, this could result in annual savings of $186 million dollars in the United States. In addition, and not calculated by Rao and his colleagues, there was the gain in lower morbidity and patient satisfaction by avoiding surgery that the patient did not need. This study is a nice example of how using high technology CT studies in situations where they had not previously been used can result in both an improvement in the quality of care and significant cost reductions in delivering that care.

(Source: Rao P et al. *Effect of computed tomography of the appendix on treatment of patients and use of hospital resources.* New England Journal of Medicine. 338:141–146, 1998.)

fessional inpatient amount of money spent on radiology amounts to approximately $12.95/member/month in the Partners HealthCare System, which is composed of the Massachusetts General and Brigham and Women's Hospital system. This is a large academic medical center, and one could argue that these costs are high for a variety of reasons. Dismiss that for a second, and assume that number should be lowered to that of Austin, Texas, where the per member per month rate for radiology is about $4. Assume now that the cost of radiology in Boston could be lowered over a five-year period to the same level of Austin, Texas. That is an annual radiology savings of about $129 million on a population of 1.2 million covered lives, which is what constitutes the Massachusetts General Hospital and Brigham and Women's Hospital network services. Assume that the quality would be improved or at least maintained. Perhaps some outcomes research done during the five years of our example would lead to savings from using more radiology and thus save money elsewhere in the system. The investment in time and data collection becomes worthwhile. An example of cost savings resulting from increasing radiology utilization can be read in the box on cost savings.

A cooperative effort between insurance companies and providers makes good long-term sense. It will improve the quality of medicine, decrease the costs, and make both patients and physicians happy. So why hasn't it been done? It is a difficult assignment, but one in which the opportunities and the challenges lead to tremendous returns.

CONTRIBUTORS

▶ **KATHERINE P. ANDRIOLE, PhD**

Dr. Andriole has been involved in various aspects of the field of digital medical imaging for the past 15 years. She is currently an Assistant Professor in the Departments of Radiology and Biomedical Informatics at the University of California at Berkeley. She also serves as the UCSF PACS Clinical Coordinator.

▶ **DAVID AVRIN, MD, PhD**

Dr. Avrin is past Chairman of both the Society for Computer Applications in Radiology and the Radiology Information System Consortium. He is a member of the American College of Radiology Committee for the NEMA Standard. His research and development activities include diagnostic workstation design/user interface issues, PACS cost effectiveness, integrated digital teaching file, prefetching algorithms, and hierarchical storage methods using compression.

▶ **GILES BOLAND, MD**

Dr. Boland has served as the Director of Teleradiology at Massachusetts General Hospital for the past seven years and is an Associate Professor of Radiology at Harvard Medical School. During this period, he has been responsible for transitioning a disparate international and domestic analog teleradiology system into a seamless, fully integrated DICOM system and then into the existing PACS/RIS, with online scheduling reports using voice-activated systems.

▶ ROBERT T. BRAMSON, MD

Dr. Bramson set up a team that developed a radiology utilization management program at Massachusetts General Hospital. While at MGH, he was appointed the COO and Director of Partners Radiology, formed from the merger of MGH and Brigham and Women's Hospital. In addition, he was Division Chief of Pediatric Radiology at MGH. He is currently the Executive Vice-Chairman of the Radiology Department at Children's Hospital in Boston.

▶ JOHN A. CARRINO, MD

Dr. Carrino is currently an academic musculoskeletal radiologist, with a special interest in spine disorders, structured reporting, and health services research. A technophile with experience in several large-scale PACS deployments, he enjoys participating in the development of the DICOM standard as a member of working group 6.

▶ DAVID A. CLUNIE, MD

Dr. Clunie, who was formerly a neuroradiologist working in Australia, Africa, Saudi Arabia, and the United States, now specializes in digital medical imaging and information technology. He also works in industry and is the Co-chairman of the DICOM Standards Committee and editor of the *DICOM Standard.*

▶ KEITH J. DREYER, DO, PhD

Dr. Dreyer is the Vice-Chairman of Radiology Informatics at Massachusetts General Hospital and Assistant Professor of Radiology at the Harvard Medical School. He holds a BS in mathematics, an MS in image processing, and a PhD in computer science. He completed his medical school training at Michigan State University and his internship and radiology residency at Wayne State University. He holds an MRI/Medical Informatics fellowship at Harvard Medical School and is board certified in diagnostic radiology by the American Board of Radiology.

▶ STEVEN C. HORII, MD, FACR, FSCAR

Dr. Horii did his undergraduate work at Johns Hopkins University and earned his MD at the New York University School of Medicine. He followed this with a residency and fellowship in radiology at NYU as well. He is an elected Fellow of the American College of Radiology and the Society for Computer Applications in Radiology. He is a leader in the field of computer applications in medicine and has received numerous awards. He is widely rgarded as one of the leading developers of the DICOM standard and has a special interest in workstations.

▶ STEPHEN MANN, PhD

Dr. Mann has advanced degrees from the University of Maryland and the Georgia Institute of Technology. He is one of the founders of Peachtree Software Inc., MultiMedia Technologies Inc., and Pegasus Imaging Corp. His imaging projects include the poster system for the National Cente for Missing and Exploited Children and serving on the X3L# committee developing JPEG and JPEG 2000.

▶ AMIT MEHTA, MD

Dr. Mehta is the Medical Director of the advanced imaging laboratory of the Massachusetts General Hospital. He holds a special interest in informatics and computer applications in radiology. He has published extensively in this area, both in print and electronic media. He is also the author of *The Internet for Radiology Practice*, published by Springer-Verlag. He has directed multiple courses nationally on PACS and informatics and is currently pursuing interests in computer aided detection in radiology.

▶ SYRENE R. REILLY, MBA

Ms. Reilly has a Bachelor of Science degree in accounting from Boston College and a Master's degree in business administration from Harvard Business School. She is currently a project consultant for Partners HealthCare System, Inc., with a focus on Materials Management and Service Improvement. Before joining Partners, she enjoyed a successful financial career at Price Waterhouse and Trans National Group.

▶ BRUCE REINER, MD

Dr. Reiner is an academic and private-practice radiologist. He currently serves as Director of Radiology Research in the Maryland VA Healthcare System and is Associate Professor of Radiology at the University of Maryland Medical Center. His radiology private practice is at Nanticoke Memorial Hospital in Seaford, Delaware. Dr. Reiner's research is focused in a number of areas within filmless imaging, including digital image processing, radiologist/technologist productivity, economics, and workflow. In addition to numerous industry sponsored grants, Dr. Reiner has published extensively within the radiology literature and serves as chair of the educational committee of SCAR University.

▶ SCOTT M. ROGALA, BA

Mr. Rogala is the Corporate manager of Netword Engineering for Partners Healthcare System Inc., in Boston, which is the parent organization of Massachusetts General and Brigham and Women's hospitals. He was instrumental in the installation of PACS at these institutions, as well as the integration of other hospitals into the Partner's network.

▶ ELIOT L. SIEGEL, MD

Dr. Siegel is Chief of Radiology for the VA Maryland Healthcare System and Associate Professor at the University of Maryland School of Medicine. He has edited three books, including *Filmless Radiology* (also published by Springer-Verlag) and has written extensively about topics related to computer applications in medicine, particularly about Picture Archival and Communication Systems. In addition to nuclear medicine and cross-section imaging, his other interests are medical informatics and telemedicine.

▶ JOHN J. SMITH, MD, JD

Dr. Smith is a musculoskeletal radiology at Massachusetts General Hospital. In addition to his clinical duties, he is an attorney and serves as the Directory of Regularoty Affairs for the Center for Integration of Medicine and Innovative Technology.

▶ JAMES H. THRALL, MD

Dr. Thrall has served as Radiologist-in-Chief of Massachusetts General Hospital and Professor Radiology, Harvard Medical School for the last 13 years. He has been a pioneer in introducing digital technology to the clinical practice of radiology and has built a large domestic and international teleradiology practice at MGH.

▶ DOUGLAS TUCKER, PhD

Dr. Tucker holds a Master of Science in Computer and Information Sciences and a doctorate in biomedical engineering from the University of Alabama at Birmingham. He is a Diplomat of the American board of Radiology. In addition, he is an active member of several professional societies, including the Society for Computer Applications in Radiology and the American Association of Physicists in Medicine. He has authored 21 peer-reviewered articles, five book chapters, and thirty published abstracts. He has served as Guest Editor of *Medical Physics* and as Manuscript Review for that publication, as well as for the *Journal of Digital Imaging and Radiology*.

▶ HARRY ZIBNERS, MD, JD

Dr. Zibners is a member and immediate past President of the Sacramento Radiology Medical Group, Inc., in California. He is currently Chairman of the American College of Radiology Medical-Legal Committee, a Fellow of the Americal College of Legal Medicine, and a member of the State Bar of California.

INDEX